Opinions

Making Choices about Fertility Treatment

University of California Press

Berkeley / Los Angeles / London

The illustration in the chapter openings is used
by permission from Lennart/Albert Bonniers
Förlag AB, *A Child Is Born,* Delacorte Press.

University of California Press
Berkeley and Los Angeles, California

University of California Press, Ltd.
London, England

Library of Congress Cataloging-in-Publication Data

Turiel, Judith Steinberg, 1948–
    Beyond second opinions : making choices about
fertility treatment / Judith Steinberg Turiel.
        p.   cm.
    Includes bibliographic references and index
    ISBN 0-520-08945-6 (cloth : alk. paper).
    —ISBN 0-520-20854-4 (pbk.)
    1. Infertility.   2. Human reproductive technology.
I. Title.   RC889.T87   1998
    616.6'92—dc 21   97-6044

Printed in the United States of America
9 8 7 6 5 4 3 2 1

The paper used in this publication meets the minimum
requirements of American National Standards for
Information Sciences—Permanence of Paper for Printed
Library Materials, ANSI Z39.48-1984.

Beyond Second Opinions

WOMEN'S HEALTH RESOURCE CENTRE
REGIONAL WOMEN'S HEALTH CENTRE
790 BAY STREET 8TH FLOOR
TORONTO ON M5G 1N9
416-351-3716 / 3717

Beyond Second

Judith Steinberg Turiel

To my mother and father,
to Elliot,
and to Joshua, who, thanks to
     medical interventions, we almost never had

Contents

Figures

Acknowledgments

Beyond Second Opinions reflects personal and professional experiences that took place over many years, beginning long before I thought of writing a book. I will undoubtedly fail to thank many people who were helpful—personally and professionally—during those years and into the present. In the interest of privacy, moreover, I do not thank by name the women and men who spoke with me about their own fertility problems; but their willingness to share sensitive feelings, experiences, and thoughts provided invaluable insights into the world of fertility medicine, its patients, and its doctors.

For assistance and encouragement that more directly helped to generate this book, my thanks go to Howard Bern, a scientist who refused to ignore the problem of human exposure to DES and other hormones and who so warmly welcomed me into his lab and into a world of scientific exchange not usually accessible to nonscientists; Pat Cody and DES Action, not only for being there, but for being a constant source of support, energy, and information; John McLachlan, always enthusiastic, creative, and thought-provoking in pursuing the science of reproductive exposures wherever it takes him; Mary Martin, a fertility specialist who graciously gave her time and thoughts to this project; and the many other physicians and scientists I consulted along the way, especially Emily Chen, Gerry Cunha, Arthur Haney, Robert Jaffe, Michael Katz, Richard Mendius, and Beth Newman. My appreciation goes also to Cecile Lampton, who works with Resolve of Northern California to help people understand their fertility problems and find appropriate medical care. While working on health issues, I have spoken to these and other individuals in conversations as well as in more structured interviews. I have also attended many meetings and seminars. I quote people by name only where I have specific permission or if a statement was made publicly, but I generally do not provide a note citation for such statements.

For their help in shaping the book itself, I am grateful to Dorothy Wall, a re-discovered friend whose professional skills helped me form my initial ideas into the start of a book; Felicia Eth, my agent, who saw this start and found it the right editor at the right publishing house; Naomi Schneider, that unfailing reader and editor I needed, at various stages, to make the book say what I wanted it to be saying; Kristin Neff, who bailed me out of a daunting computer glitch; and Erika Büky and Ellen F. Smith, whose careful reading and wonderful copyediting ensured that this book was finely—and finally—finished.

Special thanks go to my in-house computer consultant, Joshua Turiel, par-ticularly for getting me into the Internet and out of it; and to my in-house all-purpose consultant, Elliot Turiel, for the initial push, the constant encourage-ment, and the everyday life that allowed this book to happen.

Beyond Second Opinions

1 Facing Infertility

Into the Medical Realm

At the age of thirty, an unhappy medical experience forced me to learn that ignorance is not always bliss. Following successful treatment for infertility and six ecstatic months of an apparently routine pregnancy, I delivered a premature baby who did not survive. Beyond the deep sorrow of this loss, I was thrown back upon what remained—my infertility. If my husband and I wanted to try, once again, to have a child, I must become, once again, a fertility patient.

At that time I considered myself well educated: after all, I had a doctorate in education from an Ivy League university. About my own health care, however, I remained largely ignorant, willing to leave everything to my doctors. Most of my care had involved gynecologic and reproductive problems; I had been seeing gynecologists regularly since my teenage years. First the problem was menstrual periods—mine were not happening. Then, just past my twenty-first birthday, abnormal Pap tests led to surgery that removed possibly malignant cells and a wedge of my cervix. The doctor, my mother's obstetrician-gynecologist, was puzzled. The Pap results and need for surgery, he said, were highly unusual in a woman so young. This mystery cleared a few years later, after I learned from this same doctor that I was a "DES daughter." He had prescribed the medication diethylstilbestrol (DES) to my mother when she was pregnant with me, because he believed it could prevent a miscarriage. Only in 1971—some time after my unusual Pap tests and surgery—did medical researchers begin to see the harmful effects on women who had been exposed in utero to DES.

By the time I was thirty, my doctors were specialists at a major medical center. A gynecologic oncologist examined me twice a year to be sure I was not among the small proportion of DES daughters (about 1 out of 1,000) who develop a rare, invasive vaginal cancer. A fertility specialist tested various workings of my endocrine system, trying to identify which hormones were not doing their job. My menstrual problems were probably caused by stress, he told me—stress of college, then graduate school, work, everyday life—though my case history did not quite fit the usual pattern of stress-related anovulation (no monthly release of an egg).

When I wanted to become pregnant, that first time, I was thrilled that fertility treatment to stimulate ovulation succeeded. Any ambivalence I had felt as a DES daughter about the wonders of modern medicine faded into contentment. Then the premature delivery jolted me into a different way of dealing with my reproductive problems. I ventured into the medical school library and began reading medical journals. I learned that physicians were beginning to report high rates of late pregnancy loss among women exposed before birth to DES. I learned of studies suggesting fertility problems among "DES daughters"—and perhaps "DES sons" as well. I began to realize how much my doctors did not know.

Faced anew with difficult decisions about treatment for infertility and for preterm labor, my husband and I sought further information. My initial forays into the medical library evolved into a regular routine after I contacted DES Action, the nationwide consumer organization established to educate the public and health professionals about diethylstilbestrol. Eventually, I became the organization's "research liaison." As a layperson, I had an unusual job: I was to keep tabs on relevant studies from various medical specialties and scientific disciplines, to inform people about these studies, and to encourage additional research about long-term health effects of DES exposure. This work not only kept me reading medical journals, but brought me to numerous meetings, conversations, and collaborations with doctors and research scientists. In addition, I met women and men—DES-exposed and not—who were experiencing a wide array of fertility problems.

Throughout the 1980s, my personal questions about infertility and pregnancy mingled with my professional task of educating laypeople about medical information. The decade saw terms like "partnership" and "informed consent" become common descriptions of a changed doctor-patient relationship. Yet, the partnership seemed hardly mutual and consent often less than well informed. I was struck by the persistent gap separating physicians and patients, particularly regarding the uncertainties, unknowns, and controversies swirling around reproductive medicine. I was disturbed by the influence of drug manufacturers, not only on doctors, but as providers of patient educational materials. I grew increasingly concerned that today's state-of-the-art fertility treatments, considered the best in medical care, parallel in significant ways the DES mistake of a previous generation. Beginning in the mid-1940s, the synthetic estrogen diethylstilbestrol became a widely prescribed pregnancy treatment, particularly for preventing miscarriage, and its use continued even after scientifically controlled clinical studies finally showed that it did not avert pregnancy problems. In what was essentially a large-scale human experiment, millions of pregnant women and their offspring were exposed to an unsafe, ineffective—yet highly popular—reproductive therapy.

My overwhelming reaction as a layperson who has viewed more extensively than most the world of fertility medicine was that there is a tremendous amount fertility patients are not told about diagnoses and treatments. What they are learning at the doctor's office is not the picture conveyed in medical journals and conferences. If patients could see what I have seen of the disagreements among doctors, the uncertainties, the nonmedical pressures that are shaping our medical care, they might think very differently about their infertility diagnosis and reach different decisions about pursuing medical treatment.

At the same time, I could surely empathize with people who want to have a child yet discover that, for them, it will not happen easily, if at all. I could well understand the pregnancy quest—the compelling lure of treatment, the desire to benefit from medical advances. And there definitely can be benefits. Even as my skepticism grew about many fertility interventions, I also knew that appropriate treatment can mean the difference between having or not having a baby.

In my case, a newly developed method of ovulation induction, coupled with high-risk-pregnancy care, meant my husband and I have one healthy child.

I also knew the risk of becoming immobilized by uncertainty. Awareness of unknowns and disagreement does not, in itself, mean one should never start down the medical path. This awareness may modify the pace of treatment or alter certain choices along the way or help in deciding when to stop. The unknown is but one dimension, shading whatever solid information is available, in a pursuit that may always feel tentative and unsure. In matters of one's own reproduction, I had learned, reaching a decision in full knowledge of uncertainty can be the most challenging step of all.

Informing Patients: An Unequal Partnership

In 1989 my work on DES-related health problems brought me to the nation's capital and to the First National Conference on Infertility for the Patient and the Medical Team. I joined hundreds of young women and men who sat, on a glorious Indian summer weekend, in the windowless, subterranean grand ballroom of a large hotel. The darkened room glowed with slides of smiling babies born after in vitro fertilization (IVF). The tone was upbeat, the message full of hope. Fertility specialists cited prospects for the future, when procedures just being developed would produce babies even more successfully.

The audience included but a small number of the estimated five million American couples experiencing difficulty in trying to have a baby. Doctors, nurses, and social workers also attended. The gathering was in part a celebration of the fifteenth anniversary of its cosponsor, Resolve, a consumer organization that provides infertility counseling, doctor referrals, and information. The conference's other sponsor, Serono Symposia, the educational division of Serono Laboratories, Inc., planned the medical presentations in coordination with its public relations staff and underwrote costs of the three-day event. Serono also publishes patient information brochures that are distributed by Resolve or through doctors' offices. As the manufacturer of hormones commonly used in reproductive therapies, Serono Labs happens to have cornered a fair amount of the $2-billion-a-year market that infertility creates. Its educational arm extends to patients and health professionals alike, through conferences, medical symposia, and written materials.

A conference for patients and the medical team would appear to reflect the best in health care. Patients in need seek the latest information from medical specialists who attempt to provide useful treatments. Technological progress aids the process, as do the resources of the pharmaceutical industry. Throughout the conference presentations, however, hints surfaced that all was not well with fertility medicine. There was talk of the expense of the many diagnostic tests and various treatments couples usually undergo, the vast majority of which fail. And difficult ethical issues complicate vitro fertilization, embryo freezing, surrogacy, egg donation, and genetic engineering. But overall the message was highly positive. After the final panel of experts, one physician who had been listening muttered, "The only thing they're not providing is their phone number." The data on success rates offered from the podium, he whispered, were well "massaged." Looking around him, he added, "And the audience is like warm butter."

I looked at the people listening intently to speakers, skimming patient-education brochures, signing up for small group sessions where they would give each other emotional support. I could not help thinking that these women and men might be surprised to learn that some doctors, as well as government officials, believed infertile couples were being exploited. Though more diligent than most about informing themselves, even these patients might not know how much uncertainty, controversy, and professional disagreement surround infertility practices. They might be angered to learn that agencies of the federal government, just blocks from this Washington hotel, have not helped: regulations on private industry were failing to protect consumers; and, in an ironic twist, anti-abortion forces were obstructing government support for research that might improve chances for infertile couples to have babies.

I could not help thinking, as I watched from the audience, that this First National Conference on Infertility captured more faithfully than its participants or cosponsors might imagine trends that not only reflected the decade just ending, but would also reach into the coming years. These trends are not always in the patient's best interests, yet they define in important ways the experience of women and men who are considering fertility treatments.

Suppose that patient is you. Perhaps you never thought getting pregnant would be a problem; when you wanted to have a baby, you would simply have a baby. Or perhaps you did have some suspicion that conceiving would be difficult. Either way, infertility is now a part of your life. You face a sometimes overwhelming medical world, with its array of options aimed at overcoming infertility. You may already have consulted a specialist or joined a support group of other women and men living with fertility problems. You may have read books written for laypeople, describing causes of infertility, methods of diagnosis, treatments to help you conceive or maintain a pregnancy. These treatments range from the simple—a few pills each month—to the more involved surgeries or increasingly common injections and other procedures related to in vitro fertilization (now gathered under the more general term of "advanced" or "assisted reproductive technologies"). The sheer amount of information available to you reflects, in fact, a major health care trend of the past two decades: brochures in the doctor's waiting room, volumes lining local bookstore shelves, newspapers, magazines, television, the Internet, conferences for patients and medical professionals. You join other patients who are "well informed" when they enter a doctor's office. Your interactions with the doctor are not like the old days, when doctors told patients what to do and patients did not question them. In the 1970s and 1980s, the consumer and women's health movements altered the doctor-patient relationship, particularly in gynecology and obstetrics. The long-established and paternalistic "doctor knows best" evolved into "let the patient decide."

Yet how are patients to decide about diagnoses and treatments when there is so much they never hear from doctors or the media? Books and brochures written for the public omit crucial facts of reproductive life—economic and political realities along with the biological and medical. Despite all the so-called education showered on them, today's fertility patients remain woefully *mis*informed; some treatments may actually reduce chances for a successful pregnancy and threaten a patient's existing good health. What do people need to know, beyond now easily available descriptions of various interventions, in order to reach more fully informed decisions? How can fertility patients—especially women—maintain control over an aspect of life that too often seems to slip beyond their powers?

The Bigger Picture: A Preview

First, laypeople should know of conflicts within the medical profession. The calm atmosphere of a doctor's office belies sharp disagreements that flare in medical journals, in meetings, in doctors' conversations. Patients are not privy to these intense arguments; if they were, they would be able to consider additional information and opinions that might sway their decisions about undertaking diagnostic procedures or treatments. Controversy is by no means limited to the interventions related to in vitro fertilization, which capture the most public attention; these technologically sophisticated procedures are but the tip of a very broad iceberg. Far more people—approximately 80 percent of fertility patients—are undergoing "conventional" treatments that, despite their wide acceptance, share some of the serious inadequacies of the more dramatic newcomers.

Patients also need to understand that fertility treatments are in large part a process of trial and error. Every day, in doctors' offices and clinics throughout the country, supposedly well-informed women (and, though to a much lesser extent, men) are unknowingly subjected to uncontrolled experimentation, with too little regard for their long-term health. Less directly, the trials and errors extend to their unborn offspring.

Beyond the highly experimental nature of reproductive medicine, forces remote from an individual's medical condition have a tremendous impact on the health care received. Commercial interests seeking financial gain exert a troubling influence on what doctors do. Political interests, reflected through government policy, touch every woman and man facing a fertility problem.

Everyone needs to see the bigger picture within which his or her very individual medical situation fits, but gaining this wider perspective is especially urgent in the area of reproductive medicine, which is expanding its potential clientele for increasingly technological, invasive, and costly interventions. Most people considering fertility treatments are otherwise healthy; taking on the risks of medical intervention requires special caution, since one of those risks is damage to the health they presently enjoy. Too often, decisions are made under pressure of ongoing treatment. The monthly cycle of hope following disappointment creates its own momentum, obscuring the balance of benefit against risk.

Today's patients need ways to increase the chances of receiving medical care appropriate for their particular case; they should not assume a medical intervention is always the best option. Laypeople need skills for finding and interpreting current medical knowledge. To evaluate a range of options—including the option of no medical treatment—fertility patients need to comprehend more fully the possible consequences of their decisions. Those consequences include not only whether they are likely to end up with a baby, but whether their own health or that of a baby might be harmed. Just as doctors sometimes practice "defensive medicine" to avoid lawsuits, patients may at times need to take a "defensive" stance—to avoid unproven diagnoses and treatments, unjustified experimentation, interventions that may help one person sitting in the waiting room but are of no use to the others.

For patients now inundated with information—information at times contradictory and nearly always incomplete—it is tempting to just leave it to the doctors, trusting that their expertise will find the best solution. Although trust in a doctor's judgment is important, the "doctor knows best" of past years must not be replaced by "don't confuse patients with the facts." Rather, fertility patients must contend with a frustrating paradox: state-of-the-art fertility medicine is constantly changing, yet disturbing characteristics remain stubbornly the same. To untangle the good medicine from the bad, the hazardous from the benign, patients need to determine when a physician's help is needed and which physician to choose. They need to question the safety and effectiveness of available options. At some point, fertility patients may need to take a leap of faith, making decisions in the face of uncertainty; they should also understand, however, that retaining a critical approach to this field of medicine is a positive act of moving forward, of working in genuine and productive alliance with their doctors.

A Shifting Medical Landscape

As I began writing the chapters that follow, before the ink could even dry, events dramatized the profound impact of fertility medicine's broader landscape on individual lives. These events were not medical discoveries or new research findings; that such information changed with each passing month was to be expected. Less predictable was the country's political arena, where volatile shifts substantially influenced the medical terrain. The Clinton administration seemed initially to offer a real possibility of major changes toward greater equity in health care access and financing. In addition, the new administration initiated steps to rescind Reagan-Bush policies that had significantly affected fertility medicine. By the middle of Clinton's first term, however, health care legislation had collapsed, shoving reform prospects into obscurity, and the administration's early policy steps, particularly regarding research and regulations, screeched to a halt. Reversal became the real possibility, guided by a newly elected, reinvigorated conservative Congress. During this time, managed-care health plans governed by large corporations were increasingly defining medical treatment for more and more people.

Another event occurred in a smaller arena—one of the country's most prestigious fertility clinics. In May 1995 the University of California at Irvine shut down its affiliated Center for Reproductive Health, and university officials charged the center's director and two other physicians with egregious mistreatment of patients. The director, Dr. Ricardo Asch, was one of the world's most prominent fertility specialists, the individual credited with developing a widely used reproductive technique called gamete intrafallopian transfer, or

GIFT. Dr. Asch published his research findings regularly in medical journals, wrote and consulted for Serono Symposia, and supported activities of Resolve; a much-sought speaker on the international medical circuit, he discussed in his presentations not only his research but also medical ethics and regulations. Accusations against this physician and his colleagues included the most serious ethical violations ever revealed within fertility medicine: that without patients' knowledge, physicians took eggs or embryos belonging to women undergoing in vitro fertilization or a related treatment and transferred them to other women, some of whom became pregnant. A year after the scandal broke publicly, at least sixty couples and perhaps seven children were known to be directly affected. The stark outcome of this reproductive theft was that a couple's genetic offspring (including those of some couples whose attempts to have their own baby had failed) could be "out there somewhere," born to a different family, or that a child thought to be conceived from the egg of a fully informed and consenting donor might in fact have come from a woman who never knew her eggs were being used. Even patients treated successfully at this clinic, using their own embryos, could no longer feel sure they knew the truth about a child they now enjoyed.

Additional accusations against Dr. Asch and colleagues pale in light of these most painful abuses, but were nonetheless substantial. According to staff whistle-blowers, doctors used embryos for laboratory research without patient knowledge or consent, imported and sold to patients a fertility drug not approved by the Food and Drug Administration, and mishandled and falsified insurance and other financial reports.

Attached to these accusations were powerful metaphors, chilling images of dangers underlying reproductive medicine. In stealing a woman's eggs or embryos, the physicians violated not only medical ethics but the women themselves, raising a specter that hovers unmentioned over women whose doctors speak commonly of "getting their patients pregnant." News reports described the thefts as "biomedical rape"; a lawyer characterized his client suffering, after learning of her doctor's actions, as if she had been "brutally raped."

In vitro–related treatments present in exaggerated form the vulnerabilities of patients. These procedures literally do take reproduction out of women's bodies, out of their hands, out of their control. This clinic highlighted the dangers with particular intensity. Dr. Asch was the expert; a patient searching for the best in the field would feel she had found it. Patients revered and trusted him. The violations struck at the core of trust required to put one's life and hopes into the hands of a doctor, especially given our limits on understanding medical technology and even on knowing exactly what the doctor or a laboratory's staff has done to, or for, us. In the view of Dr. Albert Jonsen, a University of Washington bioethicist, "These were big-time people who were very well familiar with the kinds of [ethical] matters we've talked about for years. . . . If this can happen at this clinic, then what are the others doing?"[1]

The story unfolding from within the Center for Reproductive Health not only reflected fertility medicine's past—the experimentation on women, pressure for success, preponderance of ineffective and often harmful interventions—but also threw a glaring spotlight on new reproductive definitions and directions. For the children of patients at the Irvine clinic, a fundamental human question—"Where did I come from?"—was now rendered unanswerable. More concretely, the Irvine story highlighted failures of regulation and oversight at all levels—the university, its medical center, state and federal government. For the public, the fact that all of this sophisticated reproductive technology proceeds without patient protections was a rude awakening. For fertility specialists, the awakening more likely came with the clear demonstration of limitations to professional self-policing. Alarming reproductive scenarios involving patients, doctors, and embryo laboratories became all the more imaginable when in 1997 embryologists in Scotland announced the first successful cloning of a mammal—a baby lamb developed from a single cell scraped off an adult sheep's udder.

What This Book Is and Is Not

In writing this book, I set out to share with laypeople what they might not otherwise learn about fertility medicine from their doctor, from patient-education brochures, from the newspaper, or from their local bookstore shelves. Patients can already obtain detailed information on various fertility problems and treatment procedures. (Appendix 1 lists some more typical "how to get pregnant" handbooks.) Although I do go into some detail on prominent diagnoses and procedures that best illustrate patterns characteristic of fertility medicine, my intent is to provide a broader view, to examine the implications of how fertility medicine is practiced today.

I take this approach in part because trying to provide the latest information in a book is a losing battle—a significant portion of that medical knowledge is outdated before it is ever read—and in part because diagnoses of infertility are often so vaguely defined. Posing a different set of questions about fertility and possible medical treatment can help people use the ever-increasing quantity of information in a way that meets their particular needs. And finally, each individual's fertility problem and decisions about treatment take place within an ongoing story of reproductive interventions, all given shape by larger social and economic forces. Laypeople need to look beyond the surface into a medical realm not generally revealed to them. With greater awareness of the overall fertility enterprise—from specific research findings to the nonmedical forces shaping this country's choices about health care—women and men can make more fully informed decisions and be more confident in their own handling of this experience.

This book asks fertility patients, at least temporarily, to turn from concentrating on details of their particular diagnosis and treatment in order to consider instead the broader sweep of issues and themes; it asks readers to focus on gaining a feel for what goes on within this specialty—where it has been, where it is going, how a patient may fit into the bigger medical picture, and how fertility treatment fits into that patient's bigger life. The aim is to use medical resources differently—to bridge persistent gulfs that separate patients and doctors and that limit informed patient involvement in medical care, to help readers make more discerning evaluations of ever-expanding medical options and of the mass of information now available.

I should therefore make explicit three assumptions about readers of this book. I assume, first, that readers have some knowledge of diagnostic and treatment procedures available to fertility patients or have access to handbooks that provide more detailed descriptions and definitions. I also assume that most people do not particularly want to read medical journals on a regular basis; however, I draw on both medical articles and comments of physicians, and quote from them frequently, in the belief that laypeople can gain from these professional sources insights not provided elsewhere. Printed sources are identified in the Notes and Works Cited, and some guidance in how to begin using this literature is given in Appendix 2. In approaching much of the medical literature, a lay reader's most important tool is a good dose of logic and critical analysis. The goal is not to become an expert on a particular technique or to know as much as doctors. A little bit of knowledge can indeed be a dangerous thing and is certainly no basis for making medical decisions. Rather, the layperson's goal can be to understand concerns within the profession, to learn what "they" are arguing about, and to generate questions about a diagnosis or treatment. Once let in on a conversation among doctors that does, after all, pertain to patients, the patients will be able to participate more fully in evaluating options.

Finally, I assume readers have at least a glimmering of the dangers patients face when considering what appear to be ever-improving medical choices. In addition to women whose fertility problems relate to their prenatal DES exposure, a good number of fertility patients during the past two decades can trace fallopian tube blockage or pelvic scarring to the Dalkon Shield, an intrauterine device (IUD) widely used during the 1970s. Falsely promoted by its manufacturer to doctors (and, through them, to patients) as a modern, superior, effective, and safe contraceptive, this dime-sized plastic IUD seemed a good choice, especially given increasing concern about the safety of that era's birth control pills. No regulations covered the testing of such medical devices or their insertion into women's bodies. By the time the manufacturer—A. H. Robins Co., Inc., a large pharmaceutical company—pulled the Dalkon Shield off the market in 1974, more than 2 million women in the United States alone were using this type of IUD. The damage—including pelvic infections, infertility, spontaneous septic abortions, and death—was already done.[2] More recently, disfigurement, pain, and illness suffered by women with silicone breast implants have become the focus of public attention, as well as of scientific controversy. While researchers try, after the fact, to prove or disprove a cause-and-effect relationship, the fact of unregulated experimentation on women is clear. How could such a procedure become widespread in the face of, at best, great uncertainty about safety? Who was supposed to be protecting the patient? And who benefited—who reaped the profit—from these procedures?

I also offer some caveats about my role. First, I am not medically trained and do not give medical advice for any individual's situation. My extended involvement with medical and scientific questions relating to infertility stemmed initially from personal experiences as a woman with fertility and pregnancy problems. One way I dealt with these problems was to seek information, a process that included delving into medical journals. I was also fortunate to live in an area where women's health organizations kept the larger social and political dimensions in view. This book reflects my sifting through these diverse perspectives on reproductive medicine. Second, though I am keenly aware of the sadness, frustration, anger, and other complex feelings that can accompany fertility problems, I do not attempt to address these personal reactions in this book. Resources do exist to help women and men gain emotional support during this difficult time in their life (some are listed in Appendix 1). Resources also exist for people interested in adopting a baby, an alternative not discussed in this book on medical interventions.

Finally, although I hope there is much here of interest to physicians, researchers, and the general public, my main purpose remains to help the individual fertility patient become truly informed in making decisions about diagnosis and treatment. These personal decisions about available choices are a different matter than essential, long-avoided questions for society as a whole about the direction and allocation of medical, scientific, and technological resources, although I raise these questions in the context of how they affect fertility medicine and patients' choices. And I do not explore the powerful social pressures, especially on women, that reinforce desires to have a baby, no matter the personal or financial cost. For the most part, I do not ask *why* people want so badly to conceive a pregnancy and have their own biological child, but take as a given that many people do.

The Chapters Ahead: An Overview

Chapter 2 looks through the lens of one woman's experience to introduce themes that reappear throughout this book. Her story is not sensational, not the most dramatic, but is one person's own—as is every patient's. Her story takes place in the 1980s, a decade that saw fertility medicine take off, hurtling ahead with new reproductive interventions used on an expanded clientele, leaving crucial questions unexamined and still unresolved as the century's final decade reaches its end.

The next three chapters look more specifically at diagnoses and treatments fertility patients have been hearing in the 1990s. Chapter 3 focuses on assisted reproductive technologies that have followed from the first successful human in vitro fertilization birth in 1978, a birth that announced fundamental changes in fertility medicine as a whole. Chapter 4 discusses several types of fertility problems (including luteal phase defect, male infertility, immunologic infertility, repeated early miscarriage, and unexplained infertility) and treatments (including surgeries, fertility drugs, inseminations, gamete micromanipulation, immunotherapies). This chapter dwells more extensively than others on medical journal reports, not to convey technical information, but to reveal patterns of fertility medicine that greatly affect people's options and outcomes. Chapter 5 examines one cause of infertility newly emphasized in recent years, a "diagnosis" shared by all women and carrying far-reaching reproductive implications—growing older.

Chapters 6–8 explore more fully themes central to understanding the present and immediate future of fertility medicine—understanding that can help patients obtain appropriate, beneficial care. Chapter 6 considers differing types of scientific evidence that could push fertility medicine beyond the unsystematic trial-and-error approach characterizing much of its daily practice, the tendency of doctors and patients to "do something" medically without adequate biological knowledge. The discussion concentrates on the three basics of any decision within this specialty: research, risks, and resources. Chapter 7 takes up the question of how laypeople become informed patients and how the sources of information—doctors, the pharmaceutical industry, the media—may skew decisions about medical options. Chapter 8 steps back from the diagnosis and treatment picture to ask an all-encompassing question: How can women and men be protected from incompetent or unethical fertility treatment? Included in that discussion are implications of the trend toward "managed care," which too often puts cost-cutting ahead of comprehensive and appropriate health care. This chapter describes fertility medicine's pressing need for better safeguards in the form of regulations, monitoring, government-supported research, and an enlarged lay-professional dialogue.

Chapter 9 is a summing up, returning the focus to individuals who are trying to have a baby—how they can maximize the benefits and minimize the harm possible when diagnosing and treating fertility problems.

Throughout the chapters there are set-offs that serve as a kind of embellishment to the main text. They offer additional details, commentary, and other useful (and sometimes entertaining) material that help illustrate my main arguments. Although all terms are defined when they are introduced in the text, the Glossary provides a useful reference and reminder. And because information about specific conditions and treatments is dispersed throughout the chapters, readers should use the index to guide them to topics of interest.

•

I close this introduction with some comments on terminology. Although I often refer to "couples" (meaning a man and a woman)—the most common relationship among fertility patients—considerations raised throughout this book pertain also to women with no male partners attempting to conceive using donor sperm (from an acquaintance or anonymously from a sperm bank). I also use the pronoun "he" most often for doctors (unless referring to an actual female doctor), since most fertility specialists are male. And in the interest of privacy, I have changed the names and certain details about patients in descriptions based on real cases.

More significantly, in this book I deliberately use the terms "reproductive therapy" or "intervention" or "fertility treatment" instead of "*in*fertility treatment." Although the medical practices discussed target the "infertile"—self-defined and/or doctor-diagnosed—the label is vague, the category flexible. Moreover, current "infertility" procedures are increasingly being adapted in ways that create options for anyone pursuing a pregnancy. In vitro procedures make possible a variety of prenatal testing and gestation choices. The biological clock is even being reset: with donated eggs, a regimen of hormone drugs, and in vitro fertilization followed by transfer of embryos, women who have passed menopause can now become pregnant. The explosion of biotechnologies applied to human genes holds potential for barely imagined options in the not-so-distant future. Such developments add to the urgency for laypeople to become more truly educated about reproductive interventions. I write this book, then, not only for those who are now experiencing difficulty conceiving a pregnancy, or who suspect they will face such problems, but for anyone considering pregnancy or interested in reproductive issues. And I write it for anyone who must someday make difficult medical decisions—a fate that few people avoid. Reproductive medicine illustrates boldly the common threads that weave throughout American medicine, giving shape to the experience of every individual who, at some point, must enter the medical realm.

2 A Couple Decides

What Informed Patients Do and Do Not Learn

On a damp, wintry night in Seattle in 1987, the night before she was to undergo
pelvic surgery, 35-year-old Anna sat alone in a motel room, hundreds of miles
from her California home. Following surgery early the next morning, she
would take a taxi back to the motel to recuperate alone until she felt strong
enough to travel. She was in Seattle because that was where she found a specialist in microsurgery. She was alone because the expense of a trip for her husband
as well was more than they could manage. This pilgrimage marked an escalation
of efforts toward what Anna described as her goal for this time in her life—to
become pregnant. The past five years had already been consumed by gynecology
appointments, fertility tests, medications, artificial inseminations, and one conception—an ectopic pregnancy that lodged within and ruptured her one normal fallopian tube, nearly killing her.

You might think Anna is a composite, created with poetic license to dramatize an array of fertility problems and the impact they have on people's lives, but
she is not. Like most fertility patients, her case history presents a tangle of contributing factors and possible remedies. Like most patients, her story veers
away from a medical ideal of identifying reasons for a problem, then determining which treatment best eliminates the problem without causing unacceptable
side effects. Anna and Tom had chosen not to attempt in vitro fertilization, a
treatment that was no longer a novelty by the mid-1980s. Instead, they were
gambling on surgery performed with the aid of a microscope, meticulously
stitching back together the ruptured fallopian tube—ranging from an eighth to
perhaps a half an inch in diameter—in the hope that an egg could one day travel
through it.

Anna did not arrive easily at the decision that brought her to that motel room. She had gathered information, obtained second and third opinions, located a surgeon reputed to be one of the best. But like most patients, she did not know that for each difficult decision she faced at each step along the way, medical journal articles rumbled with disagreement and disenchantment. This chapter retraces Anna's steps, counterposed here with concerns expressed among doctors and scientists, the untold conflicts behind this patient's and others' stories.

Five Little Pills

The initial fertility treatment prescribed to Anna was simple: clomiphene citrate, one pill per day, from the fifth through the ninth day of her menstrual cycle. (Clomid is the best-known brand name; Serophene is another widely used brand.) This monthly regimen is a common first therapy for women who are trying to conceive. So common that these women discover friends at work, a cousin's wife, the next-door neighbor have all been given the fertility drug by their gynecologists. So common that women often feel "everyone takes Clomid." Or, as one physician put it, that "Clomid is given out like water." According to some fertility specialists, these impressions are uncomfortably close to reality. Dr. Melvin Taymor, writing not long after Anna considered this treatment, describes Clomid as "one of the most widely used medications in infertility practice and, unfortunately, probably the most abused."[1]

What are the problems that, in the view of this Harvard Medical School professor and other critics, might well be called "fertility drug abuse"? First, when gynecologists prescribe clomiphene as the first approach to infertility, they often do so without investigating why a woman has not conceived. Many physicians neglect simple tests of her partner's fertility. The only clear benefit of clomiphene—and the use for which it gained Food and Drug Administration approval in 1967—is that it can stimulate release of an egg in some women who do not otherwise ovulate; for these women, clomiphene provides one step essential for conception. Yet, even when appropriate tests are done, with results indicating a woman does ovulate, gynecologists routinely prescribe clomiphene; in fact, for two decades, physicians prescribed this medication at a steadily increasing rate, without evidence that such treatment helped.[2] Only in more recent years have fertility specialists conducted studies to determine when use of Clomid might be appropriate for a woman who does ovulate. These studies suggest that Clomid (used for no more than six treatment cycles) may improve pregnancy rates for women with unexplained infertility of three or more years' duration. If these findings are confirmed by further study involving greater numbers of women, it will be important to identify more precisely which categories of patients can benefit.[3] As Dr. Robert Jaffe, of the University of California at San Francisco, comments, "I'm not sure that infertile patients with normal ovulatory cycles can be shown to benefit [by] clomiphene citrate, although I know this is a common practice. . . . There seems to be little to gain. . . . In fact . . . it may even be detrimental on occasion."[4]

A second problem is dosage. Clomiphene should be started at a low dose, writes Dr. Taymor, which should be increased only if ovulation does not occur. Too often a doctor's automatic response if a woman ovulates but does not *conceive* after taking this drug is to give her more. Dr. Jaffe goes further in criticizing this routine escalation, even suggesting the opposite approach: "Some clinicians feel that if a little is good, a lot must be better. However, particularly with clomiphene citrate, others maintain that if a little does not work, try less."[5]

Concern about improper dosage leads directly to a third problem, when clomiphene is successful in causing a woman to ovulate, yet she still does not conceive. Her doctor may simply increase the dosage without attempting to determine why the woman is not becoming pregnant. In fact, clomiphene can actually work against fertility. As with any medication, clomiphene brings side effects. Among the best-known side effects of clomiphene is the altering of the quality of cervical mucus in ways that hinder the sperms' journey through the cervix to meet an egg. Complicating matters further is that whatever additional interventions a doctor might recommend—whether to counteract clomiphene's side effects or to overcome other factors working against conception—bring their own problems.

A fourth concern is the common practice of prescribing clomiphene in cases of "unexplained infertility," that is, when a thorough fertility evaluation has drawn a blank. Diagnostic tests are normal, with no reason found for infertility in either the woman or the man. According to Dr. Taymor, "The most important point is that the couple with unexplained infertility . . . have up to a 34 percent chance of conceiving within six months and 76 percent by two years without any therapy. Until control studies with Clomid can come close to matching these results, the therapist is best advised to refrain from the use of fertility drugs in unexplained infertility."[6]

Clearly, physicians disagree on when or how this popular fertility drug should be used. However, the criticism and uncertainty long remained within the ranks, buried in medical journals or voiced within the confines of a professional convention, beyond the reach of patients. Anna had not heard about doctor misuse of Clomid when her doctor first prescribed it. Yet she did balk at the prospect of taking the drug. Her reasons are instructive, as are the events that unfolded for her.

Benefits, Risks, Unknowns

Even before she began trying to have a child, Anna thought she might have trouble. She knew from gynecologic exams that her cervix was "like a pinprick hole," rather than an elongated lower segment opening into her uterus. Anna's abnormal cervix was a legacy of medication her mother took while pregnant—DES. The synthetic hormone DES, intended initially to prevent miscarriage and then prescribed for a wide range of pregnancy problems, proved to be neither effective nor safe. Its side effects reached all the way to the next generation, exposed before birth. Thus, Anna was reluctant to take any drug while trying to conceive. "I just didn't want to take anything," she recalls. "It seemed rather ironic, being a DES daughter. I'm having problems because my mother took a pregnancy medication. And then it turns out I may have to do the same thing."

Anna's gynecologist did first test whether she ovulated regularly. However, the results—which can never unequivocally confirm a completed ovulation—were ambiguous. She probably did ovulate, but it was not clear how regularly: perhaps not each month or perhaps without a normal hormone response. So her doctor suggested she try Clomid. In answer to Anna's questions about safety, he cited the many years Clomid has been used without serious problems. He would check her ovaries each month to be sure they were not enlarged by cysts, the most common hazardous side effect. He did not mention that there are few good follow-up studies or other mechanisms for reporting problems with Clomid. He did not mention that no one knows just how this chemical affects the human body. Doctors do agree on one fact: while Clomid stimulates ovulation in some women, the resulting pregnancy rate is surprisingly low. Beyond its effect of lowering the quality of cervical mucus, journal articles speculate that clomiphene may alter the delicate hormonal balance required for conception and embryo implantation into the uterine lining or that the drug may impair blood flow to the uterus just as the lining's intricate vascular build-up prepares for an embryo.[7] Some studies suggest subtle damage to the egg or embryo may lessen chances for a pregnancy. [8]

Anna's concerns about safety extended beyond her own health. If she did conceive after taking this drug, could there be any effects on the fetus? For her doctor, these concerns were remote. He assured her that Clomid has a short half-life—that is, much of the drug would be out of her body in a matter of days, before she ovulated. What her doctor did not say—and might not have known—is that some scientists do worry about that other "half," particularly after repeated treatment cycles and increased dosage.[9] Some quantity of drug does linger and can build up over months of use. Animal studies suggest possible harmful effects on an embryo during the earliest weeks, those weeks most crucial for normal development. No one has studied health effects on human offspring born after clomiphene-treated cycles except to check for observable birth defects in newborns. Though present information indicates that long-term health problems seem unlikely in children of women who took clomiphene before conceiving, the possibility that this drug might have effects on the developing fetus is something physicians have not conveyed to patients.

Anna and Tom might well have decided to try Clomid even if they had learned of a possible long-term risk, since the sparse hints of harmful effects on offspring have been limited to experimental animal models. But they might have decided the drug's benefits were not certain enough to take any chance, even if risks are minimal or only "theoretical." For Anna and other patients, potential harm—the unknowns—must join known risks weighed against the benefits provided by a treatment. This type of decision is highly individual, depending on personal views about having a baby and about taking risks with one's own health or a baby's. This decision requires full airing of the possibilities, their likelihood, the strength of existing evidence. In Anna's case, risks as well as benefits of Clomid fell heavily among the unknowns; the balance would not tip easily toward a certain direction. However, the risks her doctor did describe—side effects she might experience during the months she took Clomid—did not seem to outweigh the possible benefits. Anna decided, though with reluctance, to take the drug.

After several months on Clomid—months with mood swings her doctor had not warned her about but with no pregnancy—Anna faced the next questions. How long should she continue? Should she take a higher dose? Should they be trying something else? To counteract the deleterious effect of Clomid on cervical mucus, her doctor suggested they try adding estrogen, the female hormone that normally enhances mucus quality at the time of ovulation. To support an embryo in its earliest stages, even before a pregnancy test, they could try adding progesterone, another female hormone with a crucial role immediately following ovulation. Unfortunately, there is no good evidence that administering these hormones increases the likelihood of pregnancy. At this point, then, her doctor was ready to move beyond Clomid, but the desire to "do something" was outstripping reasons to think the something would do any good.

And what of the potential for harm? No one can say whether taking estrogen posed special risks for Anna, exposed in utero to the synthetic estrogen DES; however, scientists who study long-term effects of hormones have expressed concern about prescribing hormonal drugs to DES daughters.[10] Even more compelling to Anna was that her doctor's suggestions sounded rather like the DES regimen her mother was given, the pregnancy treatment that brought Anna to this point in the first place. She remained concerned about effects all of these medications might have on a developing fetus if she did conceive and decided against taking additional hormones.

Questions about Risks

Questions about risks for women taking Clomid and other fertility drugs emerged publicly in 1993, with reports of a possible link to ovarian cancer. One epidemiological study of women diagnosed with ovarian cancer suggests that use of Clomid for more than one year may increase an individual's chances of later developing this disease.[1] Pointing out the large proportion of women in the study who took Clomid even though they did not have ovulation problems, Dr. Robert Jaffe cautioned, "If additional carefully performed and controlled studies also point to the possibility of increased risk of ovarian malignancies in infertile women who undergo repeated attempts at ovulation induction, clinicians should be circumspect in their use of [fertility drugs]. At the very least, the sometimes thoughtless, profligate, and often prolonged use of clomiphene citrate, particularly in women with normal ovulatory cycles, should not be perpetuated."[2] By the mid-1990s, fertility specialists were more commonly recommending that women try Clomid for not more than three to four treatment cycles, perhaps alternating months with no treatment.

Lack of knowledge about how Clomid affects the human body extends further than a woman's reproductive tract. In 1994, an ophthalmologist reported on a woman taking clomiphene citrate who developed a dark area in one eye; her vision was seriously impaired and had only partially improved months after stopping the drug. Noting that Clomid, like other hormonal drugs, can reduce blood flow to the eye and that vision problems are common with Clomid, he cautions that this medication should be stopped and a patient's eyes examined if she experiences any changes in vision.[3] While only a case report, it does raise questions: first, whether gynecologists read and pay attention to an eye doctor's cautions, and second, whether they inform women who are deciding whether to take Clomid about this potential side effect.

Another interesting case report, given patients' common reports of moodiness or depression while taking Clomid, describes psychotic symptoms in a woman shortly after she started treatment. The authors suggest that clomiphene—in combination with the physical and psychological stress of undergoing fertility treatment—may trigger such a reaction in some women. They recommend that physicians inform patients "in detail about the possible psychological effects of clomiphene"; if a patient has previously experienced psychiatric illness, ovarian stimulants such as Clomid should be prescribed "with particular care."[4]

1. Rossing, Daling, and Weiss 1994.
2. Jaffe 1995a.
3. Lawton 1994.
4. Seidentopf et al. 1997, 707.

Escalating Treatment

Now Anna's doctor presented another strategy. They could bypass the cervix altogether with a procedure called intrauterine insemination (IUI). Unlike the more commonly performed artificial insemination in which sperm are placed in the vagina at the cervical opening, Tom's sperm would be placed directly into Anna's uterus with a long syringe. As Anna's doctor explained, IUI does bring more risk than a vaginal insemination. Besides painful cramping caused by the procedure, there was the chance of uterine infection. Bypassing the vagina and cervix means also bypassing a natural barrier that helps protect the uterus from harmful bacteria. If infection did develop, it would not only threaten a conceived pregnancy but would also further jeopardize Anna's chances of conceiving in the future. (The risk of uterine infection has diminished with more recent technical improvements.)

Anna and Tom decided they would take the chance. For Anna, this decision meant driving three hours from their home in the country to her doctor's office, Tom's semen in a vial wrapped in a paper bag on the car seat beside her; then undergoing the insemination procedure on the examination table, feet in the stirrups; and then driving the three hours home. This routine, centered on Anna's menstrual cycle, became the focus of this couple's life for six months—until their wish came true. No period, a positive pregnancy test, morning nausea. But then came the intense pain shooting up Anna's arm, the anxious three-hour drive to her doctor's office, and a diagnosis of ectopic pregnancy within the fallopian tube, which ruptured before they could reach the hospital.

Anna was left with only one fallopian tube. Although women do conceive with a single fallopian tube, her remaining tube did not appear to be normal in an X-ray examination. Her doctor now raised new choices. They could try to circumvent that tube with in vitro fertilization (IVF). Eggs and sperm would be joined in a laboratory dish; if fertilization was successful, a doctor would place embryos directly into Anna's uterus where, they must hope, one would implant. Or they could try surgery to repair Anna's ruptured tube, increasing chances that an egg could travel the usual route from her ovary through the tube for an "unassisted" conception. Either choice increased her chances for yet another ectopic pregnancy—a risk already elevated with her history of DES exposure, fertility problems, and a previous ectopic pregnancy.

Anna and Tom once again faced a crucial decision. Once again, Anna sought information. She talked with her own doctor, with surgeons who could perform the microsurgery, and with IVF practitioners. She asked them about percentages—the likelihood of being able to reconstruct her fallopian tube, the success rates for IVF—and about side effects she might experience with each of the two options. She consulted the *Physicians' Desk Reference* (PDR), a bulky volume in which drug manufacturers list the uses and side effects of their products. She wrote for information directly to the manufacturer of drugs used during IVF and received copies of studies that support use of these drugs. Like most patients, however, Anna was not reading medical journals on a regular basis. There she would have received an education that would have shed quite a different light on her choices.

A View from Within

During the mid- to late 1980s, as Anna and Tom became consumed with the pursuit of pregnancy, a stream of critical journal articles on the diagnosis and treatment of fertility problems began to appear. Defying physicians' strong tradition of refusing to criticize colleagues, a few fertility specialists expressed alarm at practices they were observing within this field of medicine, a situation they believed was moving from bad to worse. Established, widely prescribed procedures popular with doctors had never been shown through scientific study to increase significantly the likelihood of pregnancy. New techniques were being adopted in the absence of evidence that they were better than the

old. What doctors often cite proudly as their "armamentarium" for fighting infertility was built largely of unproven weapons. Caught in the cross fire, deciding among these old and new procedures, were fertility patients. Unbeknownst
to them, a battle was brewing within the profession over the very recommendations these patients were offered daily at the doctor's office.

As Anna deliberated microsurgery to fix a ruptured fallopian tube, she did
not see an editorial entitled "Anything You Can Do I Can Do Better . . . or Differently!" Published in *Fertility and Sterility*, the journal that specializes in reproductive medicine, this article zeroed in on tubal surgery as an example of gynecologists' growing tendency to leap onto the latest technological bandwagon.[11]
The author decried his colleagues' "premature" declarations of success for new
surgical procedures on the fallopian tube. They had no numbers yet on the rate
of pregnancy after such procedures; an operation might "succeed" in removing
an obstruction, for instance, but the patient still might never have a baby.

Nor did Anna see the next month's editorial, "What Is Efficacious Infertility
Therapy?" Its author did not find many examples of "efficacious" therapy among
the therapeutic standbys. Rather, he saw doctors prescribing treatments out of
habit or faith alone. Once suggested, treatments "seem to generate a momentum independent of their demonstrated benefit, assisted by the lay medical
press and well-meaning practitioners who are personally convinced of their
value."[12] Yet a doctor's personal belief is a far cry from scientific evidence showing that pregnancy rates increase as a result of a medical intervention.

The author reminded his colleagues of an essential fact of reproductive life:
most fertility problems fall along a continuum. Individuals may be at the low
end, that is, below the normal fertility range; in most cases, however, spontaneous pregnancy—conception without treatment—is possible. A proportion of
less fertile couples will conceive with no medical intervention, though they
may take longer than more fertile couples. Too often, credit for a pregnancy
that would have occurred anyway is awarded to a treatment that happened to be
employed.

Such undeserved credit was abundant during the three decades when millions of women, including Anna's mother, were prescribed DES to "save" their
pregnancies. Today's overzealous use of Clomid in women who do ovulate
means numerous conceptions will be attributed to a fertility drug that was
probably not needed. Artificial insemination with the partner's sperm—a procedure also in vogue for many years—may also frequently receive undeserved
credit for pregnancies. Couples who undergo this intervention (for example, to
overcome "inadequate" cervical mucus or "unexplained infertility") commonly

have intercourse during the same months. If conception occurs, who knows which activity was efficacious?

There is also uncertainty about the usefulness of the fertility tests that guide the course of treatment. Do they actually identify less fertile individuals who are likely to benefit from medical intervention? As with treatments, old and new diagnostic procedures have drawn criticism within the profession. The long-established postcoital test (PCT), for example, is all too familiar to couples experiencing fertility problems. The woman hurries to her doctor's office following intercourse that has been unromantically timed around ovulation and appointment hours. The doctor peers into a microscope to see whether sperm are wriggling robustly through mucus he has swabbed from her cervix. If the sperm appear sluggish or immobile, the mucus is described as "inadequate" (or downright "hostile"), likely to destroy sperm before they can reach the egg. Most patients don't know, as they wait anxiously for the results, that the postcoital test's value for predicting pregnancy has been questioned in medical journals.[13] In many cases, whatever the doctor observes about cervical mucus and sperm tells little about whether the couple will conceive. Not only are patients subjected unnecessarily to these tests, but treatment may proceed on the basis of useless results.

Newly developed techniques can also yield questionable diagnoses. For example, physicians now test patients for immunologic problems that may cause infertility. However, the immune system is notoriously complex; its role in conception, implantation, and pregnancy remains a scientific enigma. Not only is it difficult to diagnose problems in a system doctors do not understand, it is impossible to know what harm they might cause by tinkering with the fine workings of that system.

And, after all the tests are done, there remains that amorphous diagnostic category labeled "unexplained infertility"—a diagnosis by default with disturbingly flexible boundaries. These patients (that is, the women in couples with unexplained infertility) are barraged with treatments. For many couples, however, particularly if they have been trying to conceive for less than two years and the woman is not yet nearing forty, a conservative approach—waiting for a spontaneous pregnancy—is at least as likely to succeed; the woman can avoid risks of a medical intervention that must be a shot in the dark, where no one even knows the target.

Were patients to read medical journals, they might be surprised to find that physicians apparently need to review the basic facts: that many diagnoses are ill defined and many common practices unproven; that many fertility patients will conceive spontaneously, with no treatment; that results for most treatments have never been compared to spontaneous pregnancy rates; that, lacking evidence of significantly improved chances of pregnancy with a medical intervention, the patient may be better off without it.

Testing Fertility Tests

Most fertility tests are not themselves tested on fertile women and men in order to compare results. One recent small study that did make such a comparison found that a surprising 70 percent of fertile couples had at least one abnormal result, compared to 84 percent of infertile couples. Several commonly used tests identified a "cause" of infertility at the same rate in the fertile couples as in the infertile. Only tubal blockage and endometriosis were significantly more frequent among infertile couples; the two groups did not differ in results for semen analysis, tests for cervical infection or mucus (PCT), luteal phase defect (endometrial biopsy), or immunological or uterine abnormality.[1]

Not only do these abnormal results become the reason for a treatment, but they add greatly to a couple's anxiety and stress, which may in itself lower their chance of conceiving. Argues one critic about the postcoital test (PCT) in particular: "The most important reason for not using [the postcoital test] is the frequency of meaningless abnormal results. In six clinical studies, 45 percent of the test results were abnormal. Postcoital tests are simple and commonly used, but the test can be a harrowing performance evaluation for infertile couples, and for those with abnormal results, the potentially negative impact is unwarranted by the questionable value of the results."[2]

A Dutch report argues that the postcoital test can provide useful information about a couple's chances for conceiving without treatment within the following year—but only if intercourse occurs nine to twelve hours before microscopic examination of the cervical mucus and if the woman has normal ovulation and fallopian tubes. Using a newly proposed system for classifying observed movement of sperm in the mucus (negative, nonprogressive, progressive), estimates ranged from a nearly 50 percent chance of conceiving within one year (with the most favorable PCT results, characterized by sperm progressing through the mucus) to a 15 percent chance (with negative results, or no moving sperm). While such predictions may help some couples decide whether to undergo treatment now or wait before intervening medically, the actual use of postcoital tests by most gynecologists is not likely to meet this study's stringent requirements.[3]

One recent overview places diagnostic tests into three categories, based on whether an "abnormal" result identifies a condition that actually impairs fertility and can be improved by treatment:

Abnormal results are associated with infertility that requires treatment—semen analyses showing no sperm; hysterosalpingogram or laparoscopy showing both fallopian tubes blocked; blood tests of hormone levels indicating the absence of ovulation.

Abnormal results are not consistently associated with impaired fertility—postcoital test; laparoscopy showing mild endometriosis; hysteroscopy; sperm/hamster egg penetration assay; antisperm antibody tests.

Abnormal results do not presently appear to be associated with impaired fertility—endometrial biopsy; varicocele assessment. [4]

1. Guzick et al. 1994.
2. Collins 1995, 1161.
3. Eimers et al. 1994b.
4. ESHRE Capri 1996.

The Risk of Exploitation

Unfortunately, these basic facts are not the whole story. Patients would be chagrined to learn the depth of problems characterizing fertility medicine. Step back now from Anna and Tom to view what they and other fertility patients were missing. In the late 1980s, criticism within the profession came to a head. Eleven prominent specialists coauthored a highly unusual editorial titled "Are We Exploiting the Infertile Couple?" With a title like that, appearing in a medical journal, you know the answer is "yes."[14]

The authors begin, "As experienced practitioners in the field of reproductive endocrinology and infertility, we feel obligated to address a problem that is creeping into American gynecology: the exploitation of the infertile couple." These fertility specialists claim that exploitation is often unintentional, for most physicians think their prescribed therapies are appropriate. The editorial does state in no uncertain terms, however, that improper physician actions too often result in "substandard or unnecessary medical care." Few fertility treatments, lament the authors, "have withstood the test of time" or the test of careful scientific scrutiny. And these insiders clearly see more than faulty science and inadequate physician knowledge behind patient exploitation. A doctor's recommendation is too often geared toward personal or corporate gain, at the expense of patients rather than in their best interest.

Where might patients detect signs of exploitation? Perhaps in affiliations listed on a letterhead or in certificates hanging on an office wall—medical "credentials" that imply infertility specialization. Most obstetrician-gynecologists are trained to conduct a general fertility evaluation of a couple. Expertise in more sophisticated diagnoses and in more complex fertility therapies requires substantial additional education—at least two years of training in reproductive endocrinology following an ob-gyn residency. Physicians can join a professional society, such as the American Society for Reproductive Medicine, and display this membership on office stationery, but membership in such societies does not indicate certification or expertise in this field.

Numerous short courses on infertility topics are offered to physicians. Course brochures often advertise "certificate suitable for framing"; yet these courses do not provide adequate training in appropriate use of particular therapies. Patients viewing certificates on walls may well assume the gynecologists have thoroughly proven their competence. The eleven authors of the editorial, in contrast, perceive deceptive credentials displayed by weekend-course participants who, for example, "may return to their community and begin to do microsurgery or laser surgery without an appreciation of the appropriate selection of patients or a thorough understanding of the limitations of the procedure or potential for complications."[15]

Beyond spurious credentials, doctors and clinics may claim inflated success rates. Before deciding to undergo treatment, patients need to know the likelihood that medical intervention will increase their chance of having a baby. Too often, however, patients receive only false advertising; physicians manipulate numbers, definitions of success—and their patients—to paint an overly optimistic picture of expected results. A physician may give numbers more favorable than his own—the nationwide average or, even more misleading, the highest success rate published in medical reports from the most experienced fertility clinic. Patients learn nothing about the experience and skill of this doctor—how many times he has attempted a particular procedure in cases similar to their own, the resulting pregnancy and birthrates, the rate and type of complications. This doctor's success stories may bear little resemblance to the case of the inquiring patient. Treating primarily younger women and couples with less severe fertility problems—patients who have the best prognosis—can also inflate a physician's rate of success.

Most basic of all is what the doctor means by "success." When considering treatment for fertility problems, the ultimate success is the birth of a healthy baby. Clomid's success in stimulating ovulation is far more impressive than its success in achieving pregnancy. Microsurgery might successfully reunite a ruptured fallopian tube or remove an obstruction. But what happens next? How many conceptions follow the operative success? And how many of those embryos implant within a repaired tube rather than within the uterus, where they can develop into a successful pregnancy? (Definitions of success are nowhere more troublesome than in claims made for assisted reproductive technologies, the focus of Chapter 3.)

All in all, the authors of the editorial concluded, gynecologists are too quick in recommending expensive, highly invasive procedures. They fail to investigate systematically the causes of a patient's infertility, and, if a treatable cause is revealed, to tailor the therapy to it. The least invasive tests should be used first and, if results so indicate, the least invasive treatment. Wait a reasonable amount of time for pregnancy to occur, these authors urge their colleagues, before proceeding to the next more expensive and invasive steps.

Fertility Treatment for Endometriosis

Mysterious Condition, Elusive Success

Endometriosis, frequently diagnosed in women who are trying to conceive, is a condition in which tissue from the uterine lining migrates, attaches, and grows outside the uterus. For many years, doctors have prescribed hormonal medications (danazol or nafarelin) that can reduce the aberrant endometrial tissue. However, by the 1990s, critics were questioning this widespread treatment. One noted that existing studies proved only that these drugs can successfully decrease the amount of tissue visible during a laparoscopy and lessen the pain endometriosis causes some women. There was no evidence that this success translates into increased fertility. In an editorial written for medical colleagues, this physician comments, "Apparently it has been taken for granted by almost everyone until recently that a drug which makes the endometriotic implants less visible at second look laparoscopy should also increase the patient's fecundity [the statistical likelihood of conceiving per month]."[1]

The editorial then summarizes a review of nearly 300 medical journal reports on endometriosis therapies published between 1982 and 1989. Remarkably few adequately designed studies actually looked at the fertility of endometriosis patients, "and none of them has proven the superiority of any treatment of endometriosis over placebo." Of the fifteen studies that did meet scientific standards, only seven included a control group receiving either no treatment or placebo; the others compared a different medication and/or surgery (none of which had themselves been shown to increase the likelihood of pregnancy in women with endometriosis). Of the seven studies that did compare treatment with no treatment, only four reported pregnancy rates. The others measured patient discomfort and/or the amount of tissue visible to the gynecologist during pelvic surgery.

The four studies that did include pregnancy rates reported "no significant differences between the treated . . . and non-treated or placebo-treated groups of patients. If anything, the pregnancy rates were higher in the no-treatment groups in three of the four studies." In the fourth study, the rate of pregnancy was nearly identical among those using medication and those receiving placebo. In sum, doctors were prescribing these medications, with their considerable side effects, without evidence of improved chances for pregnancy.

A more recent study, analyzing pregnancy rates and including a no-treatment group, concluded that laparoscopic surgery by a skilled surgeon is the most beneficial treatment for infertile women with moderate or severe endometriosis who do *not* have abnormalities of the fallopian tubes and/or fimbria (the wavy fringe lining the entrance to the fallopian tubes). Noting the risk of adhesions forming after removal of superficial, minimal, or mild endometriosis, the authors caution that "careful consideration of this potential complication is imperative before performing this operation, especially in younger patients or those with short duration of infertility. No treatment may be the best approach in these patients."[2] Another study, focusing specifically on minimal or mild endometriosis, reached a different conclusion. During diagnostic laparoscopy, surgeons randomly assigned patients with this condition to treatment (surgical removal of observed endometriotic tissue) or no treatment (the diagnostic laparoscopy only). After a 36-week followup, the cumulative pregnancy rate in treated women was 30.7 percent, compared to 17.7 percent in those with no surgical treatment, an approximately 70 percent difference. (During this time patients knew whether or not they had received treatment, introducing the possibility of a placebo effect.) Put another way, the authors concluded that one in eight women with minimal or mild endometriosis would benefit from surgical removal of tissue at the time of laparoscopy.[3] These surgeons do note that treatment did not restore fertility to normal range, indicating that unidentified factors remain. It should also be noted that such studies cannot provide comparisons with women who do not undergo laparoscopy but in fact have a similar condition and who receive no treatment or treatment with medications or IVF. A larger research project has been gathering data from several treatment centers and may provide more solid comparisons of surgery, medications, and no treatment for mild, moderate, and severe endometriosis.

Women desiring pregnancy (rather than relief from pain) may not have much choice among treatments in years to come, as doctors increasingly direct patients with various fertility problems, including endometriosis, to in vitro fertilization (IVF).

However, a 1996 study compared cumulative pregnancy rates after three years in 118 women diagnosed with endometriosis who underwent IVF or received no treatment. This study found significantly better outcomes with IVF only in women over the age of thirty-one, particularly if the condition was at an advanced stage. The authors advise their younger patients—especially those for whom mild or moderate endometriosis is the only fertility diagnosis—"to postpone treatment a few years, explaining that they have a comparable probability of achieving pregnancy without IVF during that period."[4]

In 1997, the American Society for Reproductive Medicine (ASRM) declared that its long-standing and widely used system for classifying the severity of endometriosis does not correspond with impairment of fertility. A study commissioned to evaluate, for the first time, the relationship between the stages of endometriosis and prognosis for successful pregnancy after treatment found no significant differences in pregnancy rates across the four ASRM stages. Describing the relationship between infertility and endometriosis as "an enigma," the study's authors suggest that the classification system's predictive failure stems from "our meager understanding of the pathophysiology of infertility in women with endometriosis."[5]

In fact, no one knows why women develop endometriosis or how this condition, which ranges widely in its severity, affects fertility. The underlying cause of endometriosis—not just the observable tissue that is the condition's symptom—may itself directly interfere with becoming pregnant. Thus, it is not surprising that treatment successful in lessening a symptom may not provide equivalent success rates for attaining pregnancy, if the original cause of the symptom remains. Studies in baboons, as well as in fertile women undergoing tubal ligation, suggest that mild endometriosis may be a common condition unrelated to fertility; the procedure of laparoscopy to detect the tissue may even worsen an otherwise harmless condition, perhaps by aggravating an inflammatory process.[6] One theory receiving increased attention is that endometriosis reflects a physiological response to environmental pollutants such as dioxin.[7] Clearly, until further research solves the basic mystery of what endometriosis is and how the condition relates to lowered fertility, doctors will lack therapies that specifically target that relationship and lack strategies aimed at preventing it.

---

1. Evers 1989. See also Bayer et al. 1988; Hughes, Fedorkow, and Collins 1993; Hull, Moghissi, and Magyar 1987.

2. Adamson et al. 1993.

3. Marcoux et al. 1997.

4. Kodama et al. 1996, 978.

5. Guzick et al. 1997, 827. See also Schenken and Guzick 1997.

6. D'Hooghe et al. 1996.

7. Mayani et al. 1997.

For Anna and Tom, treatment choices narrowed to IVF or fallopian tube surgery, each with its own risks and with inadequate information on outcomes. In Anna's case, however, chances of conceiving without treatment, following the ectopic pregnancy, were very low. Although glad to have choices available, her decision on pelvic microsurgery felt like selecting the lesser of two evils. "I wasn't afraid of the IVF procedure," she explains, "but of the trappings surrounding it. The heavy-duty hormones . . ."

If Anna hesitated before taking Clomid, she was even more wary of the IVF hormone regimen used to "shut down" a woman's own menstrual cycle, then "superovulate" her (that is, cause several eggs to mature and be released), then nourish the replaced embryos into a sustained pregnancy (a procedure described more fully in Chapter 3). The information she obtained from doctors, from the consumer organization Resolve, from the *Physicians' Desk Reference* and drug manufacturers could not ease her qualms. "Not that I was eager to have surgery. . . . But I found a surgeon who was supposed to be the best and just felt more comfortable with that. I decided I'd rather go under the knife." Anna can smile now at the memory of this choice.

And so Anna journeyed to Seattle for pelvic microsurgery. The operation repaired her ruptured tube. Two years later Anna did become pregnant and delivered a healthy baby. Whether she would have conceived before those first Clomid pills, if she and Tom had tried a while longer, can never be known. After several years of attempting to become pregnant again, Anna and Tom adopted a second child. Throughout those years, however, thousands of other couples were choosing in vitro fertilization. By the 1990s, IVF was outstripping microsurgery as the treatment of choice for most tubal problems—except in cases where a woman's health insurance would cover only surgery.[16]

3 Assisted Reproductive Technology

A Modern Fact of Life

"Whatever we went through was worth it," Sharon affirms now unequivocally, gazing at her daughter, a happy, healthy-looking baby who does all the things babies do. What this doting first-time mother and her husband went through included fertility drugs, which made Sharon feel sick and depressed, then two variations of in vitro fertilization. That was after Jeff's surgery to reverse a vasectomy, the legacy of a previous marriage when he thought he would never want more children. Although Sharon had no reason to suspect she would have problems conceiving, she was in her late thirties, past the age when women are most fertile. And although Jeff's fertility test showed sperm swimming energetically—evidence that his vasectomy reversal was successful—there was the risk of what the doctor called "male factor problems." Faced with these potential difficulties, Sharon decided after only three months of trying to conceive that she would begin fertility treatment. For six months she took clomiphene citrate. Their life revolved obsessively around the moment of her ovulation: Would it be today or tomorrow? Should they have intercourse before going to work or later that night? Had they missed the best time, had they lost the month? Could Jeff go on a business trip next month?

When Sharon's doctor advised a more aggressive approach, they plunged ahead. First, Sharon took stronger fertility drugs so that her ovaries would produce many eggs, which the doctor then extracted for in vitro fertilization (IVF). To maximize the likelihood of pregnancy during these cycles, her doctor performed two differing embryo transfer procedures at the same time. He inserted two embryos through her vagina into her uterus; and, through a small abdominal incision, he placed one embryo at the entry of each fallopian tube.

All the while Sharon and Jeff continued their intense schedule of sexual intercourse.

Sharon's doctor, a fertility specialist, keeps a tally and tells patients his success rates for various treatments. Asked which manner of conception her doctor would list as successful in her case, Sharon jokes, "Both." In every joke, of course, is a grain of truth. For the burgeoning category of fertility treatments known as "assisted (or advanced) reproductive technologies"—shortened perhaps too suggestively to the term ART—that grain can be large indeed. Reports on the success of these interventions have been inadequate and, in some instances, deceptive. As Sharon and Jeff's experience illustrates, moreover, physicians' tallies often ignore another explanation for successful pregnancies. Perhaps their low-tech, at-home process of sexual intercourse actually resulted in the pregnancy. Now, with Rebecca in tow, they do not really care which process did the trick. But for other couples—and for the specialty of fertility medicine—the question is crucial.

Today's fertility patients decide about their own treatments based on numbers from cases such as Sharon's. No patients—even the majority who do not initially undergo assisted reproduction—are untouched by these technologies, which have become pivotal for fertility medicine today and for the field's future directions. Fertility specialists now recommend some form of in vitro fertilization to nearly any woman who does not become pregnant with less invasive treatments. While helpful for some patients, these reproductive technologies highlight dangers in the ongoing expansion of fertility interventions. Only rarely do these dangers erupt into public view as egregious ethical violations.

The less extreme but far more common problems, however, are woven of the same cloth. This chapter traces the growth of assisted reproduction and of its controversies, not only as information important in itself, but as background for what follows in subsequent chapters. Understanding the array of fertility treatments now available to women and men requires an understanding of ART. Understanding ART, in turn, requires taking a broad view that encompasses doctors who are doing too much to too many patients, politics that make for strange reproductive bedfellows, government that abrogates its responsibilities, and technology that in the words of one prominent fertility specialist "is running away from us."

New Forms of Conception

Since the birth of the world's first IVF baby in 1978, the basics of the procedure have become familiar to the public, though medical details may remain vague. At the time of ovulation, doctors remove at least one mature egg (also called an ovum or oocyte) from a woman's ovary. This process involves passing a long needle through the vaginal or abdominal wall, puncturing fluid-filled ovarian follicles, sucking out (aspirating) the follicular fluid, and examining this fluid with a microscope to see whether it does, in fact, harbor an egg. Sperm, gathered through masturbation, meet egg in a specially prepared laboratory dish, where they bathe in nutrients intended to promote conception.[1] If a sperm does fertilize an egg and cell division proceeds to a stage and quality the embryologist considers adequate, the embryo is removed from the dish and placed into a catheter, which the doctor injects through the vagina and cervix into the woman's uterus, where, it is hoped, the embryo, released from its catheter, will burrow into the uterine lining and grow normally.

In a medical specialty too often characterized by exaggerated claims, IVF did mark revolutionary changes in fertility treatments and human reproduction itself. Most profound was moving egg, sperm, and conception from the body to a laboratory; sexual intercourse was no longer required. A second major change evolved after the earliest attempts at in vitro fertilization, as in vitro programs attempted to increase the likelihood of conception and successful pregnancy by removing more than one egg from the ovary and transferring more than one embryo per menstrual cycle. Normally, a single egg matures each month, bursting through the ovary's wall in the process of ovulation. To force maturation of several eggs in one cycle, the woman takes a combination of hormones, in most cases by daily injections that she or her partner can give, in a regimen known as controlled ovarian hyperstimulation—also known as "superovulating" the woman.

Initially, IVF was intended for the relatively few women with blocked or absent fallopian tubes whose naturally ovulated egg cannot otherwise reach the uterus. Although the chances of a successful IVF pregnancy were always small for these women (hovering between 10 and 15 percent in the more experienced programs during earlier years, up to 15–20 percent by the mid-1990s), they were better than nothing. If the woman did become pregnant, the IVF procedure—bypassing the problematic fallopian tubes—was responsible. Birth of a healthy baby could rightfully be called an IVF "success." Once physicians and the public have access to a procedure like IVF, however, its use extends beyond the original target population. Doctors offer the new treatment for a broader range of conditions—wanting to "do something" when no better medical alternative exists—without systematically evaluating the outcomes. The number of patients and types of diagnoses indicating "need" for a treatment grow independently of biological rationale or scientific data. Doctors were soon trying IVF on women with conditions other than intractable tubal problems, prescribing this technique for patients with endometriosis, ovulation disorders, and "unexplained infertility." IVF even became a treatment aimed at *male* fertility problems that may lower a couple's chance of conceiving. By the 1990s, the American Society for Reproductive Medicine (ASRM) deemed IVF an appropriate treatment for anyone who had failed in attempts with conventional therapies (i.e., fertility drugs, surgery, inseminations). "The primary medical indication" for IVF, according to the society's rather broad definition-by-default, was "failure of conventional therapy to provide a pregnancy for the infertile couple."[2] One fertility specialist, chagrined but not surprised at the growth of IVF, put it succinctly: "If all I have is a hammer, the whole world looks like a nail."

The original in vitro fertilization process, with transfer of embryos to the uterus, has engendered variations that have, in turn, expanded in use (see Figure 1). For example, as with IVF, gamete intrafallopian transfer (GIFT) entails retrieving eggs from the ovary and combining them with sperm. In GIFT, however, the doctor places eggs and sperm (the female and male gametes) through a small incision near the woman's navel into the fallopian tube for fertilization, rather than into a laboratory dish. If conception occurs, the fertilized egg must then travel to the uterus in the usual, unassisted manner. GIFT is possible only if a woman has at least one open fallopian tube; the hope is that a more natural fertilization, within the tube, will allow for more successful embryo growth and

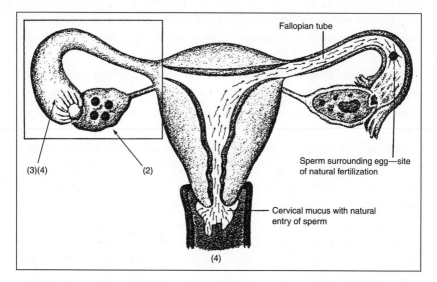

Figure 1. The assisted reproductive technologies. In this illustration of the female reproductive tract, the natural process of fertilization is shown to the right, with sperm entering at the cervix and proceeding through the uterus to meet a released egg in the fallopian tube. On the left, the sites of ART interventions are indicated, corresponding to the steps listed.

Step 1: (not shown) Ovarian hyperstimulation to mature several eggs.

Step 2: A needle puncture (usually ultrasound-guided, through the vaginal wall) to aspirate eggs from mature follicles (usually 4–20 per cycle).

Step 3: Each egg mixed with prepared sperm for fertilization—done in individual laboratory dishes for 1–5 days for IVF, TET, ZIFT; for GIFT, eggs retrieved by laparoscopy are returned to fallopian tubes immediately, along with prepared sperm.

Step 4: Return of embryos vaginally to uterus (IVF) or during laparoscopy to fallopian tube (TET, ZIFT). For intrauterine insemination with controlled ovarian hyperstimulation (IUI/COHS) women undergo Step 1, followed by the injection of the hormone human chorionic gonadotropin (hCG) to trigger ovulation; prepared sperm are then placed through the cervix into the uterus. For intracytoplasmic sperm injection (ICSI, a micromanipulation technique) a single prepared sperm is injected directly into each mature egg (as adjunct to Step 3); if fertilization is achieved, resulting embryo is then transferred to uterus and/or fallopian tubes. (Illustration based on C. Harkness. 1992. *The infertility book: A comprehensive and emotional guide.* Berkeley, Calif.: Celestial Arts.)

implantation. Less commonly used variations transfer eggs fertilized in vitro into a woman's fallopian tube. The specific timing of this transfer procedure aims at catching the most opportune embryonic stage for entering and implanting within the uterus. Zygote intrafallopian transfer (ZIFT) uses one or more fertilized but undivided eggs, and tubal embryo transfer (TET) uses fertilized eggs that have undergone cell division. Additional spin-offs of the in vitro procedure include cryopreservation, the freezing and storing of unused embryos, which can be thawed and transferred during a later attempt at pregnancy; micromanipulation techniques, which assist the actual fertilization process by helping sperm enter an egg (see Chapter 4); the use of "donor eggs," usually from younger women, for transfer after fertilization into women nearing or beyond menopause (see Chapter 5); and combining donor sperm and/or eggs in various types of surrogate gestational relationships, during which one woman carries a pregnancy for another.

More Specialists, More ART

One decade after the first IVF birth, the American Society for Reproductive Medicine formally broadened the in vitro field to encompass numerous interventions employing laboratory-related conception techniques and direct retrieval of eggs from a woman's ovary; in the society's medical journal, *Fertility and Sterility,* the section previously entitled "In Vitro Fertilization" became "Assisted Reproductive Technology." Not long before, the same journal had published the editorial expressing concern over "exploitation" of infertile couples that was discussed in Chapter 2. This unusual editorial gave voice to increasing discomfort among some fertility specialists at how their colleagues were using fertility treatments, a discomfort magnified by the rapid growth of assisted reproduction.

By the late 1980s, concern over ART in particular spilled beyond editorial comment. At the society's annual convention in 1989 the professional dispute simmering in the journals gained greater exposure. True to medical convention form, the days were filled with presentations, honored speakers, prize papers, commercial exhibits, and hallway conversations. As participants packed into daily sessions on "clinical assisted reproductive technology," one could readily believe the society's description of infertility as the fastest growing subspecialty in medicine. Yet underlying all this activity was the disturbing sense of an Alice-in-Wonderland world in which the medical specialty was scrambling to catch up with events and people. Even as this conference churned out more physicians who would return home to practice newly learned procedures, one officer of the organization was decrying the steadily increasing number of doctors performing an expanding "alphabet soup" of untested IVF-related therapies.

In fact, anyone who graduates from medical school and obtains a state license can perform any reproductive procedure—IVF, GIFT, freezing embryos, laser surgery—if he or she has the resources. Not only is any physician permitted to perform fertility treatments, but ob-gyns were attracted increasingly to these therapies by a peculiar set of incentives. The perception that no harm is done serves as one lure. In the words of another officer of ASRM, "People are more courageous in treating patients, since the ultimate side effect is not as obvious." In fact, injuries, and in rare cases deaths, have resulted from fertility treatments; but the perception of safety leads doctors to proceed more freely with these interventions. With assisted reproductive technologies, lack of success also encourages, paradoxically, more interventions. While critics were assailing deceptive, inflated pregnancy claims, a low rate of success—hovering around 10 percent nationwide for IVF—was becoming acceptable. As Dr. Martin Quigly, a specialist who performs these treatments, stated bluntly at the 1989 convention, "The expected result is failure." He went on to recommend counseling patients to cope with this reality.

With failure the norm, practitioners gained two significant payoffs. First, a physician's reputation and ability to attract patients could withstand considerable lack of success with IVF. Second, since failure could not easily be attributed to improper practice, physicians gained protection from a double-edged threat—malpractice lawsuits and soaring insurance rates. During the 1980s, according to fertility specialists, malpractice became a powerful economic force behind doctors' eagerness to perform new reproductive therapies. Malpractice insurance rates were rising most precipitously for obstetricians, since serious injury can occur during labor and delivery. To keep their insurance rates lower, many ob-gyns abandoned obstetrics altogether. To increase their gynecologic practices, they offered specialized fertility care, though few had special training. The costs of this venture—for example, investment in an IVF laboratory (or laser surgery machine)—could be recouped when patients were attracted and the equipment employed. This trend would be reinforced in the 1990s as managed care whittled down insured reimbursements for other ob-gyn services and physicians sought fertility patients, who generally pay out of their own pockets.

The sheer number of doctors hanging out fertility shingles with inadequate training exacerbated an absence of oversight typical of American medicine. No mechanism existed to oversee the explosion of fertility treatments performed in offices and clinics throughout the country, to evaluate whether doctors employ such procedures in appropriate cases and with the necessary skill. Unlike other types of medical laboratories, those handling embryos are subject to no mandatory regulations; federal legislation passed in 1992 set up a *voluntary* laboratory certification model, to be implemented by late 1994. (As of 1997, however, there was still no funding for implementation.) The American Society for Reproductive Medicine promulgated minimum standards for IVF and GIFT and published cautionary editorials, but these efforts carry no power of enforcement whatsoever. As the organization's officers made clear during their convention, this voluntary professional society is not a regulatory body and will not become one.

Like other physicians, fertility specialists hold tenaciously to their independence, resisting surveillance or regulation. With regard to one type of oversight, however, a novel chorus of medical grumbling about government inaction could be heard by 1989 over convention lunches, at press briefings, in hallway conversations. The government, complained these doctors, refused to fund research on IVF and related therapies. While the federal government is a major source of support for research on a range of medical therapies, it had removed itself from the area of assisted reproduction. Yet scientific study not only generates essential information about a medical treatment; it also provides more generally some degree of scrutiny, review, and discussion that can guide a treatment's development.

The government's position did not reflect a deliberate decision that reproductive technologies are not a medical research priority for limited government resources. Initial deliberations among government officials, medical professionals, ethicists, and lay citizens had occurred at the federal level more than a decade earlier, and the recommendation then was to go ahead with government funding. How the opposite prevailed, a story in itself, is told in Chapter 8. Suffice it to say here that the Reagan and Bush administrations, prodded by the anti-abortion movement, instituted and maintained a de facto moratorium on IVF research because embryos might be destroyed in the process. In a strange ideological alignment, "pro-life" forces were pitted against—and were triumphing over—women and men seeking to have babies. Stranger yet, these anti-abortion conservatives found themselves allied with those feminists who see the new technologies as robbing women of control over their reproductive lives rather than creating greater control and choice.[3]

Government noninvolvement did not, of course, halt the expansion of ART, though it did stymie research. The lack of government funding for research, coupled with lack of regulations, gave economic forces a freer rein, leaving development of these therapies exclusively to the private sector; this development would, in turn, directly affect what happened to individual patients.

"What you see here are two forces—entrepreneurs versus the academics," explained Dr. Robert Stillman, then a George Washington University fertility specialist. As he surveyed participants spilling out of a 1989 convention session on "transfers of frozen-thawed human embryos," he worried that "everyone" was doing procedures that should be tested at a few special centers, to be improved or discarded. Proven procedures could then become more widely practiced at clinics throughout the country. Presenting the reality as a stark question, Stillman asked, "Why have them do forty patients wrong before they have a success?" And patients do bear the burden. They are the material on which a new IVF clinic develops its skill. Established IVF practitioners try new techniques on patients. Patients are not only paying for the cost of IVF equipment, personnel, and labor; they are essentially paying to be experimented upon, in a trial-and-error fashion, by individual doctors. Evaluation of these clinical experiments is impossible.

Stillman views his specialty's entrepreneurial direction as a "national tragedy," driving good scientists out of research as well as hurting patients. "The situation is grim," he commented in 1989. "Certain areas of medicine just shouldn't be free market." But free market it certainly was. In the absence of government-mandated quality control, fertility clinics proliferated and flourished. Rather than improve the product, stiff competition was increasing its quantity and cost, a dynamic that would become more apparent throughout the medical marketplace as the country embarked on health care reform efforts during the next decade.[4] As the 1987 *Fertility and Sterility* editorial on patient exploitation put it, "Unfortunately, in a consumer-driven medical care system, the physician is often in a precarious position of having to offer premature or indiscriminate therapy to those who demand it, or risk losing the patient to a more accommodating competitor."[5]

Certainly, some individual physicians saw their income swell as they performed more and more assisted reproductive treatments. Also profiting handsomely were manufacturers of various fertility drugs integral to the various new technologies. For-profit corporations, and their public relations agencies, soon entered the field of assisted reproduction. National and international chains of IVF clinics appeared, opening their doors and soliciting patients from local communities. Whether consumer- or provider-driven—or some combination thereof—women and men already susceptible to exploitation from physicians, for whom money is *not* supposed to be a primary motivation, entered a competition that required success to be measured in financial returns.

As the 1980s ended, fertility specialists faced an uncomfortable quandary, pushed largely by developments in assisted reproduction: How could medical standards be monitored, improved, and maintained without stepping toward the precipitous slope of government regulation? Some ART practitioners perceived a need to rein in the technology, in part by restraining certain of their colleagues. The IVF industry could "self-destruct" without regulation and research, said the director of one prominent ART program. The profession's lack of accountability and tolerance of low success would "come back to haunt us," warned another. At the same time, the American Society for Reproductive Medicine concluded its 1989 convention with one officer, Dr. Quigly, thanking congressional critics for "the impetus to police ourselves," and the society's president asserting in his closing statement to gathered participants, "If we don't take care of our own business, someone else will do it for us."

By this time, IVF and GIFT had become common medical practices, with additional variations on these techniques not far behind. In the mid-1990s, 315 fertility clinics in the United States alone offered assisted reproductive technologies. Once a treatment is established as a common practice, moreover, attempts to study it become, by definition, all the more difficult: precisely because these techniques are considered to be standard practice—no longer "experimental"—they "should" be offered to patients, as well as paid for by their health insurance. Indeed, the latter concern reinforced a very loose definition of "standard," among some physicians, as any procedure the doctor or clinic performed more than one time; only the first attempt is "experimental." Missing from these definitions are evaluation and minimal standards for efficacy and safety. To deny patients an established treatment, even as part of a randomly assigned no-treatment control group in a clinical study, would not be medically ethical. Nor are patients always eager to participate in research if they are not receiving a treatment. Yet the increasingly widespread application of an untested "standard" therapy contributes to the urgent need for scientifically controlled studies. In 1990, the ASRM issued a formal statement attempting to delineate more specifically which assisted reproductive procedures are established, and which are experimental and therefore in need of scientifically controlled clinical trials—though again the statement carried no enforcement clout.[6]

The most vicious aspect of this circle is that inadequate research on reproductive technologies has increased the risks that come with any new medical intervention. Most prominently, inadequate research on IVF-related treatments increased reliance on hormonal superovulation. Harvesting many eggs, in the hope that several embryos could be transferred during each treatment cycle, remained the easiest way to increase the likelihood of success. Yet there were no good data on outcomes of these technologies, especially compared to safer, less costly alternatives, and scientists could not determine the reasons assisted reproduction so often fails. Such data could guide development of reproductive interventions by identifying specific treatments that can provide benefits for particular groups of patients. Had the government funded research on IVF and its spin-offs, argue many specialists, large-scale, scientifically controlled studies could have helped identify what does and does not work, for whom, at what risk. Instead, the way reproductive technologies developed meant increased risks and complications—or "side effects"—for increased numbers of people.

No Harm Done?

Like other fertility treatments, assisted reproductive technologies are perceived by many doctors and patients to be generally safe, except in a few rare, unpredictable cases. Though the intervention may not result in pregnancy, they assume no permanent or life-threatening harm will be done in trying. However, these procedures are highly invasive. Beyond the physical, emotional, and financial costs inherent in any medical intervention, such fertility treatments entail certain unique risks. Chances for harm may be greater than commonly perceived.

Laypeople may understand that, basically, IVF includes removing eggs from a woman's ovary. They may not know that this procedure, repeated for each mature egg to be harvested during a particular treatment cycle, brings risks of injury and infection to the woman (for example, bleeding or infection at the puncture site in the vagina, abdominal wall, or ovaries). Initially, when IVF egg retrievals required pelvic surgery (laparoscopy) in order to see where the needle was going, the procedure also carried the risks attending all surgery. Later, IVF programs began switching to ultrasound-guided egg retrieval for most women, eliminating the pelvic surgery and its risks, as well as lowering the cost of treatment. However, the most commonly used IVF variations—transferring eggs and sperm (GIFT) or early embryos (ZIFT) into a woman's fallopian tube—do still rely on a laparoscopic surgical procedure.

More troublesome, in many ways, is the regimen of ovarian hyperstimulation characteristic of most assisted reproduction. The widespread use of potent fertility drugs on healthy women brings not only immediate risks for the woman, but also considerable questions about long-term effects on her health. Moreover, risks from superovulation extend into the next generation.

Medically Controlled Menstrual Cycles out of Control

Attempting to increase women's fertility is but one aspect of reproductive medicine's broader efforts to manipulate women's menstrual cycles. The controlled ovarian hyperstimulation of fertility treatments developed in tandem with its opposite—hormonal contraception, the Pill. Both superimpose exogenous (from outside the body) hormones upon a woman's natural hormonal cycle. In contraception, the intent is to shut down ovulation and/or prevent implantation, thereby preventing pregnancy. For assisted reproduction, the aim is to replace a woman's ongoing monthly interplay of hormones with a hyperstimulated, superovulating cycle. In this cycle, numerous eggs can mature, and the time of ovulation can be more accurately predicted and controlled. Since an egg must be fertilized within hours after ovulation, accurate timing contributes to successful egg retrievals and conception—not to mention convenient scheduling.

Most women undergoing controlled ovarian hyperstimulation receive daily or twice-daily injections of hormones to mature several eggs, each within an enlarged fluid-filled sac (the egg follicle); in some women the ovary responds to hormonal stimulation with maturation of one or two eggs, in others as many as thirty or forty. To monitor this process, women must also receive ultrasound scans of the ovaries and have blood drawn to test hormone levels. Immediate side effects of the drugs—which may include headaches, backaches, breast tenderness, bloating, nausea, insomnia, increased vaginal discharge—are generally considered a tolerable if unpleasant burden of fertility treatment.

Like the sorcerer's apprentice, however, the physician can lose control of the ovary's production of mature eggs. Instead of a single, raisin-sized egg follicle during a natural cycle, twenty or thirty or more can dangerously enlarge the ovary from golf-ball to grapefruit size and cause "weeping" of the ovaries, a condition in which the excess follicular fluid spills into the abdominal cavity. Estimates indicate that up to 2 percent of superovulated women suffer this severe form of ovarian hyperstimulation syndrome, with risk of liver damage, kidney or liver failure, rupture of the ovary and abdominal bleeding, compromised breathing or acute lung failure due to abdominal distention, shock, blood clots, and stroke. This syndrome, from which women have died, requires hospitalization and extremely careful monitoring. Another 3–4 percent experience less severe grades of the syndrome following "controlled" ovarian hyperstimulation.[7]

Beyond those side effects a woman feels in the present, beyond treatment complications her doctor must handle immediately, what of long-term threats to the woman's health? The most ominous threat lurking behind any manipulation of hormones is an increased risk of cancer. Scientists have long been aware that many cancers—particularly those affecting endocrine organs (breast, ovary, uterus, vagina, prostate, testicles) involve exposure to hormones, from both within and outside the body. Though understanding of the process remains incomplete, a biological relationship is well established. Scientists have, therefore, long been aware that cancer is a potential risk from fertility drugs. It was with good biological reason that Dr. Florence Haseltine, then director of the Center for Population Research at the National Institutes of Health, voiced this concern at the 1989 convention of fertility specialists: "Someone should be studying the women. . . . Everyone looks at risks of cancer from oral contraceptives, but what about these fertility drugs?"

These "unknown" risks, quietly discussed among a few researchers, became more plausible and more public in 1993 when the lay press reported findings of an ovarian cancer study suggesting that women who have taken fertility drugs are more likely to develop this disease than women who have not (see Chapter 6).[8] Whether a woman completes an IVF cycle or not, whether she becomes pregnant or not, most assisted reproductive technologies "prepare" women with some type of fertility drug; in fact, those who never became pregnant showed the greatest increase in risk, according to the ovarian cancer study. Nor is the danger limited to women who have undergone IVF-related treatments. Though this group grows ever larger and attracts the greatest attention, it still represents a minority of fertility patients, one segment of a much larger population of women given fertility drugs.

The Dangers of "Success"

The reliance of assisted reproduction on ovarian hyperstimulation has increased risks of a more evident "side effect," inhering in the very "success" of this one step in the process. Quadruplets and quintuplets, glimpsed now and then on our nightly news, are the public faces of an array of medical complications brought on by "multifetal" pregnancies. Development of IVF-related fertility treatments has centered on a technical dilemma: How many eggs retrieved and embryos transferred will give the best chance for ending up with a healthy baby? Practitioners of assisted reproductive technologies experiment with these numbers, aiming to improve their ultimate "take home baby" rate.

The trade-off is clear. Too few eggs retrieved and fertilized means fewer embryos transferred and lower chances of implantation, ongoing pregnancy, and delivery of a baby. For each embryo placed in the uterus during an IVF cycle, pregnancy rates rise about 8 percent—thus giving rates on average of 8, 16, 24, and 32 percent for one, two, three, or four embryos.[9] Reported increases are higher with GIFT and ZIFT. With many embryos transferred, however, too many may implant and grow; the average rate of multiple gestations resulting from assisted reproduction is about 25–30 percent of the total pregnancies.

For the pregnant woman, health risks increase with each fetus, jumping substantially with triplet and larger pregnancies. A typical journal article listing of maternal risks with multiple fetuses includes increased incidence of pre-term labor requiring medical treatment (which can itself bring life-threatening side effects such as cardiac failure and pulmonary edema), preeclampsia, pregnancy-induced hypertension, gestational diabetes, anemia, uterine rupture, placenta previa, abruptio placentae, thrombophlebitis, polyhydramnios, and serious postpartum hemorrhage, including the need for transfusion, which itself has carried risks of HIV and hepatitis.[10] In addition, women face a greatly increased risk of simply not being able to carry the pregnancy long enough, even with treatment of pre-term labor. The ultimate result may be no baby at all or several extremely premature babies risking the myriad problems of prematurity—including respiratory failure, brain hemorrhage, cerebral palsy, and eye damage. Other fetal risks include growth retardation, umbilical cord accidents, and congenital anomalies. Even twins, whether low birthweight or not, appear to have increased incidence of cerebral palsy—a risk that may not be explained to people considering fertility treatments.[11]

While an ART program may count these multiple newborns among their "successful" outcomes, many of the severely premature babies will die weeks or months later, or will survive with severely damaged health, a "side effect" of assisted reproduction that becomes the pediatricians'—and the parents'—problem. Media coverage of a septuplet birth in California in the mid-1980s did not follow the case. One year later, only three of the babies were still alive, at least two of them suffering severe, possibly long-term mental and physical handicaps. Less dramatic, but more typical, was a triplet birth, fifteen weeks pre-term, each baby weighing less than two pounds. After ten weeks of newborn intensive care, all the babies had vision problems; one, who suffered brain damage, was still attached to an oxygen tank at home nearly one year later. Dr. Louis Keith, director of the Chicago-based Center for the Study of Multiple

Births, describes the public picture as "buffed, toned, air-brushed, and made to look wonderful. What distorts the issue is that the press is very eager to do a story on a mother of quints all of whom are 4 pounds or more, but they don't find it very newsworthy to describe the cases where the babies are born very prematurely and die one by one."[12]

Nor does the public hear about high levels of stress and depression reported in parents caring for multiples when they do make it home from the hospital.[13] With fertility clinics pursuing higher success rates, the trade-off was not lost on some within the profession. A 1991 recommendation of the American College of Obstetricians and Gynecologists' Ethics Committee urged doctors to counsel fertility patients, prior to treatment, of the "dire consequences" of large multifetal pregnancies. As one specialist commented in the pages of a medical journal, "There is no question that grand multifetal pregnancy is a serious risk to the mother and fetuses. . . . [Such a] pregnancy secondary to poorly monitored reproductive techniques is not a therapeutic triumph."[14] Another notes that, contrary to depictions in the media, most of these pregnancies bring "suffering you can't imagine."[15]

By the mid-1980s, medical reports were beginning to reveal initial attempts to eliminate this major side effect of assisted conception—too many fetuses—by eliminating several of the fetuses conceived. The aim was to save a viable number of babies and protect the pregnant woman's health. The reports were soon appearing regularly, presenting hundreds of cases in which a woman pregnant with triplets, quadruplets, quintuplets, or more underwent "selective fetal reduction" (sometimes called "selective termination"). While a similar procedure had previously been used in spontaneous pregnancies with a fetal anomaly (e.g., one of a set of twins, especially when the abnormal fetus jeopardized survival of the other), the pressing concern now was an iatrogenic condition (i.e., caused by medical intervention) endangering mother and offspring. In these increasingly frequent instances, a number of normal fetuses must be terminated. The medical literature described various procedures and outcomes, as practitioners sought the best method for ending physiologic activity in some fetuses of a multifetal pregnancy without injuring or losing all. Early results were not encouraging; too often, the outcome was loss of the entire pregnancy. Practitioners altered their reduction techniques. They tried varying the number of fetuses eliminated, the number left to grow. Starting with six or eight, should they reduce to three or four or two? They discussed timing. Performing the procedure a few weeks later might allow spontaneous reduction to occur through miscarriage, a winnowing that brings fewer complications. However, if this natural process did not occur, delay might ultimately bring greater physical risk and psychological cost. And with six or more fetuses, two or three reduction sessions might be required.

Soon came the inevitable warnings to colleagues about the need for experience in order to perform this procedure successfully. Such warnings could only hint at the number of botched attempts becoming common knowledge within the medical community. "The literature fails to provide readers with appreciation of technical nuances this operation requires," one specialist cautioned with impressive medical tact, citing a "learning curve" of improved results as practitioners improve their skills.[16] By 1996, a report on 400 pregnant women would show that approximately 8 percent lost their entire pregnancy when fetal reduction was performed by experienced practitioners.[17]

The technical dilemma that created multifetal pregnancies through assisted reproduction translated immediately into an ethical debate. Although legal, abortion was a highly charged issue during the Reagan-Bush years—and remains so today. Beyond arguments against terminating any fetus, however, were concerns more pertinent to selective reduction. The idea of "choosing" which of several normal fetuses to eliminate was troublesome; with the choice determined by physiologic and technical considerations alone, many practitioners eliminated "selective" from the vocabulary. More difficult were questions of benefit and harm during these much-desired pregnancies, many of which followed years of fertility treatments. A 1988 *Lancet* editorial on selective fetal reduction identified as ethical issues "the risk of damaging the surviving fetuses; the degree to which complications of multiple pregnancy are resolved by selective reduction; the effect on the mother both during pregnancy and after the birth; social and economic considerations for the children's well-being; and the effects of information about selective termination on attitudes and feelings of the parents and surviving children." The authors note the "dearth of reports on the outcome of fetal reduction, particularly the occurrence of complications for the mother and remaining fetuses and any lingering mental or physical effects after birth." Not only is this procedure performed "more frequently than is apparent from published reports," but the ethical issues "have not been discussed widely, and the public are largely unaware of the technique of fetal reduction or the medical reasons for it."[18]

The medical conundrum of fetal reduction gained sharpest focus at the hazy borderline of triplets. The threat of causing total pregnancy loss—and the agonizing balance of fetal and maternal well-being—hangs heaviest over three. Should large multifetal pregnancies be reduced to triplets or fewer? Should triplet pregnancies be reduced to twins? Advances in high-risk obstetrics and newborn intensive care mean that triplets have a good chance of surviving, though with significant risks from prematurity and low birthweight. Risks to the woman pregnant with triplets remain considerable. One study in France, comparing triplet pregnancies that were and were not reduced, reported as "one of the most important results" the finding of "life-threatening maternal complications" among only the forty-eight women who chose not to undergo fetal reduction: spontaneous rupture of the liver complicating severe preeclampsia; hemiplegia (paralysis of one side of the body resulting from stroke) during the sixth month of pregnancy with incomplete recovery; and massive pulmonary embolism following cesarean section, requiring cardiac intensive care, despite preventive measures.[19]

Journal descriptions of fetal reduction portray in cool clinical detail the spiral of increasingly complex, invasive, and expensive technology spinning from those initial experiments with IVF. The medical literature documents the growth of this offshoot of a serious iatrogenic problem into a medical intervention in its own right, with its own specialists—and its own critics. Indeed, critics within the ranks began turning responsibility back onto the profession. Creating multifetal pregnancies in infertile patients is "a tragic irony of immense proportions," wrote one group of physicians and ethicists. "Many cases of iatrogenic multiple pregnancy are probably avoidable by more diligent management of infertility drugs. Many of the currently known instances of grand multiple pregnancies should never have happened. Selective termination should be viewed not as an end it itself, but as a provisional approach, appropriate until improved medical care obviates the need for its use."[20] A 1993 Belgian study of triplet pregnancies concluded: "The fundamental ethical problem the medical community has to solve is not whether to reduce triplet pregnancies but whether to continue to induce so many high-rank multiple pregnancies." The authors' warning of potential "banalization of embryo reduction" echoes the *Lancet* editorial's concern that fetal reduction "not become the management method for ovulation induction, IVF, and related techniques."[21]

More strongly and broadly put, a letter to *Obstetrics and Gynecology* asks: "Where is the duty to the woman before she is pregnant, a duty that must include protecting her from 'iatrogenic' multiple gestations that could threaten her life? Where is the duty to human life itself, a duty that must dictate not creating life that has little chance for a reasonable existence. . . . The ethics of selective termination must be paired with the ethics of infertility treatments: If obstetricians are willing to 'gamble' on the possibility of grand multiple gestations, they must be willing to provide some remedy for the harm they cause. Any ethical guidelines pertaining only to selective terminations further victimize the woman and her fetus(es). . . . If there is a clear 'wrong' . . . it lies in the unexamined enthusiasm for infertility treatments, not in the management of a woman's subsequent pregnancy."[22] Clearly, the ethical debate over selective reduction encompasses more than the imperative to minimize complications through more skillful fertility treatment. For women facing selective reduction, the added ethical irony is that better research might have meant less reliance on superovulation and transfer of multiple embryos—research stymied still by anti-abortion politics. Given that IVF and related technologies are often used inappropriately, on women who do not need them, the additional question is: How many women are undergoing this attempt to correct a "complication" of treatment that should never have been performed in the first place?

The Next Round

Amid the swell of journal reports describing the latest variations of ART and the increasing number of categories of patients on whom these variations were tried, a different type of argument appeared. With mounting evidence of serious side effects—actual and potential, immediate and long-term—and with persistent concern for cost, physicians began acknowledging that assisted reproduction literally reaches the point of diminishing returns. Creeping into the fray were titles such as "A Simplified Approach to In Vitro Fertilization," and "In Vitro Fertilization in Unstimulated Cycles." Practitioners of ART were now experimenting with less invasive protocols, suggesting fewer fertility drugs, describing nonsurgical techniques. Depending on which fertility specialist you were seeing, you might now be offered a much less onerous—and less risky—option than just a year or two before.

The pattern is familiar in fertility medicine, yet patients rarely perceive this medical progression that can so greatly alter the course of their treatment. Obtaining the latest information about a particular fertility condition—important as such knowledge is—reveals only a slice of the medical here and now. The current state of the art reflects developments that reach back into medical history and across specific medical conditions. Assisted reproductive technologies illustrate more vividly than most fertility treatments that the professional "learning curve" is more convoluted than a simple progression toward increased experience, skill, and, therefore, success. This curve may eventually turn downward, toward moderation in therapeutic zeal. With assisted reproduction now a possibility for all fertility patients, they need to stand back and ask where these treatments fit into medical trends. They need to view this option—or any fertility treatment—as an intervention with a history that could significantly affect their care.

Consider the trends in development of assisted reproductive technologies and the potential impact on individual patients. Announcement of the first IVF baby unleashed an explosion of attempts throughout the world to create more "high-tech" babies. A 1989 World Health Organization survey identified 708 IVF-ET clinics in 53 countries.[23] In such clinics, large and small, physicians and technicians experimented with various steps of assisted reproduction, seeking to bump up stubbornly low success rates. Initial reports focused on quantity. They showed an increase in eggs retrieved and embryos transferred, along with some increase in pregnancies conceived, thus forging the link between ART and ovarian stimulation. However, the increase in egg fertilization and pregnancy did not translate as successfully into healthy "take home babies." Fertility specialists began to speak of limits, both on the number of eggs and embryos and on the number of attempts.

The 1988 *Lancet* editorial on selective fetal reduction was one of the first calls for less aggressive fertility treatment:

> Given that the problems of premature delivery, very low birthweight, and perinatal mortality in IVF pregnancies are exacerbated by the high frequency of multiple pregnancies, there is a good case to reduce further [below three or four] the number of eggs and pre-embryos replaced. Some IVF and GIFT clinics continue to replace large numbers of eggs and pre-embryos in their patients. The reasons for this practice vary . . . [but none] is a reasonable excuse for putting a woman or her babies at risk of the severe complications of quintuplet or larger multiple pregnancies, and there are even grounds for concern about triplet and quadruplet pregnancy. . . . Instead of replacing large numbers of eggs and pre-embryos, IVF practitioners should carefully consider the reverse trend of replacing fewer eggs and embryos.[24]

During the ensuing years, more physicians reassessed their procedures. ART programs more commonly reported outcomes with fewer rather than more embryos, searching for an optimal number that would better balance increased births with decreased medical complications, psychological stress, and financial cost. By the early 1990s, many doctors recommended transferring no more than three or four embryos in any one attempt. By 1997 the large number of triplet pregnancies, and their risks, led Dutch specialists to argue that transferring only two embryos results in acceptable pregnancy rates. Other European specialists suggest this limit is particularly warranted for women younger than thirty-seven who respond well to ovarian stimulation.[25]

In the same years, physicians began suggesting another type of limit—on the number of unsuccessful ART attempts patients should endure. A 1989 letter to the *New England Journal of Medicine* raised the question, "How Much Is Enough?" The authors write, "Medical technology offers almost endless hope for infertile couples; however, when to stop has become a difficult question to answer. When the treatment offered is in vitro fertilization, determined couples may initiate many cycles with the hope that with one more try they will succeed in having a child." However, among the first fifty women who conceived and delivered a baby in their IVF program, 84 percent of the births occurred after two IVF cycles, and "births were extremely unlikely after the fourth IVF cycle. . . . We conclude that the overwhelming majority of couples who will achieve pregnancy as a result of IVF do so within a relatively short period of time. Couples who do not achieve a viable pregnancy after four to six IVF cycles should be counseled that success with this technique is unlikely and should not be encouraged to pursue IVF further."[26]

Again, the concern was physical and psychological hardship, as well as expense. These IVF practitioners were seeking a cost-effective number of in vitro cycles, particularly as compared with such alternatives as major abdominal surgery for tubal abnormalities (most of which have low success rates) or extended non-IVF treatment. Three or four IVF cycles might keep stress and cost at reasonable levels while offering at least equal chances for success as other methods.

In addition to seeking limits, a second trend evident by the early 1990s was toward reducing invasiveness. One approach was to wean assisted reproduction from ovarian stimulation. Some doctors began prescribing a lighter fertility drug regimen for their patients or use of only clomiphene citrate instead of the more potent Pergonal (brand name for hMG, human menopausal gonadotropin), particularly in women younger than forty with fertile partners. A 1993 study described "a novel ovarian stimulation protocol," using reduced drug dosages on fewer days of an ART cycle,[27] in order "to lower the escalating costs of assisted reproduction and decrease the extent of patient discomfort and disruption of life-style without sacrificing success rates." Commenting that "the history of ART illustrates how the pendulum of medical therapy can swing from one extreme to the other," the study's authors conclude that their "minimal stimulation" protocol "is easy to administer, requires less intensive monitoring, fewer medications, and virtually eliminates the risk of ovarian hyperstimulation syndrome."

By the mid-1990s, physicians would also acknowledge fertility patients' and egg donors' concern about ovarian cancer risk. In 1996, one group of specialists stated their own concern about this danger and about "as yet unrecognized factors in these complex and powerful endocrine treatments" that could, for example, adversely affect women's menopause; they communicated with other physicians in an editorial written "as practitioners in assisted reproduction who are increasingly concerned about current approaches to ovarian stimulation"— particularly "increasing reliance on complex treatment protocols resulting in large numbers of oocytes." [28] In this echo of the editorial on exploiting fertility patients written nearly a decade before, these specialists contend that such protocols "may help to organize the activities of the clinic," but "could be injurious to women's health." Fertility treatments should entail milder stimulations based on greater understanding of—and connection to—a woman's natural menstrual cycle. Simpler and milder stimulations that produce "relatively minor modifications of the natural cycle" could be tailored to individual patients "who could self-administer two or three injections per cycle rather than the daily injections that have become routine." They criticize especially the many doctors who emphasize the sheer number of eggs and embryos as a sign of successful ovarian stimulation when the goal should be to stimulate the fewest follicles necessary for the individual patient's treatment needs.

Compared to earlier years of reproductive technologies, patients now had new options and trade-offs. The pregnancy rate following milder ovarian stimulation is lower for each retrieval cycle, but so are the health risks and emotional stress. And, as fertility specialists admitted, the lowered cost achieved by minimizing use of fertility drugs provided many infertile couples with "their only financially sound access to ART." [29] Other ART programs backtracked even further, eliminating fertility drugs altogether. They retrieved patients' naturally ovulated eggs during unstimulated cycles, to be mixed in vitro with sperm. This latter approach was not "novel" at all, but rather swung the pendulum back to the original IVF birth in England, achieved during the mother's natural menstrual cycle. [30]

Further modification of IVF downgraded the high technology by eliminating both fertility drugs and fertilization in a laboratory. In 1992, a Harvard-affiliated

ART program described a treatment tried on forty-five women that combined natural cycle egg retrieval with "intravaginal fertilization." In this "simplified approach" doctors retrieve a spontaneously matured egg from the ovary. The egg is then placed with sperm and nutrients into a sealed capsule, rather than a laboratory dish as in standard IVF. The capsule goes into a special sealed envelope, which is inserted into the woman's vagina for two days. If fertilization occurs, doctors transfer the embryo to the woman's uterus. Advantages, according to the physicians, include elimination of fertility drugs, simplicity of monitoring egg maturation and retrieval, and lack of need for expensive laboratory equipment. This method, they suggest, "may prove appropriate for those women requiring IVF who fear multiple pregnancies, have side effects from controlled ovarian hyperstimulation, or cannot afford standard IVF." Their report concludes, "Pregnancy rates . . . may never equal those achieved with standard IVF. However, for some patients the marked advantages and reduced costs [approximately one-third standard IVF] . . . may outweigh the small reduction in the percentage of success."[31] They speculate that patients might be willing to repeat this easier and less expensive process more often than standard IVF, resulting in nearly the same number of women who eventually become pregnant.

Finally, the assisted reproduction trend revolved full circle. For some women with open fallopian tubes, egg retrieval itself could be eliminated, along with laboratory fertilization. Instead, the doctor might suggest trying less invasive and less costly intrauterine insemination of sperm, but with controlled ovarian hyperstimulation (called stimulated IUI). The theory was that *something* about superovulation—perhaps increased numbers of egg and sperm at the fertilization site—contributes to the success of assisted reproductive technologies; as with many fertility treatments, just what that something is could, perhaps, be determined in future studies. The trade-off here, of course, is that women still face the risks of ovarian hyperstimulation.

The journal article that proposed this alternative raised a stir among fertility specialists. Describing 148 stimulated IUI cycles in 85 couples, the authors reported pregnancy rates "approaching that of normal women and comparable to reported results with GIFT and IVF-ET in couples with . . . endometriosis, idiopathic [unexplained] infertility, or cervical factors." Of pregnancies conceived, 29 percent were multiples—five sets of twins, one of triplets—a proportion similar to IVF and GIFT.[32] Tagged onto the end of this article was an unusual, italicized comment from the journal's editor: "The decision to publish this controversial manuscript has been made with the intent of stimulating debate. The referees feel strongly that, before advocating IUI during hMG-stimulated cycles, a prospective controlled study with critically evaluated infertile patients is mandatory. The advocating of this essentially empiric therapy cannot be supported by the rather meager retrospective data presented. . . . Clinicians should be discouraged from applying this therapy until controlled prospective studies can support this approach." While the editor may have been legitimately concerned that an unproven treatment with proven risks would become widely used, the comment failed to acknowledge what the article's authors point out—that GIFT and IVF in women with these same diagnoses had themselves never been properly evaluated. Yet clinicians were surely applying these therapies "empirically"—that is, based on trial and error and their personal observations, rather than on systematic, scientifically controlled studies.

Proposing superovulated intrauterine insemination as an alternative to egg retrieval, fertilization, and transfer of IVF or GIFT blurred the very definition of "assisted reproduction." Amidst the turmoil engendered by IVF-related treatments, however, one thing was clear: ART had become a fact of life. Though most fertility patients initially undergo "conventional" treatments involving medications, insemination, and/or surgery, assisted reproductive technologies have grown to be far more than a last resort for patients and doctors. These treatments are now the ever-present backdrop for doctors' recommendations and patients' decisions. ART is a benchmark within fertility medicine, an option with which conventional alternatives are compared if not combined. Moreover, these techniques are vehicles for future reproductive developments, particularly in combination with new genetic tools. At the same time, public interest in ART, the technology's media appeal and relative visibility, would eventually help throw light on inadequacies with fertility medicine more generally—the preponderance of unproven therapies, the questionable value of many diagnostic procedures, the potential for patient exploitation and harm, and the absence of guidelines or regulations for reproductive interventions. In addition, there is another fact about these interventions: disagreements among doctors translate directly into treatments of differing invasiveness, risk, and benefit for their patients. To the individual woman and her partner, these differences may make all the difference in the world.

Claims of Success

Among many nagging questions surrounding expansion of assisted reproduction, none has been more persistent than claims about success. None is more important for fertility patients to understand: Will these substantial medical interventions increase their chances of having a healthy baby? For women with completely blocked or absent fallopian tubes, in vitro fertilization can be an effective treatment. Without treatment, the chance of pregnancy is virtually zero; through the IVF procedure, some of these women will conceive. The proportion of treated women who end up with a baby provides a fairly good measure of IVF success in overcoming this particular fertility problem.

As assisted reproduction expanded beyond this original use of IVF, however, the question of effectiveness became less clear-cut. The development of ART has been accompanied by controversy over just how successful these therapies are. The main complication is that most of the newer "indications"—the conditions for which a doctor might prescribe ART—bring respectable rates of spontaneous pregnancy; that is, the women thus diagnosed can conceive without treatment, though they may require a longer than average time to do so. As the uses of ART grew, so too did the numbers of women who became pregnant while on an ART waiting list.[33] To determine the success of medical intervention for this broader range of fertility problems, the spontaneous pregnancy rate—the "background rate"—becomes a key comparison. The question becomes whether the pregnancies result from the treatments. For the individual woman considering assisted reproduction, the question is whether her likelihood of pregnancy is appreciably greater with treatment than with no treatment or with a less invasive and costly one.

Success rates reported for GIFT provide a good example. If a woman has at least one functioning fallopian tube in which to place eggs and sperm for fertilization, her doctor may recommend GIFT, pointing to higher success rates than with standard IVF. However, because she does have at least one good fallopian tube, she also has a better chance of becoming pregnant without treatment. One ART program's description of "the ideal GIFT candidate" seems also to describe women who may well conceive spontaneously: "a woman who has previously proven her ability to fertilize her eggs (by IVF or a previous pregnancy), who has no tubal disease, is free of sperm antibodies [an immunologic factor that some doctors think reduces fertility], and who has a fertile partner; prime indications therefore include 'unexplained infertility' and non-immunologic cervical mucus hostility." At least a portion of the greater success attributed to GIFT, therefore, may result from its use on women who are relatively more fertile to begin with and will conceive more easily than, say, women advised to undergo IVF. And if these women have sexual intercourse during a GIFT cycle, there simply is no way of knowing whether a pregnancy was a result of treatment.

Aside from the very basic question of whether a treatment was responsible for a subsequent pregnancy, controversy over assisted reproduction reflects a confusion of definitions and profusion of methods for calculating success rates. Attempts to evaluate IVF-related procedures have been plagued, first of all, by misleading definitions of "success." The ultimate measure of a successful fertility treatment is birth of a healthy baby who would not otherwise have been born. While this definition may seem obvious, many IVF clinics stretched the meaning of success to improve their reported track record. As with surgery declared "a success, but the patient died," assisted reproductive treatments have too often been labeled "successes," but without, in the end, a baby.

A clinic might boast an impressive pregnancy rate, for example, but include in its tally *biochemical pregnancies*—transient elevations of the "pregnancy hormone" beta-hCG, detected through a very early blood test. A rise in this hormone level can indicate first stages of a pregnancy; however, results may also be only a temporary "positive" from the effect of hormones administered around the time of ovulation as part of the fertility treatment itself. In contrast, an actual pregnancy, known as a *clinical pregnancy,* can be more directly observed. To be counted as an established, clinical pregnancy, at least one gestational sac within the uterus must be seen by ultrasound examination (a count that thus excludes ectopic pregnancy, which must be removed). This pregnancy rate will, of course, be lower than the tally of biochemical pregnancies.

ART programs sometimes report their *implantation rate*—the proportion of embryos transferred that appear as gestational sacs during the initial ultrasound exam. Patients may want to know how successful an ART program is at getting embryos to implant, as one measure of technical ability. However, a relatively low implantation rate may instead reflect a relatively older patient population, since this step appears to be where pregnancies frequently fail in women nearing forty.

A fertility program's reported pregnancy rate will be higher than its success in producing live, healthy babies. Of ART pregnancies confirmed through ultrasound, the number of living newborns is approximately one-quarter to one-third lower, due to miscarriage and complications of multiple births. Even definitions surrounding births can be unclear. ART programs report live deliveries, defined as the birth of at least one living infant. Again, since multiple pregnancies are more common with ART, the number of deliveries will differ from the number of babies born alive. Some premature newborns never make it home from the hospital's intensive care unit; the number of babies born alive, therefore, will be higher than the total of "take home babies." Unfortunately, the description "healthy" too often disappears entirely from medical definitions and calculations of success. The rate of successful live deliveries tells us only that at least one baby was born alive, not that a baby went home in good health.

As IVF clinics proliferated during the 1980s, prospective patients needed also to be wary of an additional confusion—whose success rate were they hearing? Over half the clinics performing IVF in 1987 had failed to produce even one live birth. To inquiring patients, these clinics might quote a nationwide success rate or, more egregious still, rates for the country's most experienced programs; the patients would never know that for this particular clinic, the success rate was zero. The new Boston branch of a worldwide chain—IVF Australia—advertised "the program's" 236 live births, these impressive numbers culled from the entire IVF chain. By the 1990s, freezing extra embryos (cryopreservation) had become a common procedure, allowing women to attempt additional embryo transfers without undergoing additional risk and cost of hyperstimulation and egg retrieval. On the one hand, a clinic might boast that it offers cryopreservation, without mentioning to inquiring patients that not one of this program's frozen embryos has ever thawed into a successful pregnancy. On the other hand, clinics that limit the number of fresh embryos transferred—for example, to minimize multiple gestations—may achieve successful pregnancies from later transfers of patients' thawed embryos that are not reflected in standard success reports.[34]

Claims of success for ART have not been clouded solely by deceptive jiggling of numbers. Researchers do not always agree on how best to evaluate and compare outcomes of ART programs. What patients considering assisted reproductive technologies most need to know is the "take home baby" rate following treatment; yet this information can be more or less optimistic—intentionally or not—depending on how the proportion of live infants is calculated. Pressured by undeniably deceptive success claims and by growing congressional awareness of them, specialists in assisted reproduction began searching in the late 1980s for a precise measure of the likelihood that treatment would result in a living baby. The American Society for Reproductive Medicine helped establish a voluntary registry that gathers yearly reports from ART programs in the United States and Canada. The registry's first report, published in 1988, included overall data accumulated from forty different clinics. In 1991, after much internal argument, the registry began documenting success rates on a clinic-by-clinic basis—essential information for people choosing an ART program.[35] By mid-decade, this registry was reporting success rates for 267 ART programs. The most recent years show small increases in success overall, with women's age and male fertility problems as key factors affecting rates of success. However, among ART practitioners debate about these reports continued; now that individual programs could be identified, registry participants were particularly concerned with protecting their own program's favorable standing in the growing ART competition.[36]

What Patients Should Know

While physicians argued over competing definitions of success, a "best" measure remained elusive. The need that emerged most convincingly was for a broad accumulation of information that could shed light on two separate but interrelated questions: What do the numbers about a particular reproductive technology reveal about its effectiveness for treating a particular fertility problem, when performed at its best? And where is this treatment performed at its best? That is, what do numbers from specific ART programs reflect about their skill and success with this intervention, compared to other programs?

For fertility patients, these general questions translate directly into decisions about whether a treatment is worth trying and, if so, where to seek care—a choice (assuming they have a choice; this issue is discussed in chapter 8) of obvious concern to providers of these treatments as well. In attempting to answer these questions, different calculations provide information about different aspects of a multistep process. Patients should understand that each method of calculation—while contributing to the overall picture—has limitations in what it can reflect about treatment success. Adding to the complexity of reported success rates are the varying characteristics of patients and of the assisted reproduction process that influence success or failure at each step along the way; some of these characteristics are known, others mysterious.

Most success rates now reported by ART programs present the number of live deliveries (i.e., at least one live newborn) as a percentage of a total number of attempts to achieve this goal during one year. This proportion of successful outcomes, however, depends on which step in the ART process is used to define the number of "attempts." Some calculations inflate the degree of success because they do not include all of the women who began a treatment. In fact, a crucial dimension underlying measures of success is an ART "attrition rate." Patients drop out at each stage of an ART cycle for a variety of reasons, physical, financial, and/or the stress of it all.

Some patients drop out after the first step of egg maturation and monitoring for the approach of ovulation. The vast majority of ART programs use hormonal hyperstimulation, which can cause side effects requiring the treatment be stopped. Whether the cycle is stimulated or natural, the treatment cycle is canceled if ultrasound monitoring shows no enlarged egg follicle. Measures of follicle size (indicating egg maturation) and hormone levels (indicating readiness of endometrium for an embryo) may not meet requirements doctors consider to be properly synchronized for successful implantation, resulting in cancellation of the egg retrieval. If at least one egg does mature, the practitioner may not be successful in the second step, aspirating it (or them) from the woman's ovary. The ART process may falter at step three, the meeting of egg and sperm; fertilization may fail to occur or may not produce an embryo deemed suitable for transfer.

Since at least one embryo must be transferred in order to complete an ART cycle (although with GIFT, it is the eggs and sperm that are transferred to the fallopian tube), medical reports often use this fourth step—the embryo transfer procedure (referred to as ET)—as the basis for determining the likelihood of a live delivery *if* a woman completes the treatment. This success rate, then, reflects the proportion of live deliveries out of all embryo (or gamete) transfer procedures performed, but it does not include women who started treatment but never got as far as the transfer stage. Patients considering assisted reproduction, however, also want to know the likelihood of success for a woman who *starts* treatment. This calculation would compare the number of live deliveries to the number of egg maturation and monitoring procedures (or, if no hormonal stimulation, the total number of natural treatment cycles started).

One Clinic's Results

This summary of a hypothetical fertility clinic's in vitro fertilization–embryo transfer results in a single year, based on representative figures in the annual SART Registry, gives some insight into success rates—and into important questions that need to be asked. The report covers sixty women under the age of forty whose male partners have normal fertility.

  60 women begin a total of 100 attempts at ovarian hyperstimulation; 14 of these attempts are canceled before egg retrieval because of dangerous side effects or lack of enlarged follicles

  86 egg retrieval procedures are performed; approximately 12 percent of the procedures result in no viable embryo for transfer

  76 embryo transfer procedures are performed

16 "clinical" pregnancies are confirmed by ultrasound (at least one gestational sac within the uterus); this represents a 16 percent pregnancy rate per initiated treatment and a 21 percent rate per embryo transfer procedure

12 deliveries with at least one live baby result; this represents a 25 percent miscarriage rate, a 12 percent success rate per initiated treatment, and a 15.8 percent success rate per embryo transfer procedure

Overall, 20 percent of the women treated that year achieve a live delivery

These results leave a number of questions unanswered:

How many attempts did individuals go through before a success? Before a decision to stop trying?

Under what conditions do these doctors cancel a treatment before embryo transfer?

How many embryos were transferred during each cycle? What was the rate of multiple gestations? Of these, how many twins? Triplets or more? How many multiples survived out of all delivered? How many multiples went home healthy? Did this clinic employ fetal reduction for large multiple gestations? If so what were the results (i.e., number of healthy newborns after reduction from what number of fetuses before the procedure)?

Out of all babies born alive (singletons and multiples) how many went home healthy?

What were the complications of treatment (including of fetal reduction, if performed)? In what proportion of cases did complications occur?

What are the results for women older than forty? For couples with male fertility problems?

Does this clinic offer cryopreservation? If so, what are the results after transfer of frozen embryos (i.e., no ovarian stimulation has occurred during transfer cycle)? How many additional women take home how many healthy babies?

In evaluating a report, a prospective patient should be sure the results are for a completed year (not the best week, month, three months, or predicted future). If results include ongoing pregnancies, a final success rate will generally be lower due to pregnancy loss.

A somewhat different calculation is also important: the number of clinical pregnancies (i.e., observable through ultrasound) out of all treatment attempts or embryo transfer procedures. Comparing this proportion to the eventual rate of live deliveries helps determine the likelihood of pregnancy loss after successfully conceiving. This information, in the words of one group of ART evaluators, "provides couples with a realistic understanding that not every pregnancy progresses to delivery."[37] In reality, 20–25 percent of ART pregnancies end in miscarriage. Approximately 5 percent of ART attempts result in ectopic pregnancies and must be removed immediately; these should not be counted as clinical pregnancies.[38]

Understanding of ART success rates is not likely to be "realistic" if based solely on percentages of outcomes and procedures. Any such proportions can be only gross measures that require considerable explanation and that should be accompanied by data describing additional aspects of a complex picture. A multitude of characteristics about the patients treated and the process performed complicates all success calculations. Only the composite of many small pieces allows some grasp of relevant likelihoods—the likelihood of pregnancy, of pregnancy loss, of multiple births, of time and money, of a healthy "take-home baby." Despite the risk of information overload, this composite approach may avoid what the director of one prominent IVF clinic describes as "the major risk in interpreting reported outcome data . . . that of oversimplification."[39]

What prominent factors emerge, then, from ongoing medical debate as significant influences on success of an assisted reproductive technology? First, are the characteristics of patients undergoing treatment—most significantly, *the woman's age* and *the couple's diagnosis.* Fertility in women generally declines after the mid-thirties, a pattern reflected in both natural and assisted reproduction. As ART programs extended their age range and experimented with various egg donor–recipient combinations, the age of forty for women using their own eggs became a rough boundary, beyond which success rates fall to extremely low levels. For women of any age undergoing ART, the type and number of conditions that lower the couple's fertility also have an impact on success. "Male factor" problems and the diagnosis of several fertility problems in the woman and/or man bring lowest rates of success. Second, are the characteristics of the ART process—most significantly, the *number of eggs and embryos* used during a treatment cycle. Transferring more embryos (or eggs for GIFT) increases the pregnancy rate, but it also increases multiple gestations (possibly necessitating selective reduction procedures), pregnancy loss, and obstetric and neonatal complications. Reports of success need to include whether the treatment used ovarian stimulation, what particular hormone regimen was used, how many eggs or embryos (fresh or cryopreserved) were transferred per cycle, and whether procedures augmenting standard IVF were used (for example, directly injecting sperm into eggs, "assisted hatching," egg donation).

With the above characteristics in mind, additional questions help assess the amount of time, cost, and stress successful treatment may entail. Since individual patients often undergo many treatment attempts, which can extend over many years, reports of live deliveries also need to indicate which cycle resulted in this outcome. That is, how many attempts did a woman go through before the success? In addition to annual data on procedures performed for all patients, what proportion of women who entered an ART program eventually had a baby, and with how many treatment cycles over how many months? What is the "cumulative" likelihood that a woman will have a successful pregnancy after three treatment cycles? After six? At what point does success become very unlikely? When presented with a treatment's or program's cumulative success rate (i.e., chances for a live-born infant after a certain number of months or treatment cycles), patients need to ask themselves, moreover, whether they are willing and/or able to undergo that particular number of attempts. A cumulative rate after six IVF cycles is overly optimistic for a woman who will attempt no more than two treatment cycles. After fewer cycles, fewer successful pregnancies have accumulated, giving a lower cumulative rate.

Finally, comparisons among specific ART programs are crucial for patients considering treatment as well as for quality evaluations in general. Selecting and comparing only one number—such as the percentage of deliveries out of all embryos transferred—does not provide a valid evaluation of a fertility clinic. Although few clinics are significantly better or worse than average, those that perform only a small number of procedures cannot provide reliable success rates.[40] Aside from these relatively small programs (the SART Registry suggests thirty initiated cycles per year may be a minimal number for useful results), the number of live deliveries for all treatment attempts, for egg retrieval procedures, and for embryo transfers can provide a basis for comparing the degree of experience and success of different practitioners at different steps of the ART process. These numbers can help identify a clinic that performs far less well than most; however, the numbers are not useful for ranking ART programs from best to worst.[41] Differences in the patients treated—the type and severity of fertility problems that predominate, especially the women's age and couples' diagnoses—influence that program's success rate. A "highly successful" ART clinic may be treating the easiest patients. This clinic may offer IVF to many young women with relatively mild problems who have tried to conceive without treatment for only a short time—patients who stand a relatively good chance of pregnancy with or without treatment. Although clinics now report success rates for different age groups, they do not report how long their patients had been trying to conceive before beginning treatment. A clinic may select primarily patients for whom a treatment is most effective—for instance, IVF for women younger than thirty-five whose only fertility problem is blocked fallopian tubes. A clinic may offer special payment plans to "medically eligible" patients—that is, those with the best prognosis for pregnancy. Such a program's impressive success may reflect in good measure what physicians call the "patient selection factor."[42] Another clinic, with a lower success rate, might advise the "easy" subfertile patients to wait another year in order to see whether a spontaneous pregnancy occurs, and then begin with a less invasive therapy that succeeds. This clinic may be willing to treat relatively large numbers of women who are over forty or couples with severe and several problems in the woman and man, patients with previous treatment failures referred by other clinics.

Patients who do require assisted reproduction in order to become pregnant must be certain a program has qualified, experienced personnel and a track record open to public scrutiny. However, an individual patient may well receive the best care from an ART program with somewhat lower success rates than others. Individuals need to find the best match for their particular needs. Among fertility programs with longest experience and generally similar success rates, characteristics of a program's patients and procedures are essential considerations. How does the program select and reject patients? For what reasons do its practitioners advise patients to drop out before embryo transfer? At what point do they suggest escalating treatment (for example, use of donor eggs)? After how many failed attempts do they advise patients *not* to try again? How aggressive are they about superovulation, the number of embryos transferred, and use of selective reduction if large multiple pregnancies occur? In cases of selective reduction, what are the rates of healthy newborns, of complications, of total pregnancy loss? In addition, patients must ask themselves how willing they are to rely on fetal reduction if they choose a more "aggressive" ART program— and how much disruption to their daily life treatment with this program will mean. (Chapter 9 discusses additional considerations in choosing a physician or ART program.)

Unfortunately, information needed to complete the ART picture has not been systematically gathered and reported. Patients and their doctors could benefit from more numbers, sharper calculations, more insight into the medical complexities that affect an individual's outcome. Even more disturbing than the lack of adequate statistics is the absence of regulation, oversight, internal checks, and public scrutiny—with outcomes that became apparent only years after flagrant medical practices were occurring.

There is yet another complication, an additional inadequacy in the data available and in the medical treatments themselves. These technologies proceed in spite of gaping holes in basic knowledge about the reproductive process and intervention in it. For example, individual patients often try assisted reproduction many times—yet no one understands the impact of such repetition on a woman's chances for having a baby. Evidence suggests that successful pregnancy becomes less likely during later cycles, but the reasons are not well understood. Will a treatment work well for particular women early in the process if it works at all? Does increasing age, inevitable as the number of attempts increases, make later success unlikely? Does a physiological reaction to repeated ovarian stimulation and puncture for egg retrieval compromise a woman's chances in later attempts to become pregnant? Claims of consistent success rates after as many as six attempts are questionable, since they are based on the small number of couples who persist through so many failures rather than stopping out of physical, emotional, or financial exhaustion; many studies, in fact, suggest very few successes beyond four cycles.[43] More generally, fertility specialists have not learned enough about why ART has not been more successful, why progress has indeed been so slow.[44] They try new hormonal stimulations, or change the timing of embryo transfers or alter nutrients in the fertilization dish; they select embryos for transfer that "look good" in the absence of ways to more accurately identify those embryos most likely to implant and develop successfully. For the most part, however, fertility specialists have not systematically studied, and do not know, why these interventions so often fail.

Inadequate knowledge about the safety and efficacy of ART—as well as professional dispute over the use and reported success of these technologies—has continued into the 1990s. Among physicians, calls for change in the performance and evaluation of assisted reproduction ranged from mild, even congratulatory, to angered. One eminent specialist, Dr. Howard W. Jones Jr., director of the Jones Institute for Reproductive Medicine, lambasted the specialty's efforts at reporting clinic-specific success rates. Writing in late 1993, he and three colleagues noted that "in the mid and later 1980s, there was considerable consumer disquiet about what was perceived as inadequate and misleading information about pregnancy rates." This disquiet, they add, was picked up by politicians, resulting in congressional pressure to publish clinic success rates. These specialists then cited "at least 10 serious variables that cloud the Clinic Specific Report in its present form and provide an opportunity to manipulate the variables . . . with the intention of providing superior data for the [report] at the expense of what is best for the individual patient." Their conclusion: the profession's response to dissatisfaction about misleading information was generating "different but equally misleading information."[45]

By the early 1990s this specialty's arguments shifted increasingly to the issue of costs, to the need for evaluating diagnostic tests and treatments, especially expensive procedures such as ART. With the election of the Clinton administration, national health insurance loomed suddenly, if momentarily, on the horizon. Concerns about expense of tests, treatments, and resulting complications came to a head, overshadowing worries about the actual harm treatment might cause women and offspring. The prospect of limits dictated by cost and effectiveness did serve to heighten pressures to demonstrate what procedures work, for whom. But fertility patients did not as a result gain real protection from uncontrolled and controversial procedures. As the next chapter shows, the hottest areas of current clinical activity are usually connected in some manner to ART and continue to exhibit an unsettling eagerness to intervene with questionable reproductive experiments.

4 Experiments In Fertility

Mixed Results, Mixed Messages

By the 1990s a fertility specialist could find cautions such as the following in medical journals:

> The selection of a [reproductive] procedure should not be based on a belief system. Medicine is not a religious institution with blind obedience to faith and dogma. Belief in the effectiveness of a procedure without substantiating data is unacceptable and reminiscent of the science behind bloodletting.[1]

> The proliferation of certain technologies by themselves creates a bias in clinical decision making in the direction of action. Unaudited clinical experience is not enough, because it may lead to repeating the same mistake over and over, but with greater confidence.[2]

But these messages are not likely to be conveyed to a young couple arriving for an appointment at the doctor's office. They enter the waiting room and sink into a soft, comfortable couch, enveloped in a world where attention focuses on having a baby. The carpeting is thick, its pastel blue a pleasing match to the couch and to mild, soothing artwork that seems to melt into pink walls. The fragrance of fresh flowers and fresh coffee fills the room; beside the coffee urn rests a china dish with three kinds of cookies. A photograph album, strategically placed between cookies and flowers, displays other young couples playing happily with new babies. Handwritten notes give names and birth dates, and thanks. Informational brochures are fanned out on a small coffee table beside the couch.

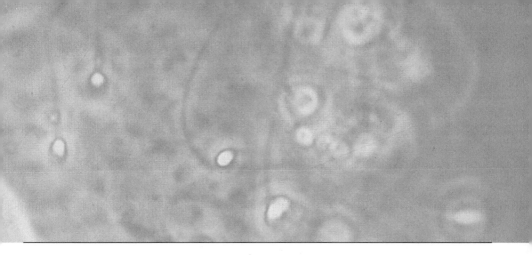

After their first appointment, the woman and man go home with several different brochures, describing various causes of, treatments for, and ways of coping with infertility. They go home feeling somewhat overwhelmed, but hopeful. Like other patients passing through the waiting room, this couple has been trying to have a baby. Month by month, they grow more anxious. Their question for the doctor: Can you help?

For most fertility patients, the answer to this straightforward question is "maybe." Anything more specific depends on characteristics of the particular woman and man, as well as abilities of their doctor. Today, when a nurse ushers this couple into the physician's office, he is sitting at his desk, skimming through a file of diagnostic test results. He interprets these results for them, tells them a diagnosis, and proposes possible treatments. The couple then goes home with decisions to make.

Relatively few patients hear a clear-cut diagnosis for which a proven treatment exists. For example, if this woman does not ovulate, she will not become pregnant without treatment that causes ovulation (though with the possibility of donor eggs, even this statement must now be qualified). If both of her fallopian tubes are completely blocked, she needs a treatment that can bypass this obstacle through in vitro fertilization or corrective surgery. If the man has virtually no viable sperm, they will need to try either artificial insemination using another man's sperm or a far more complicated assisted reproductive technology. The main ongoing consideration in such cases is to minimize risks and decide when they outweigh known benefits. Most diagnoses, however, are less certain, the prescribed treatment unproven or of questionable success. The couple may eventually conceive on their own, given only time and patience. Their decision to undergo treatment requires a more difficult assessment of pros and cons.

This chapter focuses on several diagnoses fertility patients hear and treatments their doctor may offer. My aim is not to provide comprehensive descriptions of these fertility problems and medical interventions; rather, I have selected prominent diagnoses and treatments that reveal patterns patients may never see, even as they shape in crucial ways the choices patients hear. Readers need not have the particular fertility problem or be considering the specific treatment to gain new perspective on fertility medicine or on individual decisions. I do, however, describe couples that know about in vitro fertilization but wish first to consider what their doctors call conventional therapies—fertility drugs, surgeries, artificial inseminations. My discussion leaves aside questions of the skill, judgment, or manner of the doctor and staff, important as these considerations are. A doctor may, in fact, work at the specialty's forefront, its cutting edge; his patients need to be aware of persistent concerns that emerge at this edge.

In exploring diagnoses, treatments, and the concerns they illustrate, I describe and quote liberally from a number of medical articles. My focus is not on technical details of a medical procedure or biological explanation, nor am I emphasizing any single study, which can be but one small part in a shifting aggregate of ongoing research. Rather, my aim is to convey some flavor of the controversy and uncertainty surrounding many procedures recommended to fertility patients, the hesitations and discomfort expressed by physicians themselves, among themselves. This chapter dips into the medical realm to share arguments that pass between doctors only, as if over the heads of women lying flat on an operating table or with their feet in the gynecologic stirrups.

In navigating the following discussion—with its medical excerpts and variety of diagnoses and treatments—readers should concentrate on the more general questions and broader perspective. The couple's deceptively simple question of whether the doctor can help must first be divided and rephrased: Should they undergo an *established* treatment, an intervention physicians presently accept as effective? Should they agree to a procedure that is *new*, an intervention the doctor thinks is worth trying in this case? These questions relate directly to two long-standing patterns that shape fertility medicine: *once a fertility treatment exists, doctors expand its use to an array of diagnoses, often without sufficient medical reason;* and *a named diagnosis may have no appropriate treatment, resulting in unscientific—at times dangerous—experimentation with medical interventions.*

Pelvic Surgery

That an operation can be done through a telescope does not imply that it should be.
GRIMES 1992, 1068

Long before fertility attracted so much medical attention, gynecology developed primarily as a surgical specialty. For many urinary and reproductive tract problems—unusual pain or bleeding, fibroids, cancers—surgery was the available treatment. Before hormonal medications (starting with DES in the 1940s) and the more recent assisted reproduction techniques, surgery on women was the only intervention prescribed for fertility problems as well—other than suggesting a couple relax on a long ocean cruise. Through various operations, gynecologists attempted to repair damaged fallopian tubes, remove abnormal tissue of endometriosis, or improve ovarian function.

Today, the couple seeking help for a fertility problem could face decisions not just between surgical or nonsurgical treatments; they may need to choose among increasingly sophisticated techniques for performing gynecological operations. Women with tubal damage or dysfunction—one of the most common fertility problems—must often decide whether to bypass the fallopian tubes with in vitro fertilization or to attempt surgical repair of the tube(s) and then attempt natural conception. While new surgical methods may sound good, as described by a doctor or informational brochure, most patients are not aware of the acrimony new techniques have provoked within the profession. Yet knowing about the concerns expressed by gynecologists could help patients avoid overzealous, potentially harmful surgical intervention. Two prime examples of such techniques in recent years are laparoscopic and laser surgery.

Laparoscopy is a procedure introduced initially for diagnostic purposes. Using a narrow telescope-like instrument called a laparoscope, a doctor can peer inside a patient's abdomen through a small incision at her navel to obtain diagnostic information that might otherwise require more invasive abdominal surgery. Controversy centers on what critics describe as frenetic growth of laparoscopy, beyond its diagnostic role, into a means of surgical *treatment*—growth that has accelerated without scientific assessment of risks and benefits compared to nonlaparoscopic treatments.[3]

Laser surgery uses a highly concentrated, intense beam of light instead of scalpel, electrocautery, or other surgical tools to cut and/or burn tissue. In some areas of medicine, a particular treatment of demonstrated benefit could not be performed prior to development of the laser technique. For example, an ophthalmologist can correct previously untreatable eye problems because a laser beam can reach specific structures inside the eye without damaging other tissue. For most gynecologic purposes, however, laser surgery may be no more effective, may bring more risks, and is certainly more expensive than other treatments.

To treat fertility problems, in particular, doctors have most commonly used a laparoscope in attempts to correct tubal injuries and abnormalities, and to remove abnormal tissue growth thought to interfere with conception or pregnancy (e.g., endometriosis or adhesions from previous surgery or infection). The surgical tool employed might be a laser. For the woman thinking over her doctor's recommendation, both technological innovations bring a danger not listed in forms she will sign before consenting to surgery: new operations become popular among doctors—and widely performed—with no systematic analysis, regulation, or monitoring. Manufacturers of laparoscopes and laser equipment promote them heavily to hospitals and doctors. Hospitals and doctors invest considerable sums of money in the equipment, which then needs to be used. Risks to patients are enlarged because wide dissemination means more physicians with inadequate training and skill perform the surgeries. Medications, at least, are subject to Food and Drug Administration requirements for scientifically controlled studies demonstrating safety and efficacy; even with such protections, drug manufacturers commonly promote medications for unapproved uses, and doctors at times prescribe medications inappropriately. In the case of surgeries, argues one physician, "Competitive marketing, opinion, and uncontrolled human experimentation determine what operations [patients] may receive. Unnecessary trial and error is particularly troubling in surgery because, unlike a medicine, an operation cannot be withdrawn after it has been administered to a patient."[4]

Both surgical procedures—laparoscopic and laser—have taken root in various areas of medicine, with varying effectiveness and safety. Within gynecology, advocates of laparoscopy were soon predicting this technique's eventual takeover of most gynecologic surgery. With the explosive growth of fertility medicine as a subspecialty, it is no wonder gynecologists' enthusiasm over laparoscopic surgery bubbled over into treatments for infertility. However, concerns within the profession also grew.

By the early 1990s, members of the American Gynecological and Obstetrical Society felt compelled to initiate an annual critique of medical innovations that "are frequently expensive, inadequately studied, aggressively promoted, and, perhaps, prematurely incorporated into clinical practice."[5] Laparoscopic and laser surgery were among the first to be evaluated. Physicians with "no personal or vested interest" reviewed evidence and published conclusions that are highly informative for women considering pelvic surgery to correct a fertility problem.

Although the list of conditions for which doctors perform surgery with a laparoscope was lengthening, the evaluation panel found sparse evidence to justify laparoscopic treatments. Based on an analysis of studies from 1966 on, the panel could report "fair evidence" (a grade between good and inadequate) to recommend laparoscopic surgery for a very few conditions: removal of ectopic pregnancy, ovarian biopsy, and treatment of polycystic ovary syndrome that does not respond to the medication clomiphene citrate. For treating other conditions, evidence was inadequate. A more specific focus on infertility caused by tubal injury or endometriosis found "almost no adequate studies" by which to compare pregnancy rates and complications following laparoscopy or various forms of laparotomy (surgery requiring a larger abdominal incision and not using a laparoscope). Overall, the evaluators found "very few randomized controlled trials or analytic studies," and those they did find "have methodological shortcomings."[6]

Laser surgery, according to this panel, can well be considered an "archetype," symbolizing problems in the rapid development and dissemination of new technologies. The novel, high-tech aura itself makes laser surgery an easy sell. Manufacturers can sell laser machines to doctors and hospitals; doctors can sell laser treatments to patients. The public learns of this technology—through patient word-of-mouth and the media—creating "patient demand" that, in turn, reinforces the medical marketing cycle. All this proceeds unfettered by scientific evaluation.[7]

How to slow this cycle? Patients considering laser surgery might pause were they to learn the gynecologic panel's perspective. These evaluators question whether the "net surgical outcome" for patients is any better when a laser is used than when it is not. Physicians' use of a laser requires large financial and training commitments. Few studies have attempted to identify benefits and risks, particularly regarding the healing process and potential injury when using a laser. Rather, the panel concludes, "laser technology has at times been clouded by hyperbole, illusion, and myths that have grown like Jack's beanstalk. . . . Recognizing when a scalpel or a $5,000 electrocautery knife can be more appropriate and less risky than a $100,000 laser device is pivotal to the continued success of laser technology in medicine."[8]

Whether laser beams, internal scopes, or whatever the next invention, individual patients must attempt to separate hype and generalities from their own medical needs. Obtaining current information on rates of successful pregnancies and of complications is, of course, essential to deciding whether surgery is needed and, if it is, what type best balances benefits and risks. The different types and locations of pelvic disorders, as well as the type of surgery proposed, all bring a different prognosis for significantly improving a woman's fertility. Patients can also glean crucial insights about *nonmedical* influences on their treatment by tapping into the medical discussion. Most prominently, a doctor's recommendation of surgery may be influenced in no small measure by considerations other than a patient's particular fertility condition:

Doctors trained in medical programs that emphasize surgery tend to perform surgery; and older doctors, further away from their medical training, may be more likely to recommend surgery than the younger, more recently trained.[9]

Surgical rates vary by locale; thus the "medical community" in which a woman lives may affect whether she undergoes surgery.[10]

The relative ease in performing a procedure, such as laparoscopic surgery, increases its frequency independent of evidence the treatment is needed; new treatment tools, moreover, end up in the hands of unskilled practitioners—including in outpatient and office settings, where supervision is even less likely than in a hospital—greatly enlarging risks over potential benefits. The fact that a procedure is easy to schedule and perform does not necessarily mean it will be performed well on patients who are selected appropriately.[11]

Having the equipment at hand influences a doctor's choice of treatment; once doctors or hospitals purchase a laparoscope or laser device, economic pressures encourage its use on patients who have insurance coverage or can pay themselves.

Surgical procedures have provided doctors with discrete, time-limited services that could be billed to patients or insurers. As an assured source of physician income (that is, before encroachment of capitated managed-care plans), these procedures have often become established and widely practiced with no mechanism for systematic evaluation or oversight. One physician concerned about risks of laparoscopic surgery contends that much of the impetus behind its increasing popularity among doctors was the fact that health insurance usually covers surgery but not medications, which are very expensive: "We must ask whether risking permanent impairment of a woman's fertility [for instance, as a result of scarring or adhesions] is a fair exchange for the potential cost savings."[12]

A study seeking to document complications of laparoscopic procedures reinforces such concerns, concluding that "there clearly is a low level of disastrous complications due to laparoscopy."[13] More complications occur during laparoscopic treatment attempts than when the technique is used for diagnosis only. The authors note that many such complications (which include lacerations of the colon and of arteries or veins) never appear in journal publications. They do not attempt to compare these complications to rates for conventional pelvic surgery, because the procedures are so different from each other. However, a different question arises from their findings: Was the laparoscopic procedure, or any type of surgery, necessary at all? Of the 458 laparoscopic treatments for endometriosis, 70 percent were for minimal or mild conditions. Of 322 operations to remove pelvic adhesions, nearly the same proportion (67 percent) were for minimal or mild grade, rather than moderate or severe. Given the view of many specialists that treating these milder conditions does not significantly improve a woman's fertility, any complications are excessive in comparison to the alternative of *no* treatment.

Decisions about surgery—and the operation itself—carry a sense of immediacy, but there is a longer view to consider. Many women undergo an operation when that type of surgery is gaining momentum or at its peak. Doctors not only become enamored of the latest technique, they also feel pressed by their competition: to attract and keep patients, Dr. Smith must keep up with Dr. Jones. However, as one physician states, "operations come and go." After two or three decades, a particular surgical fad may be deemed not worthwhile and eventually disappear—or it may survive and be put to futile use. While some doctors are satisfied with this medical selection process, others are critical: "Natural selection pressures may work over eons in biology so that only the best survive, but one of the principal problems in medicine is that many useless, ineffective, and occasionally harmful procedures are retained. As a patient I would not want to be innocently caught in the slow, gradual evolution of medical innovation."[14]

Women attempting to avoid being caught in a worthless operation must also contend with options other than the surgical. Many patients once considered classic pelvic surgery cases—for instance, with blocked or damaged fallopian tubes—can now attempt in vitro fertilization, which may offer them a greater chance of pregnancy or one that comes sooner. The couple discussing a diagnosis and possible treatment with their doctor will now hear a list of fertility drugs, ranging from clomiphene citrate to more powerful ovarian stimulants, as well as a list of assisted reproductive procedures. Even as gynecologists trained their new surgical weapons on the burgeoning fertility field, hormonal manipulations, alone or in combination with in vitro–related techniques, were gaining a foothold, competing with surgery in the search for applicable diagnoses.

Stimulated Intrauterine Insemination and Its Variations

Controlled ovarian hyperstimulation with IUI has been widely advocated as an effective but untested method of treating subfertile couples with patent [open] fallopian tubes and presumably normal ovulatory function when more traditional therapy has failed.   Nulsen et al. 1993, 780

A layperson reading this statement in a medical journal stops, reads again, wonders at the puzzling combination of words. How can a treatment be considered effective *but* untested? And if untested, why advocated? If critics of laparoscopic surgery worry that its relative ease increases its inappropriate use, this danger is even greater in certain nonsurgical approaches—some requiring not much more than a prescription pad.

Consider again the couple sitting in the doctor's office. Suppose the doctor suggests trying a procedure called stimulated intrauterine insemination (IUI)—that is, hyperstimulation followed by injection of sperm through the cervix into the woman's uterus rather than, more simply, into her vagina. Before agreeing to the recommended treatment, the couple asks questions. How is the procedure done? What side effects will the woman experience from fertility drugs and inseminations? Why will this treatment help? The doctor describes the schedule of pills and injections, the ultrasound monitoring of egg follicles as they grow larger, the collection and preparation of sperm, the way sperm are injected into the uterus. He tells them the most frequent side effects, which he describes as generally mild. He assures them the serious complications, requiring hospitalization, are rare. He reminds the couple that nothing else has worked and says that perhaps, for some unknown reason, the superovulation of many eggs and placement of specially washed sperm directly into the uterus will improve fertility enough to result in a pregnancy. He may stress that there are no guarantees, but his answer is unlikely to convey either the degree of controversy about the treatments linking intrauterine insemination to controlled ovarian hyperstimulation or the confusion as to their effectiveness—confusion evident inside the medical journals piled on his desk. Just as some women are caught in the wave of a surgical fad, the couple considering IUI with ovarian stimulation find themselves in a formidable tangle of diagnoses, treatments, possible benefits, and unquestionable risks.

The couple's doctor may have first read of combining superovulation with intrauterine insemination in the 1987 journal article that proposed this novel therapy as an alternative to IVF or GIFT. Drawing attention to the article was an unusual editorial comment, in italics, cautioning clinician-readers not to rush into widespread application of the unproven treatment. As if to stem a predictable tide, the editor called for "controlled prospective studies [that] can support this approach."[15] A few years later, it was clear the tide had not been stemmed. A different editor of the same journal noted ruefully: "Unfortunately over the ensuing . . . years, controlled studies have not been forthcoming. Contrary to the [earlier] editorial plea, many centers treating infertile couples have adopted hMG superovulation in conjunction with IUI for certain patients who have failed to respond to other forms of therapy and for couples with unexplained infertility." Although this editor called once again for a randomized clinical trial to determine whether this treatment actually improves chances for pregnancy, his call carried neither force nor hope.[16]

The way this widely advocated treatment arose tells much about the uncertainty surrounding it and provides a cautionary tale for patients today faced with newly developing therapies. Essentially, two distinct treatments were pieced together and performed on patients with a range of fertility problems by increasing numbers of doctors who followed widely varying protocols (the specific types, dosage, and timing of drugs; the specific insemination procedures). The two treatments were each influenced by development of in vitro fertilization, then converged as an alternative for women whose condition did not require that fertilization actually occur in a laboratory dish.

For the couple whose doctor recommends stimulated IUI, the main problem is that the unsystematic mixing and matching of procedures connected to this therapy leaves no way for doctors, let alone patients, to know what works for whom. Before deciding to undergo this treatment, the couple should understand the following:

A large number of small studies focus on various steps of IUI and ovarian hyperstimulation, performed separately and in combination; however, no systematic evaluation exists that can answer basic questions about these treatments' benefits and risks for couples with differing fertility characteristics.

If stimulated IUI does increase pregnancy rates for some couples, physicians have not known whether one component—superovulation or insemination—is responsible for improvement or whether both are necessary. Some specialists minimize the importance of artificial insemination while others downplay the value of superovulation; the most recent wisdom suggests a combined effect creates the most opportune conditions for pregnancy, by bringing an increased number of fertilizable eggs and prepared sperm into close proximity.

Stimulated IUI aims at *sub*fertile patients, whose conditions do allow for spontaneous pregnancies. However, proponents generally justify this treatment by comparing it to the high cost and modest success of assisted reproductive technologies, rather than to less invasive alternatives or to the acknowledged "spontaneous cures."

Recent reports have attempted to clarify benefits of stimulated IUI. One study of couples with long-standing fertility problems (generally over three years) and diagnosed with endometriosis, male-factor, or unexplained infertility, found that IUI with ovarian hyperstimulation resulted in higher pregnancy rates than IUI alone.[17] A 1994 report analyzed the cost-effectiveness of stimulated IUI compared to IVF, GIFT, ZIFT, and no treatment.[18] Based on combined data from several small studies of varying fertility conditions, these authors conclude that up to four cycles of stimulated IUI are as effective as, and less expensive than, one cycle of the more invasive assisted reproductive technologies. They cite these results not as a final word on the widely used treatments, but as justification for a randomized clinical trial. Similarly, a review of fertility treatments performed during one year (1992) at the University of Iowa medical school found that for women with open fallopian tubes IUI, with or without ovarian stimulation, was more cost-effective than IVF.[19]

A preliminary report from nineteen European fertility clinics looked at couples with unexplained infertility of at least three years' duration, with the women younger than thirty-eight years of age.[20] This multiclinic randomized controlled trial found that stimulated IUI, IVF, and GIFT resulted in similar pregnancy rates, which were all higher than superovulation alone; superovulation alone, in turn, resulted in a higher pregnancy rate than estimates of the chance for spontaneous pregnancy in such couples. One specialist, summarizing these and other studies, concludes the following: for couples with *long-standing* unexplained infertility and a woman *younger than forty,* the live birthrate following stimulated IUI drops below 8 percent during a third or fourth attempt. Since the IVF success rate is approximately twice as high, these couples should move on to IVF following two to four stimulated IUI cycles with no pregnancy.[21] Another overview, noting "a conspicuous absence of proper prospective controlled evaluations of assisted reproductive techniques," suggests trying no treatment initially (unless a woman's fallopian tubes are blocked), then four cycles of stimulated IUI, before attempting IVF or GIFT.[22]

The subfertile couple might begin by asking their doctor why they need artificial insemination. The most common reason for intrauterine insemination has been to bypass fertility problems localized to the cervix. For decades, a diagnosis called "hostile cervical mucus"—in which too little mucus is produced by cervical glands or the chemical balance of the mucus thwarts sperm survival—was treated with intrauterine insemination. However, for decades, IUI was, in the words of one review article, "of questionable efficacy and fraught with frequent side effects."[23] While the efficacy of IUI remains questionable, technical improvements have greatly diminished such side effects as infection and severe cramping. New methods of washing sperm (developed for in vitro fertilization) and safer instruments for inseminating the prepared sperm into the uterus altered the risks, if not the benefits, of this procedure. With lessened risks, use of IUI was extended far beyond women thought to have cervical problems. According to one recent summary of IUI studies, this procedure became "a first-line choice" among assisted reproductive treatments if the woman had open, apparently normal fallopian tubes. However, doctors' reasons for choosing this treatment have been extremely varied and inconsistently applied. The actual value of IUI has been difficult to evaluate, since couples undergoing IUI are not completely unable to conceive on their own. "As a consequence, the reported results remain controversial and there is still no consensus on its real efficacy and applications."[24]

The couple might also ask why the woman needs ovarian hyperstimulation if she does ovulate on her own. For some women who do *not* ovulate, clomiphene citrate or the more powerful hMG (human menopausal gonadotropin) can stimulate the ovary to produce a mature egg for ovulation, allowing the possibility of pregnancy. When fertility drugs first emerged on the gynecologic scene, doctors appropriately prescribed them almost exclusively to women who did not otherwise ovulate. However, during the same years that IUI was transforming, prescription of fertility drugs also expanded far beyond its initial, limited use. Superovulation became the routine preparation for IVF or GIFT. Most women undergoing these assisted reproductive technologies do ovulate but have been diagnosed with tubal problems, endometriosis, or unexplained infertility—or the male partner might have a fertility problem for which IVF is tried. Thus gynecologists became more familiar and comfortable trying these drugs on women with a variety of fertility problems—or in the case of male infertility, on women with no problem at all.

Among women whose assisted reproductive treatment had to be canceled following hormonal superovulation, without proceeding to egg retrieval and transfer, some did become pregnant. Although a proportion of these couples would be expected to conceive spontaneously, physicians speculated that perhaps the superovulation itself, without egg retrieval or laboratory procedures, was the reason. And as ART waiting lists grew, so too did pressure to "do something" for waiting patients. It did not take much to combine increasingly familiar superovulation with newly improved IUI or to suggest trying this combination for a wide range of diagnoses. The problem is that many more women would now face risks of the combined treatment—including multiple pregnancy, ovarian hyperstimulation syndrome, infection, ectopic and heterotopic (one embryo in the uterus, other or others implanted outside the uterus) pregnancy—without evidence that their chances for viable pregnancy were improved. Although proponents advocated this treatment in lieu of more invasive assisted reproductive technologies, physicians could perform stimulated IUI on even larger numbers of women who were not in line for ART. Fertility drugs would flow more freely, piggy-backed onto a safer, easier uterine insemination technique.

By the mid-1990s, medical reports were reflecting just such a development. Clinicians lacking a program for assisted reproduction described efforts to extend ovarian hyperstimulation to several categories of infertility—with and without intrauterine insemination—as an alternative to waiting for a possible spontaneous pregnancy.[25] Accumulating statistics were revealing a changed pattern of large multiple pregnancies. The main contributor was no longer in vitro fertilization but ovarian stimulation itself. While ART practitioners lowered the proportion of large multifetal pregnancies by limiting the number of embryos transferred, doctors were prescribing fertility drugs promiscuously. As Dr. Louis Keith, a professor of obstetrics and gynecology who studies multiple births explains: "The real increase in twins and triplets in the United States did not occur until 1985, when we learned how to superovulate women. Now doctors are prescribing ovulation-enhancing agents as if they were prescribing bubble gum at a children's birthday party."[26] And a specialist in fetal reduction argues that too many physicians use these medications in a "cavalier" manner, relying on "those of us who pick up the pieces when there is a 'whoops' " as their safety net. Although the prescribing physicians might consider fetal reduction to be "a relatively unimportant side effect of aggressive infertility therapy," the subsequent high rates of pregnancy loss and prematurity prove otherwise.[27]

Couples with unexplained infertility are particularly vulnerable to a "do something" medical approach and illustrate well its two major pitfalls. First, the spontaneous pregnancy rate is overlooked, the no-treatment option ignored. Following treatment such as stimulated IUI, some of the women will be pregnant. The treatment will appear to have worked. However, up to 60 percent of couples with unexplained infertility will conceive without treatment within two years; as one specialist puts it, the array of suggested therapies "probably offers no better pregnancy rate than that which exists spontaneously."[28] Tellingly, his very next statement notes physicians' tendency to recommend "costly, invasive, labor-intensive . . . and emotionally stressful IVF or GIFT." The alternative he poses? Superovulation, with or without intrauterine insemination. Another example: a study finds that IUI did not result in better pregnancy rates than "well-timed intercourse"; however, the conclusion suggests treating unexplained infertility initially with clomiphene citrate, which is cheap and easy to take, then hMG with or without IUI "before the more advanced technologies of assisted reproduction."[29] The pattern reappears frequently in the medical literature: after a token bow to spontaneous pregnancy rates, the alternative of "doing nothing" disappears quickly from the discussion.[30]

Clinician-researchers may have good intentions in trying to preempt more costly and invasive reproductive technologies they know colleagues will employ. However, treatment is not the only option. Patients must persist in remembering that doing nothing—except, of course, well-timed intercourse—brings a significant chance of pregnancy for certain subfertile couples and should always enter into the comparison.

A second pitfall is that medical intervention proceeds without adequate biological understanding. Unexplained infertility exposes treatments that are shots in the dark, across gaps in scientific knowledge about the problem being treated. The accumulation of medical reports on stimulated IUI bears witness to an approach in which a treatment is tried now, an explanation sought later as to why the treatment might work, though, in fact, without good evidence that it does. Even if stimulated IUI improves fertility in an undefined subgroup—as some preliminary studies cited above suggest—doctors do not know the reason or which patients are part of that subgroup or how great an improvement the treatment will bring over their chance for a spontaneous pregnancy. For some women who are taking clomiphene citrate, intrauterine insemination may improve pregnancy rates only because this procedure bypasses poor cervical mucus caused by the very medication her doctor prescribed; the insemination, then, is treating the side effect of a fertility treatment.[31]

"Unexplained" Infertility

Conventional wisdom, and many doctors, suggests the category of unexplained infertility is consistently shrinking. In the mid-1990s, the American Society for Reproductive Medicine placed the unexplained proportion at 20 percent of fertility patients. While 10–15 percent is a commonly heard estimate among fertility specialists, some claim a diagnosis is now possible for nearly all fertility patients. However, other specialists consider such a claim to be, as one reproductive endocrinologist put it, "presumptuous." Naming a condition—and calling it a diagnosis—does not necessarily mean that condition in fact lowers fertility; certain conditions commonly diagnosed and treated as the cause of a patient's infertility occur at similar rates in fertile couples.[1] These specialists are more impressed, moreover, with recent insights into the complexities of male fertility, the interaction of egg and sperm, and the possible impact of genetics and the immune system on a couple's fertility—all of which enlarge, rather than shrink, the category of what doctors cannot explain.

1. Guzick et al. 1994.

Well-Timed Intercourse?

Fertility medicine's pitfalls can extend, in a more general form, to any couple trying for a pregnancy. In the early 1990s, epidemiological surveys were suggesting that only 25–30 percent of women trying to conceive had a fairly good idea of the most fertile days in their menstrual cycle; pregnancy might be delayed, or even thwarted, because of intercourse that was not well-timed or not frequent enough.[1] It turns out that doctors' ideas about timing may not have been accurate either. Ob-gyns commonly believed conception was most likely if intercourse occurred during a few days before ovulation to a few days after (previously published estimates of the number of fertile days varied from two to ten days surrounding the day of ovulation). However, a careful epidemiological study of more than 200 women, aged twenty-six to thirty-five, found that pregnancy resulted only when intercourse occurred during a six-day "window of opportunity" that *ended* on the day of ovulation.[2] The probability of conception ranged from 10 percent with intercourse on the fifth day before to 33 $\frac{1}{3}$ percent on the day of ovulation. Since conception usually occurred following intercourse on the day of ovulation or one to two days before, fertility specialists were now advising couples to have intercourse several times in the week leading up to ovulation; if they waited for signs of ovulation (e.g., through commercial testing kits), they might miss the most opportune time. One can only wonder how many couples failed to conceive spontaneously, were perhaps told they have "unexplained infertility," and underwent fertility treatments—some "successful," some not—because this knowledge was lacking. Similarly, clinical research that relied on inaccurate notions of fertile days might reach inaccurate conclusions.

---

1. B. Eshkenazi, Associate Professor of Public Health, University of California, Berkeley, personal communication.

2. Wilcox, Weinberg, and Baird 1995.

Together, these pitfalls—comparing stimulated IUI to assisted reproductive technologies without considering the spontaneous pregnancy rate and intervening without sufficient biological knowledge—result in studies of little value to the medical community or its clients. Frustrated by the futility of seeking useful information from the type of research so common in fertility medicine, a journal editor comments on a study of GIFT and IUI: "To compare the results of a treatment modality the mechanism of which is unclear (GIFT) with another the value of which has previously been shown to be minimal at best (IUI) in the treatment of those women with infertility the cause of which is unknown makes it difficult to design a definitive study. . . . When will it be acknowledged that the emperor is wearing no clothes?"[32]

As with unexplained infertility, application of stimulated IUI to other diagnoses is murky. Its use for male fertility problems is particularly frustrating, though the couple faces somewhat different issues. The main problem in these cases is that doctors commonly recommend treatment in the face of negative evidence. That is, adequately designed studies are demonstrating that IUI, with or without ovarian hyperstimulation, does *not* significantly improve pregnancy rates for a couple whose subfertility is traced to sperm or semen disorders. For example, one study found "IUI with or without superovulation is completely useless . . . if male factor infertility is well defined."[33] Another found no increase in pregnancy following IUI for male infertility, leading to this editorial comment: "IUI has been the 'in' thing for almost a decade now. . . . However, numerous reports have appeared, and two extensive reviews, . . . all with the same conclusion: IUI does not improve pregnancy rates in male infertility. [This] study, I hope, is the last word. . . . The labor, expense, and psychological trauma, not to mention the inconvenience to both husband and wife, overwhelmingly outbalance the occasional pregnancy which occurs apparently unrelated to the procedure."[34]

This study was not the last word, however. More reports followed, often focusing on a particular step of the treatment—comparing, for example, one insemination per cycle to two; comparing differing types of inseminations and methods for predicting time of ovulation; comparing differing drugs for stimulating ovulation in combination with insemination. This last raises a second major problem: application of these treatments to *male* fertility problems entails superovulation of the *woman*. The clear risks to her health have no countervailing benefits for either partner. Yet it is no secret among physicians that the practice will persist. Says one specialist: "In spite of analyses . . . demonstrating the ineffectiveness of often cherished techniques, I suspect that physicians will continue to use them in spite of their costs and ineffectiveness, as many feel they must offer their patients some form of treatment, even if ineffective."[35]

Recommending stimulated IUI to subfertile couples as an alternative to in vitro–related procedures distracts attention from this treatment's own invasiveness and overuse. The crucial question for each couple remains: Does this combined approach increase our chances of conceiving, and what risks does it bring? Couples must resist the tendency in fertility medicine to try interventions indiscriminately on far too many patients. Even if further study indicates the treatment improves pregnancy rates for an as yet undefined subgroup of couples, one must still ask if the improvement is substantial enough to outweigh risks. Or might the couple—diagnosed with unexplained infertility or mild endometriosis or low sperm count—conceive after six extra months without treatment, without taking on those risks?

Most striking about treatments involving ovarian hyperstimulation and intrauterine insemination is confusion regarding the usefulness of each component and of the two combined. There may be an impressive accumulation of medical reports, but there are few well-designed studies among them, and the risks and benefits of treatment remain uncertain. There is also an impressive—or alarming—amount of trial and error and of speculation on why a particular procedure *might* improve fertility. Certainly, speculation is a necessary, often fruitful step in generating new therapeutic ideas and forming hypotheses to be tested. Treatments of demonstrated efficacy may justifiably be used before understanding how they work (for example, smallpox vaccination was proven effective before the reason was understood; and scientists still do not understand completely how anesthetics work). The biological speculations undergirding stimulated IUI are unsettling, however, because these tentative rationales have emerged after the fact of widespread use; because they are so numerous and scattered in substance, proliferating beyond systematic attempts at scientific verification; and because the theories often explain the effectiveness of interventions that may not even be effective.

Diagnoses in Search of Treatments

New surgical procedures and stimulated IUI demonstrate how the existence of treatment procedures—and the search for indications to use them—can shape what doctors recommend to patients with a range of differing fertility problems. Another pattern prominent in fertility medicine can similarly result in patients receiving inappropriate and risky fertility interventions. In these cases, clinicians have a diagnosis but no corresponding therapy. A problem is named; then comes unscientific experimentation with treatments.

Luteal Phase Deficiency

I have had the feeling for some time that luteal insufficiency as a recurring phenomenon in a given woman is often overdiagnosed. However, the definitive study has still not been performed.   JAFFE 1993, 484

Many couples sitting in their doctor's waiting room have already been initiated into one fertility ritual. Every morning, as soon as the woman wakes up, she reaches to the nightstand and places a special thermometer under her tongue for five minutes. She records this early morning temperature with a dot for each day of her menstrual cycle on graphed paper known as a basal body temperature (BBT) chart. So many women have spent so many mornings taking their temperature before doing *anything* else that the activity has become a not very private joke among fertility patients. The woman watches for a mid-cycle temperature rise indicating ovulation has occurred. If the temperature drops back before fourteen or so days, marking the end of that monthly cycle (and usually the start of her period), this woman is likely to hear a diagnosis of "luteal phase deficiency" or "defect" (LPD). Her doctor may then prescribe treatment with hormonal medication to correct this condition.

The luteal phase is the time between ovulation and the start of a woman's menstrual period, often thought of as the last half of her menstrual cycle. Luteal phase deficiency is a menstrual cycle abnormality generally defined as inadequate production of the hormone progesterone by the corpus luteum (the ovarian follicle from which a mature egg has just been released) following ovulation. If there is not enough progesterone and/or if production of this hormone does not continue over enough days, the uterine lining will not receive the hormonal stimulation needed to allow implantation of an embryo. Patients diagnosed with luteal phase deficiency need to understand two basic facts about this condition: first, the diagnosis itself is uncertain, a focus of controversy among fertility specialists; and second, this uncertain diagnosis leads to treatments that are similarly controversial.

To judge by the arguments and questions among physicians, LPD might best be considered an infertility diagnosis in name only. Some specialists dispute the existence of this fertility problem altogether, placing women so labeled within the category of unexplained infertility. Although critics might grant that a condition dubbed LPD does exist in some women, they question whether this condition lowers a couple's fertility. To be defined as a factor contributing to subfertility, the condition must be consistent and repetitive, with an impact on the woman's chance for pregnancy. Instead, LPD is sporadic throughout women's reproductive life, a condition found in normally fertile women at the same rate as in the infertile, a rate expected by chance alone. As one study indicates, LPD is often observed to coincide with common events in a woman's life—including the first years of menstruation, times of stress or of very strenuous exercise, the postpartum period, the last years of menstruation.[36] Patients need to know that critics within the profession are asking if the diagnosis and treatment of luteal phase deficiency improves the likelihood of pregnancy. So far, the answer appears to be no.

As with the elephant described by the blind men, a major problem is the absence of ways to identify accurately this entity called luteal phase deficiency. All three diagnostic tools that physicians use have serious flaws. The first and easiest tool is the basal body temperature (BBT) chart indicating whether ovulation has occurred and, if so, the length of the luteal phase. However, this daily record of a woman's morning temperature, so well known among fertility patients (see Figure 2), does not correlate well with other diagnostic techniques and does not distinguish patients ultimately thought to have a luteal deficiency.

The second diagnostic tool is a blood test measuring the woman's progesterone level during the luteal phase of her menstrual cycle in an attempt to determine whether she is producing enough of this hormone to support an embryo. Physicians do not know, however, on which day, or days, to draw a blood sample in order to gain information most useful for treating that woman. Further complicating blood tests, no matter the day, are the "frequent and rather wide fluctuations in serum [progesterone] levels over 24 hours."[37] Because this hormone is released into the bloodstream in an intermittent pulsatile pattern,

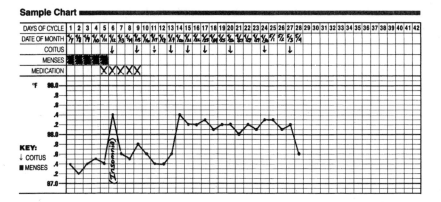

Figure 2. Basal body temperature chart (BBT). This sample chart shows a typical "normal" pattern of body temperature taken before rising in the morning. The mid-cycle rise and plateau (luteal phase) indicate that ovulation occurred. The temperature then drops if no pregnancy occurs; the next cycle begins with the first day of menstruation. If there is no sustained temperature rise, ovulation probably has not occurred. Fewer than 11–12 days of elevated temperature may be interpreted as a sign of luteal phase defect (LPD). However, basal body temperature can also be affected by such factors as insomnia or illness.

serum levels will naturally vary at different times of day and night. The level of progesterone circulating in a woman's bloodstream, moreover, may not even reflect information actually needed about hormonal stimulation of endometrial tissue. That stimulation does not depend only on amounts of hormone produced and circulating in blood throughout her body. Hormones must also interact adequately with hormone receptors—in this instance, located in the uterine lining—to achieve their needed effect.[38]

The third diagnostic approach, endometrial biopsy, is intended to analyze uterine tissue, in order to assess more directly the endometrium's preparation for implantation of an embryo. Though frequently performed, recent studies question the usefulness of this more invasive, painful, and costly test for predicting pregnancy success. Again, there are unresolved questions about when, during the second half of a woman's menstrual cycle, this test should be performed and about the need for testing on more than one day. The procedure itself can cause an early menstrual period, artificially reinforcing a picture that leads the doctor to a diagnosis of luteal phase deficiency.

At best, medical discussions of methods for identifying LPD describe evidence that is "suggestive," but not "diagnostic," of "rough approximations" rather than accurate or valid data. The incidence of LPD, many specialists now argue, is considerably lower than previously claimed on the basis of the above tests. Even more important, women identified through such tests do not appear to have lowered fertility. Simply put, one review of diagnostic methods concluded: "The diagnosis of LPD in the clinical setting remains problematic and controversial primarily because there is no practical diagnostic method that has been validated."[39] And a study of endometrial biopsy in particular found "firstly that diagnosis of LPD in both infertile and fertile women represents only a chance event; secondly, histological [from biopsy tissue analysis] endometrial adequacy or inadequacy in the cycle of conception or in previous cycles is not related to the outcome of pregnancy in infertile patients. Finally, treatment of LPD does not improve pregnancy outcome in infertile women. Thus, luteal phase evaluation [through biopsy] of the endometrium is not worthwhile."[40]

This final conclusion points to the crucial added problem attached to the diagnosis of LPD: *diagnosis does lead to treatment.* Not only do women undergo unpleasant, often painful, and costly tests that are not worthwhile, but these tests then become the basis for undergoing treatments never demonstrated to be worthwhile. Doctors commonly prescribe progesterone supplements following ovulation, yet there is no evidence this treatment improves pregnancy rates. Doctors try pre-ovulation clomiphene citrate in an effort to attain a "better" ovulation that will produce greater amounts of progesterone, though some specialists advise that clomiphene should *not* be given to women who ovulate.[41] After clomiphene, the doctor may prescribe the more powerful, difficult, and risky hMG; however, this treatment can itself shorten the woman's luteal phase. Confusion has come full circle—a treatment is tried on women to correct a particular condition whose very existence is a bone of contention; the treatment may cause symptoms of the diagnosed condition and must certainly obscure what is cause, what is effect, why the woman is not pregnant.

All such interventions bring risk—in these cases, with no known benefits. And, there is the further risk of initiating a self-perpetuating cycle of worthless diagnoses and futile treatments, with women and their doctors caught by the irresistible momentum of doing something. One can well imagine the following scenario: a couple has now accumulated three months of basal body temperature charts. One month the elevated dots cover thirteen days, another month ten, then thirteen again. The doctor orders a blood test for progesterone, which measures in the low-normal range. The doctor prescribes progesterone. After several months, he adds Clomid. Two months later the woman comes to the office for an endometrial biopsy, a procedure far more painful than the nurse described when she advised the woman to arrive well-dosed with Motrin. A shorter luteal phase follows. The doctor escalates to hMG injections; the woman must schedule her days around the injections and frequent ultrasound monitoring of her ovaries to check for ovarian hyperstimulation syndrome. Still not pregnant, the couple asks, "What now?"

There is no good way for the couple or the doctor to answer this question. From the very first step, the months of BBT charts, the missing element was knowledge about the biology of this woman's fertility problem, if indeed she has one. Without such knowledge, no specialist can determine whether any treatment will help the woman conceive. As matters now stand, patients and their doctors are dealing with what the American College of Obstetricians and Gynecologists officially describes as "a term applied to a poorly understood group of subtle hormonal alterations."[42] The diagnosis encompasses a heterogeneous group. Some women have never conceived, others miscarry very early in pregnancy. Some women ovulate regularly, others do not. Hormonal evaluations show varying patterns of various hormones. For some subgroup of women, medical intervention may improve fertility, but there is no way of knowing for whom or with what intervention.

The entity called LPD illustrates the need for more concise and discriminating diagnostic methods *before* applying treatments to individual women, as well as for treatments that target more specifically an identified fertility problem. In the meantime, the large, heterogeneous group of women diagnosed with LPD undergoes the same therapies when, in fact, their underlying physiological conditions call for differing medical treatment—or perhaps none at all. Indeed, this particular diagnostic label may become a historical remnant in this era of cost concerns. In the words of one specialist, LPD will be a "so what?" diagnosis. Why perform tests at all—especially flawed, often costly tests—when women will be given the same broadscale treatments anyway? Rather than improve diagnostic abilities to better determine individual patient needs, the label will fade—but interventions will continue to engulf a number of vaguely defined fertility problems.

Although physician enthusiasm for the LPD diagnosis may wane, two areas of fertility medicine attracting active and increasing attention—male factor and immunologic infertility—demonstrate how the existence of a diagnosis fuels precipitous intervention in the absence of adequate biological knowledge. These diagnoses may eventually identify well-understood physiological conditions that impair fertility and respond to treatment in some couples, affecting more definable and limited populations of women and men than does the amorphous luteal deficiency; at present, however, male factor and immunologic diagnoses display a sense of groping in the dark and the risks such groping can bring. Patients need to be all the more cautious about new and unproven procedures on the one hand and outdated and disproven procedures on the other.

Male Factor Infertility

We currently remain in a position where clinical practice has run ahead of scientific analysis, allowing treatment of previously untreatable semen samples by means of techniques we do not yet fully understand.   TUCKER ET AL. 1993, 324

One clear sign of progress in fertility medicine during recent years is that the woman seeing the doctor is often not alone; the appointment is for a couple. The doctor will more likely order a basic test of the man's semen and sperm before recommending extensive diagnostic procedures or treatments for the woman. Although male infertility is not a new diagnosis, infertility has until recently been defined and treated largely as a woman's problem. Frequently physicians failed to check the fertility of a woman's partner even in cases of "unexplained infertility." She might undergo years of medications, pelvic surgeries, and inseminations, unaware that the explanation resided with him. Knowledge about male fertility remained meager, as did treatment options. Now, specialists generally describe fertility problems as divided fairly evenly between the woman and man (approximately 40 percent each), with both partners contributing to lowered fertility in many couples trying to conceive. Indeed, the most common cause of infertility involves some type of sperm abnormality, many of which may *not* be detectable through sperm counts.[43] Physicians continue to characterize this area of fertility medicine as "frustrating," an "enigma" with treatment results that are "discouraging"; by the 1990s, however, male fertility problems could no longer be ignored. In fact, male factor infertility had engendered its own subspecialty among urologists: *andrologists* now join the ranks of fertility specialists, along with their gynecologist colleagues.

This greatly increased attention to male fertility is yet another spin-off of in vitro fertilization. With attempts to join egg and sperm in a laboratory dish, physicians observed before their very eyes numerous instances in which apparently normal sperm were unable to fertilize an egg. Conversely, successful fertilization came as a surprise in some cases where sperm or semen characteristics predicted failure according to standard diagnostic tests. Experience with assisted reproductive technologies enhanced appreciation of the complexity of sperm and of the sperm's interaction with an egg. New data forced doctors and scientists to rethink the fertilization process. At the same time, the growth of assisted reproduction opened new possibilities for overcoming male infertility through the use of various in vitro techniques. "Assisted fertilization" became a substep of assisted reproduction and the focus for a cascade of new fertility interventions. News reports began announcing triumphs with new treatments for male infertility.

Certainly, newfound medical interest in male fertility holds potential for expanded biological understanding and effective treatments for some conditions. If the history of fertility medicine is any guide, however, patients will need to avoid an equal potential for widespread unscientific experimentation with and dissemination of medical procedures claimed to solve the male fertility problem. Particularly during these initial years, during the first flush of professional enthusiasm over changing concepts of male fertility, doctors and patients may be all too eager to attach some kind of treatment to the reformulated diagnosis.

Enthusiasm needs to be tempered by the recognition that the diagnosis itself brings the first frustration. Physicians have few reliable methods for answering the most basic question of whether a man is fertile. Even watching a man's sperm perform with his partner's egg in a laboratory dish does not always answer this question; a failed in vitro fertilization one month may be followed by conception—in vitro or in vivo—the next. At the same time couples could read front-page newspaper articles lauding rapid development of high-tech treatments, they were almost certainly not reading a 1994 review article in *Lancet* stating that "the truth is [that male] diagnoses in most cases cover up our ignorance."[44]

Furthermore, proponents are pushing costly and invasive interventions despite major gaps in knowledge about the problem treated or the impact of these new treatments. The mainstay fertility test for a man uses a microscope to observe the number, shape, and movement of sperm in a semen sample. A low sperm count or immobile or "sluggish" sperm have portended bleak prospects for pregnancy, as did some other semen characteristics (e.g., presence of white blood cells). However, men with poor results on standard semen analysis can have normal fertility; men whose semen test appears normal can have sperm disorders that severely impair fertility. According to one overview of fertility treatments, this basic, ubiquitous diagnostic tool "is at best only a weak predictor of fertility."[45]

During the 1980s, specialists tried to develop a test of sperms' ability to fertilize an egg. Though now widely used, recent studies suggest this popular fertility test (the sperm penetration assay, or "hamster egg test," measuring how successfully a man's sperm penetrate this animal's egg) does not accurately discriminate fertile from infertile men.[46] Naturally conceived pregnancies occur for men whose sperm failed dismally with the hamster's egg in this laboratory test.

Reliance on the common diagnostic tests means that couples spend time, money, and emotional resources gaining unreliable information about their chances for a pregnancy. Test results "inform" their decisions about whether to undergo fertility treatment and the type of intervention to consider. And because the tests do not accurately identify men who are or are not fertile, ineffective treatments may be given credit for subsequent pregnancies, reinforcing use of the treatments for more and more couples. In reality, the discouraging status of diagnosis for male infertility is matched by a discouraging treatment picture.[47] No therapy for men—including surgery, hormonal medications such as clomiphene, or steroid medications—has effectively restored fertility when sperm disorders are accurately identified. Nor has intrauterine insemination or standard IVF overcome fertility problems in men.

No therapy can be adequately evaluated, because the definition and diagnosis of male infertility are so questionable in the first place. Conditions once thought to impair fertility probably do not (e.g., asymptomatic varicocele, a testicular vein varicosity), and some (certain types of white blood cells found in semen) may actually play a fertility-enhancing role.[48] The in vitro spotlight on male contributions to infertility displayed vividly how mysterious sperm and the fertilization process remains. Male infertility became all the more enigmatic as the heterogeneous nature of sperm disorders became evident. Ironically, how little is known about male fertility is revealed most dramatically through experimental interventions that are particularly troubling because they are performed with such little biological knowledge. The approach presently attracting excitement among fertility specialists is *micromanipulation*.

Although the couple asking a doctor for help might never put it this way, they may be asking a brand-new question if the diagnosis is male infertility: Can you help our sperm get into our egg? In this post-IVF era, micromanipulations (procedures requiring use of a microscope) of egg and sperm are experimental treatments that attempt to do just that. Driven by the observation that some sperm— including some with no apparent defect—just cannot fertilize their partner's eggs, fertility specialists have been trying to assist this process more directly. One approach uses chemical and/or mechanical procedures to thin or cut through the zona pellucida surrounding the ovulated egg. This approximately 4-micromillimeter-thick corona-like barrier must be traversed by sperm before entering the egg cell itself. The hope was that sperm that for some reason cannot otherwise navigate successfully could follow the laboratory-created path of least resistance and that one would penetrate the egg for fertilization. Greater assistance takes the form of injecting sperm under the zona pellucida (called subzonal or underzonal insemination). The microscopic manipulation that currently has the most potential for achieving fertilization, especially with severe male problems, injects a single sperm past all barriers into an egg (called intracytoplasmic sperm injection, or ICSI). Held at the tip of a needle, the sperm is "introduced as atraumatically as possible into the egg" with the hope it will remain lodged inside the egg after the needle is withdrawn.[49] As this country's most experienced ICSI practitioner bragged, "The presence of just a few, weakly twitching spermatozoa in the semen is all that is required" of men with extremely low sperm counts.[50] Indeed, by the mid-1990s, the injected sperm need not even come from an ejaculated semen sample or have completed its maturation process. For men with no sperm in the semen (azoospermia) due to an obstruction, the mere head of an immature sperm could be withdrawn from the epididymis or from testicular tissue. And specialists were beginning to "tackle the problem" of infertility caused by "maturational arrest"[51]—a failure of sperm to develop fully, often traced to a defect on the Y chromosome. Specialists predict that someday assisted reproduction will require only the man's genetic material, which could be taken, for example, from blood cells.

Medical reports during these early years of micromanipulation leave no doubt that physicians and their patients are forging ahead into uncharted territory.[52] The fertilization process remains a black box, medical intervention a stab into its darkness. No matter how far from understanding, however, treatment proceeds. According to a 1992 summary of assisted reproduction, the few existing comparisons between micromanipulation and standard in vitro procedures suggested that, for most people, there is "little or no benefit [from] extreme attempts to facilitate entry or inject spermatozoa through the zona pellucida."[53] This summary concluded that such attempts should "be focused on only the most severe cases" and that varying micromanipulation techniques should perhaps be applied to differing sperm disorders. Unfortunately, this conclusion immediately raises two problems. First, it brings us right back to the unknowns in defining and diagnosing male infertility of varying types and severity. And second, even if these technologies do prove, through scientifically controlled trials, to benefit certain severe types of male infertility, prospects for limiting their use to these certain conditions would not seem good. Judging from past experience, the more likely outcome is blanket application to diverse but poorly understood fertility problems, followed by unsubstantiated claims of success.

In 1994 the American Society for Reproductive Medicine issued revised ethical guidelines for use of ICSI and similar new technologies. The aims of the guidelines are "to prevent the exploitation of procedures" for personal gain or of procedures that pose significant risk to patients and to offset confusion and distortion produced by intense media coverage. The society's ethics committee stated these major reservations about micromanipulation: low probability of success; possible damage to gametes, which may result in abnormal offspring; and potential for exploitation and abuse because results are difficult to measure.[54]

International alarms also sounded. In 1995 French medical ethicists investigating the impact of ICSI on assisted reproduction wrote to Lancet: "The potential risks related to the implementation of ICSI should not be neglected—the genetic risk, the risk linked to abnormalities associated with male infertility, the risk of penetration of the oocyte, and the risk of introducing foreign material. Many are concerned about the uncertainty surrounding the fate of children born by means of this technique. . . . Injection [of immature sperm] has made this uncertainty even greater. A review of published work shows that ICSI constitutes human experimentation not preceded by adequate work in animals . . . done without any ethics committee approval of research, as provided for by [French law] . . . and its implementation has not been accompanied by any national evaluation protocol to follow the biological risks and societal effects, nor by any epidemiological surveys."[55] Similarly, Italian specialists warned that "application of [ICSI] is burgeoning and we think that this progression has been premature: there is an absence of experimental and clinical evidence for the safety of this technique." Of particular concern is "the risk of fertilisation by abnormal sperm."[56] Swedish physicians, reporting on another use of ICSI (re-inseminating an egg as a last-ditch effort *after* a standard in vitro fertilization failure), concluded that "considering both the extra work involved and the potential genetic risk, it is doubtful whether [this use of] ICSI should be recommended as a routine procedure."[57] They also noted that attaining pregnancy during a subsequent IVF cycle did not always require ICSI.

If micromanipulation of egg and sperm has aroused some skepticism, this emerging technology—like previous innovations in fertility medicine—also has strong advocates. In the 1990s, a new vocabulary proliferates in reports on male infertility: zonal drilling, partial zonal dissection, subzonal insertion, microinsemination, microsurgical epididymal sperm aspiration (MESA), testicular sperm extraction (TESE), direct egg injection, re-insemination, assisted hatching. The reports are mixed—some claim improved fertilization, others do not. Most of the experimental treatments lack scientific controls. Once again, interventions are becoming "established" so rapidly and unsystematically that there will be no way to determine what benefits exist and for whom.

Early results after use of ICSI are leading advocates to claim success rates for infertile men that are comparable to standard IVF in couples with no male fertility problems; early reports claim no increase in birth defects or chromosome abnormalities as well. [58] An American group reporting on ICSI pregnancies—after cautioning that this advanced procedure should be limited to cases of severe male infertility—also expresses "hope" that understanding the relevance of sperm disorders to fertility will follow the clinical success already being claimed for this reproductive intervention.[59] And, in a generally enthusiastic overview of ICSI in 1996, specialists from one of this country's largest fertility clinics acknowledge that "further investigation must address several major concerns: (1) oocyte damage; (2) the arbitrary selection of gametes; (3) the genetic integrity of the embryo; and (4) ensuing healthy live birth." They conclude, however, that success with the "one egg–one sperm" approach to treating severe male infertility "suggests that in the future ICSI may enjoy wider application in all IVF related treatments."[60]

Other specialists are less sanguine about the early results; regarding offspring, in particular, one group notes that "normal appearance does not preclude infants' carrying significant genetic defects that may not be clinically apparent until adulthood." [61] Indiscriminate and widespread use of ICSI—especially without improved diagnostic abilities—is eliminating the opportunity for properly designed studies to determine which men need this extreme assistance to attain fertilization and to document the long-term outcomes for offspring. Also neglected will be research into causes of male infertility and development of treatments aimed more directly at restoring male fertility and of strategies to prevent at least some of these problems in the first place. [62]

What is certain is that neither patients nor doctors can ignore this technology. They can, however, be wary. They can be wary first of testimonials, based on personal observations and vague descriptions, that substitute for rigorous evidence. For example, a 1993 report echoes refrains heard time and time again about fertility treatments, phrases that did not bode well for patients in the past: doctors' impressions and patients' hopes are disturbingly prominent, hard data and potential risks barely evident. The published article opens with mention of unknowns as basic as identifying "which spermatozoa are capable of fertilization on a consistent basis." Then—turning from these unknowns with a quick "be that as it may"—the authors launch into a description of their clinic's experience treating seventy-three couples by subzonal insemination and/or direct injection of sperm into an egg. Acknowledging that "these approaches may seem unwarranted" and that "we can be accused of being overzealous in our reporting of these procedures," the authors assert that "for many couples these techniques are their only hope for successful fertilization." With hope raised, however, reliance on the practitioners' clinical observations and impressions, rather than on any scientific evaluation, becomes evident. "Because of the conflicts of clinical and scientific interests [i.e., deciding on treatment for individual patients rather than randomly assigning patients in clinical trials], well-controlled comparisons with conventional insemination techniques are not feasible." They do conclude, however, that micromanipulation has been "of great value to many of the couples reported here."[63]

By the final paragraph, this nebulous claim of great value for many patients takes on additional troubling dimensions. Not only do the authors dismiss potential risks, but they encourage dissemination of these untested (and in their view untestable) technologies. Although not simple, the procedures "are well within the grasp" of most IVF laboratories—the necessary equipment is not prohibitively expensive or exotic; personnel can be easily trained. Although the "lax and lack" of knowing which sperm to select for injection might result in too many genetic disorders in the offspring, counseling and prenatal screening will be the answer for many couples who see these assisted fertilization techniques as "their only chance for pregnancy using their own gametes."[64] These clinicians are in effect telling their colleagues, "We think these treatments work, at least for some, but they cannot be scientifically evaluated. Sure there are unknowns and there may be adverse outcomes . . . but you can do it too."

No doubt they will, and no doubt there will be some pregnancies that would not have otherwise occurred. Fertility specialists are learning as they are doing. Whether investigators report positive results with assisted fertilization or no improvement, they agree that results do not correlate with traditional semen analyses and sperm tests; therefore, doctors cannot identify which couples do require this extra, and extra costly, procedure in order to use the man's sperm for IVF. Long-held notions about sperm, the fertilization process, and the diagnosis of male infertility are crumbling. One specialist noted the "dogma" refuted by the initial Belgian study reporting high rates of fertilization and embryo implantation after directly injecting single sperm into single eggs. Existing wisdom might have predicted the technique could not work—that sperm must undergo various physiological changes in the woman's reproductive tract before fertilization is possible, and that semen characteristics influence the fertilization process. Though impressed by these revelations, this commentator does convey some ambivalence, sardonically predicting another likely outcome of this study: "Members of assisted reproductive technology groups from around the world will be flocking to Brussels to learn this technique as if it were Lourdes."[65]

In fact, a pilgrimage of doctors to Brussels—and of patients seeking treatment—was already under way. As the decade progressed, more and more fertility clinics added ICSI to their treatment repertoire. With preliminary studies showing greater fertilization success than did the earlier attempts to assist sperm entry into an egg, ICSI has become the only micromanipulation specialists recommend. Ironically, ICSI's great popularity may actually turn male infertility into another "so what?" diagnosis; development of less invasive therapies for male infertility may be thwarted. Fertility specialists do not know why fertilization fails either in vivo or in vitro. In some IVF cycles, a problem with the ovarian stimulation or other unknown transient factors may adversely affect the egg-sperm interaction. Yet, although a failed in vitro fertilization is sometimes followed by success during the next cycle, many clinics now proceed to ICSI after fertilization failure. And others are jumping to ICSI even sooner, directing all couples straight to IVF with ICSI. [66]

Better understanding of sperm maturation and the interaction of egg and sperm could lead to new targeted treatments, such as hormonal or other types of medications for men that improve sperms' ability to fertilize an egg (though researchers seem to experiment more gingerly with hormones for men than for women). Men would avoid treatments that cannot improve their fertility— e.g., surgery to remove varicoceles—and women would avoid undergoing IVF with or without ICSI.[67]

Considerable doubt must therefore surround the potential benefit of current directions for overcoming male infertility. The search for treatments to match this diagnosis illustrates particularly well—almost in caricature—four significant issues of fertility medicine more generally, issues demanding additional wariness.

First, treatments presently generating the greatest interest among fertility specialists are all linked with IVF and superovulation of a man's partner. Infertility may no longer be attributed primarily to women, but women bear the burden of treatment, even for male fertility problems. These treatments are presented to subfertile couples as the choices they have, and many women agree to try. Early efforts with ICSI already place responsibility for treatment success upon the woman: proponents define the major determinant of ICSI success in terms of egg quantity and quality.[68] That is, by injecting a sperm in an egg, previously abysmal success rates for treatment of severe male infertility can be brought up to rates for IVF with a fertile male—*if* a woman is willing to undergo superovulation and embryo transfer and if she does not have "defective eggs" (due primarily to age) or is willing to use donated eggs. No other proven option exists, except artificial insemination with donor sperm—in fact, a more successful procedure that is much simpler and safer for the woman.

Second, early medical reports place more emphasis on how micromanipulation is done—and the relative ease of learning the techniques—than on determining when such extreme interventions are necessary for conceiving a pregnancy. In the absence of knowing how to predict which couples need ICSI in order to achieve fertilization, women again end up bearing the burden of diagnosis. IVF has become the ultimate diagnostic determinant of male fertility—by observing in a laboratory dish the sperms' ability to fertilize an egg—a diagnostic method that already involves superovulation and egg retrieval. Although several studies suggest couples can conceive on a next try following an in vitro fertilization failure, that failure becomes the reason for escalating to ICSI.[69]

Third, as with assisted reproduction for other conditions, treatment to bypass male infertility brings crucial questions about "success." Achieving "successful fertilization," or even embryo implantation, following gamete micromanipulation is not equivalent to achieving a successful pregnancy. Once again, a healthy "take home baby" who would not have otherwise been born is the outcome of ultimate concern. Valid claims of success require evidence that the intervention was responsible for the birth. Without better understanding of male fertility, and scrupulous attention to the type and severity of a couple's subfertility, patients offered sophisticated and expensive micromanipulation might do just as well with standard IVF; patients offered IVF might conceive on their own.[70]

Finally, if of less immediate impact on today's patients, is a broader dimension characterizing male fertility treatments—a dimension that in the long run affects many more women and men than those presently seeking reproductive assistance. Medical attention, resources, and technology now focus on individual sperm. From a specialty that usually deals with sperm by the millions, a sophisticated therapeutic arsenal aims at guiding a single sperm into a single egg. This approach is consistent with the emphasis of American medicine. While scientists have learned that male fertility can be significantly lowered by such environmental factors as chemical exposures (occupational and environmental), cigarette smoking, heavy alcohol consumption, and recreational and therapeutic drug use, resources allocated to *preventing* sperm disorders are pitifully meager. While researchers investigate a decline in sperm counts internationally, perhaps caused by man-made chemicals in the environment, the medical emphasis in this country remains a highly technological and invasive fix that may benefit only a few, after the widespread damage to men's fertility is done.

Immunologic Infertility

Early claims [about immunology and infertility] were magnified because of unreliable assays and naïveté concerning the complexities of the immune response. . . . The dearth of well-designed and controlled experimental studies and the lack of effective therapy resulted in confusion [over immune processes] in human infertility.   NAZ AND MENGE 1994, 1001

By the mid-1990s, some fertility specialists could recognize and acknowledge earlier "naïveté" about ways the immune system might contribute to infertility. How any pregnancy manages to succeed has long been an intriguing scientific question. After all, a woman's immune system normally attacks "foreign" cells or tissue—whether a viral or bacterial invader, or a transplanted organ. That an embryo can implant and grow without provoking a similar rejection is something of a mystery. Equally mysterious are reasons the normal reproductive process sometimes falters—yet it certainly makes biological sense that an immune response may be implicated. For any woman, sperm or embryos are different from her own body tissue. What if a woman's immune system reacts against them? Some breakdown of a special immunologic relationship that normally prevents this reaction may be the reason for a portion of unexplained infertility and of the agonizing cases in which women, for unknown reasons, suffer repeated early miscarriages.

Today, as in past years, patients receive treatments, the dearth of scientifically controlled studies and lack of effective therapy notwithstanding. Many couples with unexplained fertility problems visit the doctor innumerable times, devouring months, then years, with all manner of diagnostic tests and treatment attempts. They may be more likely than other fertility patients to try new therapies—anything that might, for whatever reason, remedy their mysterious condition. But today's patients need to ask whether new diagnostic tests can accurately determine if an irregular immune response is lowering their fertility. Are therapies the doctor is now recommending likely to overcome this problem, increasing chances for having a healthy baby? Or, in years to come, will today's immunologic information look naive, the interventions prescribed unjustified?

To assess the current moment, it helps to understand how diverse medical developments reinvigorated both clinicians' excitement about the diagnosis of immunologic infertility and their experiments with treatments—for patients are susceptible to both enthusiasms. Although relatively few couples are directly affected and although the following discussion of this complex, rapidly changing field must be limited to basic concepts, this diagnosis provides an illustration of the general need for caution in order to avoid premature, potentially harmful reproductive interventions.

As with increased attention to male fertility problems, development of IVF also spurred interest in the broad phenomenon called immunologic infertility. These technologies divided the reproductive process into discrete, observable steps, with each step holding the potential, at least in theory, for an immunologic stumble that might thwart pregnancy. If male fertility was considered enigmatic, male and female entwined—a couple's immunologic fit in vitro or vivo—appeared all the more so.

A faulty immune response may impede the earliest steps in which sperm travel through a woman's vagina and uterus to reach and penetrate an egg. If an egg is fertilized, an embryo's initial growth may also require certain immunologic responses, although the physiology of such a process is not yet understood. The next steps seem to be of critical importance. The embryo must establish itself in the uterine lining—as a "transplant" of sorts—accepted and nourished there throughout the months of fetal development until birth. As IVF practitioners and their patients learned all too well, even following a "successful" in vitro fertilization and transfer of embryos, some women consistently miscarry. With known causes (e.g., chromosomal anomalies, uterine structure defects) ruled out, immunologic "rejection" of the fetus became a prime if inscrutable suspect.

Assisted reproduction was not the only medical development fueling interest in the immune system's impact on fertility. In the 1980s two complementary explosions in knowledge and biotechnology reverberated throughout the medical world. First was the AIDS epidemic, which focused scientific and medical resources on the immune system, trying to delineate how it works and how it breaks down. In the wake of AIDS came new research and diagnostic tools aimed at unraveling immunologic mysteries. At the same time, study of human genes—particularly as culprits held responsible for specific health problems—yielded additional research techniques. Soon these new techniques were filtering into diverse medical specialties, including fertility medicine, allowing specialists to observe and measure previously hidden facets of the immune system as it participates in conception and pregnancy.

Numerous laboratory tests now generate numerous measures of various immune system activities. Measurements of differing types of antibodies (protein molecules the body produces to fight organisms or tissue not recognized as one's own) circulating in a woman's bloodstream may reflect an immune response to sperm, embryo, or fetus. DNA analyses can identify genetic characteristics that might influence a couple's fertility. Translation into safe and effective reproductive treatments, however, is not a foregone conclusion. Certainly, any such progression will not be quick or easy. As medical reports accumulate, their more immediate results translate into problematic choices for patients whose doctor suggests a diagnosis of immunologic infertility.

A first problem is the variable quality of laboratories now jumping into the lucrative business of immunologic testing and the still early stage in the development of the tests themselves. For the couple seeking a doctor's help, diagnosis relies on a series of assays run on samples of their blood. However, different laboratories come up with differing measurements on the same blood test; out of the many labs to which doctors send blood samples, few have a reliable track record for measuring the immune activities in question.[71] Laboratories define results as normal or abnormal differently, according to their own arbitrary cutoff points. To appreciate how difficult the technical issues involved in newly evolving immunologic tests are, remember that quality control has been a serious and ongoing problem with the long-established, standard Pap test for cervical cancer. Yet laboratories promote their services to doctors—for example, through journal advertisements—despite significant technical problems, not to mention vast unknowns regarding what these tests might reflect about fertility. Some advertisements suggest conditions for which antibody testing has been "recommended" although these recommendations are a focus of medical dispute (see Figure 3).

This lack of knowledge about the immune system's role in fertility is an even more basic concern. Tests now exist, but tests—even accurate, reliable ones—must be interpreted. With tools already in hand and continuing to develop, specialists are now debating just what the tests are measuring, what the numbers mean, what relevance the measures have to a couple's likelihood of pregnancy. Confusion surrounds the origin and function of particular antibodies circulating in a woman's bloodstream and, most important, whether they affect her chances for pregnancy. Little is known about the normal distribution of these antibodies in women who do not have problems with conception or early pregnancy loss. Nor has research determined whether such antibodies are a cause of infertility or a result. Elevated levels could be physiological residue of

LEADERSHIP IN AUTOANTIBODY TESTING

If your patients require autoantibody evaluations, consider **CHR Laboratories.** We not only provide the most comprehensive autoantibody profile for the evaluation of autoantibody-associated reproductive failure, but we also offer (if you so desire) a clinical interpretation of laboratory results with treatment recommendations by our clinicians. Our clinical staff is available for telephone consultations and, best of all, these clinical consulting services are provided as a courtesy. You just have to ask!

AUTOANTIBODY SCREENS*

Anticardiolipin Antibody. IgG, IgM and IgA isotypes

Phospholipid Antibody Screen. IgG, IgM and IgA isotypes of 6 antiphospholipid antibodies, inclusive of anticardiolipin

Histone Antibody Screen. IgG, IgM and IgA isotypes of 5 antihistone and histone subfractions

Polynucleotide Antibody Screen. IgG, IgM, and IgA isotypes of 4 antipolynucleotides

Complete Nonorganspecific Autoantibody Screen. Inclusive of phospholipid, histone, and polynucleotide antibody screens

Thyroid Antibody Screen. Inclusive of antithyroglobulin and antimicrosomal antibodies

Figure 3. One laboratory's ad seen regularly in ob-gyn journals, seeking physician customers for diagnostic tests that remain controversial. A list of conditions for which these tests have been "recommended" appears in fine print at the bottom of the ad (not shown here), including unexplained infertility, endometriosis, and IVF prescreening—all hotly disputed recommendations.

the earliest stages of a previous pregnancy—including unrecognized conceptions—or of the miscarriage process itself.[72]

Two Laboratories, Two Doctors, One Baby

In November 1995 a couple arrives at the office of Dr. A, a fertility specialist. He takes the woman's medical history (which includes a normal pregnancy and birth less than two years before) and orders a large battery of laboratory tests. All results are negative (i.e., normal), except for "strongly positive" anti-phospholipid antibodies. Dr. A's interpretation and recommendation: an autoimmune problem is probably contributing to the couple's fertility problem, requiring immunotherapy—heparin and aspirin (both of which act as blood thinners, said to counteract adverse effects of these antibodies on implantation, circulation, and the developing placenta), and intravenous immunoglobulin (IVIG). With such intensive and expensive treatment for the underlying immunologic problem, the couple should probably undergo IVF now as well. It is a more successful procedure than intrauterine insemination with hMG; and doing as much as possible in one treatment cycle may avoid the need to repeat immunotherapy later if the insemination fails and they then chose to try IVF.

Unsure about following this recommendation, the woman consults two months later with Dr. B, another physician in the community. He sends a blood sample to a different laboratory, specialists in the relationship between anti-phospholipid antibodies and pregnancy loss. That laboratory's results show all autoimmune antibody tests "convincingly negative." By this time, moreover, it is clear that the woman does not have a fertility problem: she is eight weeks into a naturally conceived pregnancy.

In September 1996, she delivers a healthy 10-pound baby, a sister for the couple's now 2½-year-old son. Comments Dr. B, "It is my contention that this testing should never have been performed, much less interpreted as a rational reason why the patient was not conceiving"—and even less as a reason to undergo any treatment, let alone such intensive, potentially harmful, and expensive ones.

The lag in knowledge leads easily to overdiagnosis and overtreatment of patients as the new techniques gain popularity among doctors. Since test results themselves may not be reliable, the diagnosis given to patients by their doctor may not be accurate. The sheer number of diagnostic tests now available raises the likelihood of some abnormal result. The more tests run, the more chance of an inaccurate positive finding (a "false positive"). Or a measurement will fall outside the range a particular laboratory defines as normal yet not, in fact, affect the couple's fertility. One outcome of diagnosing and treating an immunologic fertility problem without adequate knowledge is that the intervention will be futile, a waste of time, energy, resources. Even if a couple does have some type of immunologic problem, treatment may be ineffective because it targets poorly understood immune processes.[73]

Futility might seem a minor concern, however, compared to the very real potential for harm. Beyond the risk any medical procedure brings are additional risks from tinkering with a physiological system that is central to the overall health of a woman and her desired offspring. Troubling questions arise, first, about assisted reproductive technologies now frequently recommended for women diagnosed with either immunologic or unexplained infertility who do indeed have some mild, perhaps symptomless immune system irregularity. Procedures such as IVF or intrauterine insemination following superovulation expose women to unusual concentrations of sperm and/or early embryos; these exposures could aggravate conditions involving abnormal immune reactions. No one knows the immune response to repeated hormonal superovulation or punctures of the ovary during egg retrieval. In addition to jeopardizing a woman's health, such intervention may jeopardize her best chance for pregnancy—conceiving spontaneously, though it may take her a longer than average time. Each treatment attempt brings a high likelihood of miscarriage and may further exacerbate the problems she is experiencing.

More direct immunotherapies attempt to alter responses between maternal, paternal, and fetal components of an intricate, but poorly understood, immunogenetic relationship. One prominent treatment is based on the idea that the woman's immune system is not adequately mounting the response that normally protects an embryo from immunologic rejection. According to this theory, the problem may be that the woman and her partner are too similar in some genetically crucial way, a "compatibility" reflected in the combined genetics of an early embryo. To stimulate the needed protective response, the woman is injected with white blood cells (leukocytes or lymphocytes) drawn from her partner. If this "paternal lymphocyte immunization" fails to provoke an adequate response, white blood cells are added from a less genetically compatible donor. Immunization begins before attempts to conceive and—depending on periodic test results—may continue at intervals throughout the first two trimesters of pregnancy.

Genetic Match

Genetic tests can determine the degree to which male and female partners share genetic patterns that may affect immune responses to pregnancy. Patients may then receive treatments to alter immune responses said to result from too great a genetic similarity. However, the danger of intervening without adequate biological knowledge is clear. Specialists are still debating the very premise underlying the treatments: Does genetic "sharing" apparent in immunogenetic tests actually reflect a treatable immunologic problem? Proponents of immunotherapy contend that if the match between certain of the partners' genes is too close, the woman's immune response will not "accept" a pregnancy. Treatment aims at neutralizing the destructive immune response caused by an excess of genetic "compatibility." Recent studies of genes and reproduction, however, suggest a different explanation of the pregnancy failures. The "shared" genes that have been identified may be flags or "markers" of a subtle genetic defect that undermines successful conception and/or fetal development. The responsible genes are close (linked) to these observable markers, but have not yet been identified. It is not the degree of sharing—with a resultant immunologic rejection—that causes infertility or repetitive miscarriage. Rather the problem is the particular combination of genetic contribution from the woman and man—a combination of recessive lethal genes or of deleted genes that are crucial for normal fetal growth and development. The result of this genetic defect is not a baby born with an abnormality, but a pregnancy failure, often at a very early stage. Since the failure does not stem from an immune response, immunotherapy will not help this couple; they may have a successful pregnancy, given chance genetic combinations, after several untreated attempts.[1] Greater understanding of why some women suffer repeated early miscarriage is the key to decisions couples must make about treatment. If the reason is immunological, therapy that modifies the immune system may be effective. But if the explanation is a genetically abnormal embryo, argues one specialist, "counseling would be the most appropriate choice of treatment at this stage of our knowledge, and active therapies that may not be specifically effective could be avoided."[2]

The next several years will undoubtedly bring increased attention to the genetic factors in both normal and abnormal reproductive processes. Already fertility patients are more frequently offered chromosome analyses, not only in cases of repeated miscarriage but also in conjunction with ICSI for male infertility. How to apply test results to current treatment decisions—particularly regarding genetic findings that are not yet well understood—will be perplexing for doctors and patients alike. For example, genetic testing at one ICSI program revealed a surprising number of chromosome abnormalities in women of couples being treated for infertility in the men.[3]

---

1. Plouffe et al. 1992.
2. Gill 1992, 1. See also Coulam, Stern, and Bustillo 1994; Cowchock, and Smith 1992.
3. Mau et al. 1997.

A different treatment gaining attention in recent years is based on different test results, and attempts to subdue a different immunologic process—an *excessive,* "autoimmune" attack in response to a developing embryo. The woman receives a cocktail of aspirin, other blood-thinning and, perhaps, steroid medications to dampen her immunologic response and ameliorate its damaging physiological consequences. Some specialists start this treatment before conception, while others begin treatment when pregnancy is confirmed. Another therapy of unproven efficacy and safety attempts to supply a woman directly with immune system proteins that might improve her response by infusing immunoglobulins at regular intervals during pregnancy (for example, every three weeks until the final month): each unit of blood products required for this process (intravenous gamma or immunoglobulin therapy, IVIG) is pooled from approximately eighty anonymous donors.

Although these specific interventions vary, each brings its own dangers. In many instances, not only the woman but, if she does conceive, a developing fetus will be exposed to treatment. Certain risks are well documented and can be life-threatening to the pregnant woman—for example, bleeding problems and bone demineralization from blood-thinning medications (e.g., heparin, aspirin); viral contamination from intravenous immunoglobulin; ulcers, diabetes, and bone demineralization from corticosteroids (as well as the possibility of fetal abnormalities). Questions also loom about any manipulation of an individual's immune response. No one knows whether immunization with a different person's lymphocytes, for example, may have long-term consequences for the woman or an exposed fetus. As with other fertility treatments, most patients considering immunotherapy are women whose present good health could be compromised. A subgroup of women may have a mild or latent irregularity that these procedures could aggravate—a condition that may or may not be lowering their fertility. Even if it is, preliminary data indicate that, at best, present immunotherapies might improve chances of successful pregnancy for a very small proportion of these women. With no reliable tests to identify which couples are likely to be helped, many more women than can actually benefit will be taking on the risks of treatment.[74]

In addition, explanations of immunologic infertility are noticeably fluid. Factors once described as significant in lowering fertility—for example, anti-sperm antibodies or genetic "sharing"—do not appear to be as important when investigated more thoroughly.[75] At this still early stage in understanding the diagnosis called immunologic infertility, specialists are saying, in very loose translation, that there does seem to be something going on here, at least for a small percentage of couples, but we can't yet grasp what that something is or identify who those couples are. Yet the immunologic diagnosis continues to expand, now reaching back to explain the failure of fertilization or implantation, as well as repeated miscarriage, during the first or second trimester. In earlier years doctors typically recommended immunologic approaches only after a woman's third miscarriage; the wait has now been chiseled to two losses, or one, or none (sometimes called "subclinical" autoimmunity, a diagnosis based on test results alone). Obviously, no one wants the experience of miscarriage to be a diagnostic requirement before receiving treatment, if that treatment is beneficial. However, the immunologic tests, themselves controversial, now bear a greater diagnostic burden. Not only is the chance for misdiagnosis enlarged, but the relationship of abnormal test results to fertility remains uncertain. Increased reliance on the tests means that yet again more and more women end up receiving unnecessary, unproven, and risky treatments.

In years to come, research will undoubtedly contribute to more sophisticated and accurate explanations. The persistent need for caution about interventions that proceed while knowledge is lacking or in considerable flux is reflected all too well by women who have experienced repetitive early miscarriages (also called recurrent spontaneous abortions). During the 1990s, "IVF failures" joined the diagnostic pool of couples offered treatments for immunologic infertility. Assisted reproductive technologies helped to reveal early miscarriages that can occur before women know they have conceived. However, couples hearing an immunologic explanation for their difficult and perplexing experience of several miscarriages should know that this long-recognized condition has resisted an extensive list of therapeutic efforts. Treatment prospects may sound different to couples who know that longer story, particularly if they also hear today's critics echoing the same cautions expressed in the past. A 1984 letter to *Lancet* warned: "Thirty years ago chaos arose from unscientific use of hormones. The only clear results were the tragic effects of diethylstilboestrol and virilizing progestagens [synthetic forms of progesterone] on surviving offspring. Now with immunological approaches, a new generation may fall into the trap of unnecessary treatment; for, even without specific therapy, women who have had a sequence of unexplained abortions have a good prospect of carrying a child to [term]. Immunological measures may be justified in some cases, but evaluation must be conducted at the highest level of academic stringency."[76] The main difference with today's immunotherapies is the passage of a dozen and more years.[77]

Faced with this history and with the introduction of ever-changing and ever more biologically sophisticated tests and therapies, what perspective can patients maintain on the diagnosis and treatment of immunologic infertility? They can remember, first, that more couples are now labeled with this diagnosis, on the basis of immunologic testing, often when no other cause can be identified. This whittling away of the "unexplained" category during the past ten to fifteen years, however, has not been matched by improved pregnancy rates.[78] Giving infertility an explanation, however valid, does not mean an effective treatment exists. A major problem with claims of immunotherapy success is that even after three consecutive first-trimester miscarriages, a substantial proportion of couples, possibly as high as 70 percent, will go on to have a successful pregnancy without treatment. This comparison becomes all the more important as clinicians shortcut the wait, testing and intervening in couples who may have had at most one early miscarriage (a relatively frequent natural occurrence).

Another complication is the intriguing suggestion that immunotherapies may be particularly susceptible to placebo effects. That is, when the therapies do improve pregnancy outcome, it is some psychoimmunologic boost from the act of intervening itself, not its medical content, that accounts for success. Several studies report similar increases in pregnancy rates with psychotherapy, "tender loving care," use of a placebo (injections or pills that appear the same as the medical therapy but with no active medical substance), or immunotherapy. Just as health and illness, more generally, are affected by mind-body interactions that are not well understood, so too may immunologic aspects of fertility be influenced.[79] Why psychological support might be an effective intervention remains unknown, as does the reason untreated couples follow three miscarriages with a successful pregnancy. Placebo effects are not unreal or "all in a person's mind." Measurable physiological changes do occur, but it is the support, attention, and/or individual's belief in the treatment that stimulate the physiological response. Given the risks attached to immunotherapies, it is imperative to sort out this process.

Using Medical Placebos

A *Lancet* series on the potential usefulness of placebo effects in medical practice notes that these little-understood responses are more pronounced with conditions involving hormonal control. The discussion includes advice to physicians on how to "harness" this therapeutic reaction. Several suggestions seem already incorporated into fertility medicine, intentionally or not:

Perform activities associated with doctor as "controller of events" and with patients' previous experiences of effective remedies—for example, a doctor taking the patient history and performing the medical examination, writing a prescription, using special diagnostic tests.

Express optimism about the final outcome and sympathy about a patient's previous unsuccessful medical care, which will help distance this doctor from bad experiences.

Display signs of being a recognized healer—for example, observable statements of qualifications, experience, and effectiveness.

Enlarge publicity about successes, suppress publicity about complaints (which may undermine patients' faith).

Be sure the patient has no reason to doubt the effectiveness of treatment (either the current therapy or, if necessary, a subsequent one).

Build upon a patient's existing faith by, for instance, allowing her preferences to be a major determinant of treatment choice; however, be careful not to reduce effects of doctors' authority by allowing complete patient choice.[1]

One conclusion drawn from these articles is that specific treatments, such as immunotherapies, may receive credit for successes that actually result from a different, less hazardous dimension of a patient's interaction with a physician. This dynamic can occur not only in daily medical practice but in clinical studies that are not designed to minimize placebo effects. Another conclusion is that harnessing the beneficial placebo effect does not require use of "sugar pills." A consultation during which the doctor gives no treatment can stimulate this patient response. Yet doctors "are not taught that there are a substantial number of patients in whom no firm diagnosis can be made and who require no treatment, other than contact with the doctor. . . . Doctors believe that most patients expect treatment. [One study] showed that whereas 43–52 percent of patients expected to be given a prescription; . . . most doctors thought the figure would be 80 percent or more." Doctors do not appreciate that, in some cases, the placebo effect "will be less harmful and perhaps more beneficial than a complex and incompletely understood drug. . . . A better appreciation of this power would change doctors' attitudes to the consultation and would result in the making of less illness, the prescribing of less medication, and a better understanding by the patient of his or her condition."[2] Unfortunately, although fertility specialists may already harness aspects of the placebo effect, they do so in conjunction with—rather than in place of—unproven and risky medical interventions.

---

1. Chaput de Saintonge and Herxheimer 1994.
2. Thomas 1994, 1067.

The various immunotherapies also require scientifically controlled investigation to determine whether any do improve pregnancy outcomes and, if so, for what conditions. Preliminary results from adequately designed studies, performed at a few research centers, are beginning to piece together evidence that may help define immune responses that significantly impair fertility, as well as develop treatments in which benefits outweigh risks. Couples diagnosed with immunologic infertility should know they join a highly heterogeneous group; although they are offered the same treatments, the risks and benefits of a particular intervention will differ, depending on the specifics of a couple's fertility problem. Presently, medical knowledge about such specifics remains inadequate. The diagnosis encompasses abnormalities of sperm moving through a woman's reproductive tract, failure of fertilization or implantation, miscarriages, intrauterine growth retardation, and stillbirths. Not only do these conditions differ from each other, but each can itself result from a range of immunologic, genetic, endocrine, structural, and/or infectious disorders. Immunological treatment that may be promising and biologically plausible for one group (e.g., women with second-trimester pregnancy loss) cannot necessarily be transposed to another (e.g., IVF failures).[80]

Like other reproductive interventions, immunotherapies can gain a foothold and become widely adopted despite concerns and unknowns. Debate may flare within the profession over the science and its application while clinical practice proceeds on its own steam. Unfortunately, with the diagnosis and treatment of immunologic infertility, clinical excitement and advocacy, verging at times on proselytizing, outpaces demonstrable achievements. Discussion provoked by one published study offers a view of how professional debate over scientific merit coexists with advocacy of a treatment. The study compared two ways of using blood-thinning (heparin) and steroid medications aimed at suppressing a woman's immune response to a fetus: starting medications before the woman attempts to become pregnant or waiting until she has conceived.[81]

The report's authors acknowledge that "what constitutes an autoimmune abnormality in women with recurrent spontaneous abortion is not yet defined or agreed on. . . . How often the abnormalities discussed in this study are seen in normally reproducing women before and during pregnancy is unknown." Some women in their study, who show abnormal test results and experience repeated miscarriages over more than twelve years, have not had detectable autoimmune symptoms or diseases. The authors also acknowledge that, although lymphocyte immunization accompanied the study's experimental treatment of the combined steroid and blood-thinning medications, they do not know, and are only now studying, whether the immunization is helpful. Despite these limitations, they conclude that women who have experienced recurrent spontaneous abortion, with diagnostic tests showing autoimmune abnormalities, should be given both immunosuppressive and blood-thinning medications and that treatment should begin before attempting another pregnancy rather than after pregnancy is confirmed.

Comments by other physicians are included in the publication of this article. In this medical format, where etiquette tends toward complimentary and supportive discussion, the responding specialists are noticeably unenthusiastic. The first commentator notes that the "timely topic" of potential immunologic aspects of recurrent spontaneous abortion "remains a confusing and controversial area clearly in need of well-controlled studies." He clearly does not think the present study meets this need; rather, it "requires cautious interpretation" for several reasons. His criticisms could not be more basic: the diagnosis of autoimmune infertility is questionable, the study design is faulty, and the advocated treatment brings significant risks to the woman.

Regarding diagnosis, the large number of blood tests run on each patient increases the likelihood that at least one test result will be abnormal yet not reflect any condition that affects the individual's fertility. Furthermore, the study's arbitrary cut-off defining normal and abnormal levels of antibodies measured in the blood probably means that many women who could have successful pregnancies without treatment are diagnosed as having immunologic infertility.

A fundamental problem with the design of the study is that women were assigned to treatment subgroups based on consultations with physicians rather than randomly and blindly (i.e., without patients or doctors knowing who was receiving which treatment); these non-controlled conditions cast doubt on comparisons of results between the groups. The study also did not include a no-treatment group, given only placebo. In addition to these flaws, the commentator lists more than a dozen other criticisms of the way the study was conducted, the statistical analyses used, and the conclusions drawn. His own analysis, in fact, suggests the drug combination advocated may actually be less effective than a safer alternative started after conception occurs. Combining corticosteroids (which suppress immune functions) and heparin (a blood thinner) during pregnancy can cause serious complications for the pregnant woman, such as bleeding or a severe bone disorder leading to fractures. "We have recommended against this treatment in the absence of evidence that it is better than [steroids] or heparin alone. . . . The effectiveness and safety of this regimen must be clearly shown before it is widely adopted."

A second commentator echoes the concern with risks, emphasizing that longer treatment increases the rate of complications. Since several other studies show no benefit from starting treatment before conception, he concludes that "this strategy may unnecessarily expose patients to potentially dangerous therapy for longer than is needed." And there are other weaknesses. The specific group of women studied were so-called IVF failures who lost embryos repeatedly, very soon after they were transferred to the uterus (failures that can result from a range of technical and physiological causes);[82] yet the authors' conclusions take a more general form, with no further mention of this limited application.

Limitations similarly go unmentioned when one of the authors of the study speaks, eighteen months after its publication, to an audience mainly of gynecologists as part of a lecture series at a prominent hospital. This clinician-researcher is spreading the word about new techniques for diagnosing and treating immunologic infertility, as well as about his (and his laboratory's) availability for patient referrals. He displays charts and graphs tallying his patients. This presentation has none of the striking sense of criticism so apparent in the journal publication. Definitive statements—for example, "autoimmune therapy started after the pregnancy is established is far less effective than started pre-conception"—sound impressive. He does not discuss the controversy and confusion characterizing this area of fertility medicine. He does not mention risks, beyond a brief response to one question from the audience about the transient side effects of the treatment. His only allusion to critics of his work is a quotation he reads in closing: "Innovators are rarely received with joy and established authorities launch into condemnation of newer truths, for at every crossroads to the future are a thousand self-appointed guardians of the past."

Breaking Old Patterns and New Ground

The woman and man sitting together in the doctor's waiting room, their doctors, and the public at large face dazzling new developments in fertility medicine which, on closer look, repeat the long-standing patterns outlined in this chapter. However, a noticeable alteration characterizes the 1990s. Amid the usual, mostly "promising" medical reports, are fertility specialists calling more frequently than in years past for research to assess diagnostic and treatment procedures, old and new. The undeniable motivation is a nationwide concern with cost and the increasing threat that health insurance plans will simply not pay for procedures not proven effective. As one gynecologist states: "The first time [third-party insurance payers] say they will not pay for surgical procedures before the development of evidence of efficacy, we will begin to get the studies very quickly."[83]

With regard to assisted reproductive technologies, one mid-decade report puts it this way: "As the national interest in controlling health care costs grows, the need for objective evaluation of expensive therapies becomes more imperative. This is applicable particularly to [in vitro fertilization]. As more insurance companies consider limiting the number of IVF cycles covered under policies and consider imposing a lifetime limit on infertility treatment, it becomes critical that both the patient and physician have some objective means for evaluating the success of continuing a specific treatment for each patient."[84] Fertility specialists have begun to emphasize that all couples do not have a common prognosis—that, for example, some proportion of couples undergoing assisted reproduction will never end up with a healthy baby and that the specialty would do well to try identifying who these individuals are.

Knowing what questions physicians consider to be neglected and in need of systematic study can help patients think about their own treatment decisions. Among the most prominent questions posed by fertility specialists themselves:

What subgroups of patients—e.g., by age and/or type of fertility problems—can benefit from which fertility interventions? Who is likely to succeed with minimal intervention?

What subgroups of patients are unlikely to be treated successfully?

What diagnostic tests can reliably help to predict a couple's chances for spontaneous pregnancy? For success with a particular treatment?

What are the risks of treatment, and what subgroups are at high risk of complications?

How much will patients gain from treatment compared to no medical treatment or a less invasive and costly procedure? For example, does treatment greatly increase their chances of having a healthy baby or does it only shorten the time before a pregnancy that would occur anyway?

How can medical interventions be tailored to create an optimal balance of benefits and risks for individual patients?

How many attempts at particular treatments should subgroups of patients, with varying fertility problems, undergo? At what point do chances of success diminish beyond reasonable bounds?

The message about research needed to answer even these basic questions, however, is oddly mixed. On the one hand there is greater acknowledgment that much of fertility medicine is unproven and greater willingness to argue the need for scientifically controlled trials, to caution colleagues about uncritically applying medical techniques in the absence of demonstrated efficacy and safety. On the other hand the very same critiques frequently go on to suggest instances in which the very same techniques can be tried "empirically"—as if the immovable object (unproven, inappropriate procedures) must inevitably meet the irresistible force (pressure to "do something").

Fertility patients may help break this stalemate by developing a broader understanding of recommended interventions and the questions that surround them. To summarize issues raised in this chapter, patients should above all not assume "established" procedures are in fact all that well established or that a doctor's recommendation follows well-defined medical logic from diagnosis to treatment. Considerable disagreement exists among physicians about risks and benefits of procedures and the adequacy of clinical studies. Some members of the medical community fall into "camps" advocating one treatment over another. Physicians also disagree about how aggressively to intervene medically in cases of subfertility, whether to forge ahead with invasive diagnostic procedures and treatments or to take a more conservative approach, given the potential futility and harm.

Additionally, an intervention that may improve chances of pregnancy for a small proportion of subfertile couples is soon used widely on patients who do not need it, often by doctors who are not adequately trained. Many patients end up facing unnecessary risk and expense, and no one can determine the likely benefits or risks for any particular individual. Assisted reproductive technologies have become the first treatment recommended by some fertility specialists for an array of diagnoses, even though less invasive or no treatment may be appropriate, at least initially, for an individual patient.

Fertility treatments do bring the potential for harm that must be weighed carefully against benefits for patients who are essentially healthy, who may have successful pregnancies without treatment, who may not even be among the subgroup a treatment can help. For some older women, the dangers of inappropriate treatment may include passage of time, which lowers their existing fertility.

Finally, scientific knowledge that should be the basis for fertility treatments is often lacking. The tendency has been to intervene now and ask questions later.[85] Indeed, it would be a significant and valuable change in the pattern of fertility medicine to seek first a better understanding of conception and pregnancy—how these processes work smoothly, why they fail, the health consequences of medical manipulations—especially before "trying something new."

This changed pattern would increase knowledge of when and when *not* to inter-vene with fertility treatment. A doctor's oath to "do no harm"—because chances of successful treatment are too small or chances of pregnancy without treatment too great—would become more prominent in defining the ethics of fertility medicine. Increased knowledge could also inform preventive efforts that can help individuals protect their fertility and perhaps avoid medical inter-ventions (see Chapter 5).

Until there is a stronger scientific foundation for reproductive interven-tions, how should individual patients and doctors make decisions today? In ad-dition to current information patients need about their fertility problem and treatment options, what insights from accumulating research might contribute to these decisions? Two facts are important in deciding, first of all, whether a couple needs medical help and if so, how aggressive it should be. These unsur-prising and often intertwined considerations emerge from a broad range of fer-tility studies—the woman's age and the length of time the couple has attempted to conceive. Women's fertility does decline as they approach forty, though how much and how quickly varies greatly from woman to woman. And ultimately the best predictor of a need for medical intervention is the duration of infertil-ity—that is, the longer the problem has lasted, the more likely there truly is a problem. As one report from the Netherlands explained, duration—the length of "trying time"—involves a selection process. Normal fertile couples might take up to two years to conceive; the mildly or moderately subfertile might need a year or two more. Not until after five years would "nearly only severely subfertile couples or infertile couples [be] left," still trying.[86] Of course, by then the women are also five years older, which can itself lower fertility.

Given the overriding importance of these two characteristics, couples who are trying to conceive may need to shift their approach in deciding about med-ical treatment. If they are *not* among the easiest cases, in which a clear-cut ab-normality prevents pregnancy and can be effectively treated, obtaining a specific diagnosis with the limited diagnostic techniques available may not be all that helpful. Beyond the basic fertility tests (for example, to be sure the woman ovulates and has open fallopian tubes, the man has moving sperm), diagnostic findings of relatively mild or questionable abnormalities (e.g., luteal phase defi-ciency, mild endometriosis, "hostile" cervical mucus, elevated antibody levels, or moderately low sperm count) do not predict well whether a couple will ac-tually have a hard time getting and staying pregnant. For couples who have been trying to conceive for a relatively short time (between one and two years), with no identifiable fertility problem, chances are good that there is no problem and that they will conceive on their own, particularly if the woman is not yet approaching forty.

Of all recent developments in fertility medicine, none embraces more fully the complexities of gaining and applying new knowledge, the relentless experimentation on women, the ambivalence of medical progress than the question, "How old is the woman?" The next chapter focuses on this consideration, which may be bringing indelible, qualitative changes in the nature of reproduction for women and men of all ages.

5 Fertility Medicine's Older Woman

On a mild summer evening in 1992, Barbara and Alan stood on the tree-sheltered deck of their northern California home waving bon voyage to their younger son and his bride. Their older son, his wife, a houseful of family, friends, and wedding presents surrounded them. One year later, both daughters-in-law were pregnant—as was Barbara. She and Alan had tried for ten years to have a third child; after several GIFT treatments failed, they assumed it was not to be. As Barbara approached fifty, however, she read in a magazine of something new—hormonal medications, donor eggs, and in vitro procedures—for women nearing, or even past, menopause.

"They'll be like siblings," Barbara says now of her daughter and two grandchildren born just a few months apart. This baby girl, blanketed in a stroller, a pink bow adorning her fine dark hair, is already an aunt, with niece and nephew as playmates. She will grow up with the best of care and attention. Barbara looks vibrant as she pushes the stroller down the hill—a youthful grandmother to be sure. Her husband will stop at the supermarket on his way home from work, for milk, dinner fixings, and Pampers. Barbara puts it this way: "We're having a great time. We lived for seven years without children after our boys were grown and on their own. So we can compare . . . "

With medical costs and fees for a young woman's eggs added to Barbara's physical and psychological screening, IVF, high-risk obstetric care and delivery, the total cost of their postmenopausal pregnancy approaches what they would pay for a new luxury car. This couple can well afford the expense. The pregnancy and delivery went smoothly, though Barbara does wonder at times about long-term safety of the hormones she took to prepare her uterus for the embryo transfer. She wonders, for instance, if they could increase her chances of someday developing breast cancer. It is not a question she ever asked her doctor; if she had, he would not have had an answer.

Barbara's story does not make headlines or appear on television's nightly news. This family goes about its life anonymously. Neighbors were barely aware of a new baby on the block, let alone her unusual circumstances. The media go for more sensational events—the latest record breaker, a first-time mother at the age of sixty-three or the postmenopausal surrogate gestational mother of her own grandchildren, in vitro twins for her son and his wife (who had a hysterectomy years before). And we glimpse a possible future of eggs donated by women who have died, or, even more disquieting, eggs harvested from fetuses never born—or of babies cloned in the manner of a Scottish lamb.

Nor are Barbara and Alan what we generally consider an infertile couple. Across the country, in New York City, Ellen worries that she and her husband might be. Conception should not seem problematic for Ellen, who has been pregnant twice before. The first time, unmarried, she chose an abortion. More recently, after stopping birth control pills, she suffered a miscarriage. Ellen is now thirty-seven, a busy, high-powered financial analyst eager to have a baby. She and her friends hear about the "biological clock" and hear their own ticking away; they compare notes on fertility treatments their gynecologists prescribe. Through a friend, Ellen found a specialist experienced in assisted reproduction for women over thirty-five. She wanted to take the fertility drug Pergonal (hMG), just to be sure, and to sign up for in vitro fertilization, just in case. She found a doctor who affirms his patient's anxiety. "After the age of thirty-five, women *should* be worried," he asserts in no uncertain terms. "Fertility drops drastically at thirty-three or thirty-four. They should try to start a family before the woman is thirty years old. Thirty-seven is not the time to start a family."

After two cycles of Pergonal, Ellen is pregnant again. Within months of the birth of their first child, she puts herself on a waiting list not only for IVF but also for egg donation, in case she is too old to use her own eggs the next time. "It's hard to find egg donors now. I want to hold a place, if we need to go that route." Even her doctor considers this step premature, considering her recent success. She may conceive with no treatment at all, perhaps needing only to allow herself a few extra months of trying.

Indisputably, age is a significant factor in women's fertility. But when does "age" become a problem, and how much does it lower chances for pregnancy? And how should this information affect women's decisions? One specialist, interviewed on a network television news segment, counsels: "Women should have children in their twenties, or plan to have fertility treatments with good insurance coverage available in their thirties. By their late thirties they may not be able to have their own child, and may want to adopt."[1] What does this doctor's advice on family and financial planning mean for Linda, a single woman aged twenty-six, recently out of law school, and working for a large, prestigious Wall Street firm? Will she someday have to choose between career and family, or can she rest assured that modern medical treatment—and a hefty health insurance plan—will in some way allow her to have both? Should Wendy, a newly credentialed elementary school teacher hurry into marriage and childbearing, uncertain though the relationship with her boyfriend may be? Should these women consider a future that includes single motherhood?

Not all fertility specialists convey quite the same urgency. "The decline in fertility is slow," says one. "This kind of pressure could make people crazy," says another. Dr. John Bongaarts, a senior associate at the Population Council, a non-profit research organization, contends that infertility related to a woman's age is not nearly as high as some "scare" reports suggest; women in their late twenties who decide to wait five additional years will not greatly lower their chances for becoming pregnant.[2] After the age of thirty-six, according to one study of cumulative conception and birth rates for women undergoing IVF, comes a gradual decline in fertility.[3] Other researchers, however, think such conclusions understate the risk of infertility.

How to use current knowledge about women's fertility is a question of significance that reaches far beyond the relatively few women past menopause who will try to have a baby—though these cases surely rivet our focus on age. This chapter summarizes recent medical developments that are pushing age limits for childbearing ever upward, requiring women and their doctors to weigh risks with (to borrow a statistical term) an "age-adjusted" slant. A visit to an informational presentation by one medical group shows how doctors, in communities throughout the United States, are attracting customers for treatments that can only be described as experiments on a grand, if local, scale. Age as a reproductive issue is gaining momentum at a pivotal time for fertility medicine. The large baby-boom generation is growing older; during the mid-1990s, the last of these women approached their mid-thirties. Technological advances are spawning new treatments that can be used on more women and men. The following discussion suggests ways in which individuals can use evolving information about women's age to help safeguard their fertility and, if necessary, obtain appropriate care. At the same time, it reveals the inextricable link between individual, age-related decisions and questions for society at large—a society in which the current focus of health care is on setting limits, asking what should be done medically for whom.

Pushing the Limits

No one reading medical journals over the last ten years would be completely surprised by news of a sixtyish woman giving birth, following hormone treatment, in vitro fertilization, and transfer of embryos using donated eggs. During the 1980s initial case reports described success with similar techniques for women in their twenties and thirties who could not produce their own eggs for a pregnancy because of a genetic abnormality or previous radiation treatment, or for unknown reasons. It was not long before fertility specialists were asking: If women with a medical condition sometimes called premature menopause could have a baby, what about women who experienced menopause at the normal age?

Experimental treatments that could answer this question soon followed, and with each new medical report, the childbearing age of pregnant patients climbed higher. The work of a group of fertility specialists at the University of Southern California—pioneers in developing egg donation for older women— provides an example. First came a preliminary report of treatment results in a small number of women over the age of forty; this study suggested egg donation as a fertility treatment not only for the few patients who experience unusually early menopause, but for women whose ability to conceive is waning as expected with age.[4] Two years later, countering what they describe as "a general reluctance" during the 1980s to offer egg donation as a treatment for women over forty, these physicians declared nothing less than an ability to reverse the natural, age-related decline in human fertility; the trick is to fertilize in vitro eggs donated by younger women and transfer the embryos to women "of advanced reproductive age." The age of fifty then seemed to present a limit. Beyond that, the researchers acknowledged, "Little is known about the ability to achieve pregnancy or the wisdom of establishing it. . . . The question 'How old is too old?' remains controversial, as does the issue of the appropriate application of the technology."[5] Such concerns did not put a brake on the experiments, however. By the following year, this group was reporting seven successful pregnancies for fourteen couples, in which the women, all in their fifties (including two grandmothers), had all passed through a natural menopause. The USC specialists conclude: "As the average life expectancy and quality of life in our population increases, establishing pregnancy in individuals *nearing 60* years of age becomes a more rational goal" (emphasis added).[6]

Not everyone agrees this goal is rational. The question "Can we do it?" was far easier to answer than "Should we? Is it wise?" With feasibility demonstrated, advocates now argue that withholding egg donation from older women constitutes age discrimination. Neither egg donation nor postmenopausal pregnancies have been subject to public discussion, though critics include at least two of this country's most prominent medical ethicists. Dr. Arthur Caplan of the University of Pennsylvania argues that this combination is "way outside the realm of what medical ethics ought to allow"; and Dr. George Anas, a Boston University lawyer and ethicist wonders, "What is driving this?"[7] Answers to this question may help individual patients decide whether a particular new reproductive intervention is in their best interest.

To begin with, medical researchers pursue experimental avenues that interest them and that advance their careers. With three dozen postmenopausal babies delivered by 1994, Dr. Mark Sauer, then director of the USC group, described such pregnancies as " a natural extension of what I do."[8] This answer may accurately reflect the progression of his research and clinical practice; however, women's health needs—particularly the extension of their natural reproductive lives—remain a separate matter, one certainly open to dispute.

Among gynecologists more generally, the aging woman was becoming a focus of attention during the 1980s. The baby-boom generation's first wave was past its peak reproductive years and approaching menopause. This life-stage became a hot topic, not only for journalists and book authors, but also for women's physicians and drug manufacturers. Gynecologists needed to attract and keep patients who were getting older. The largest swell of patients was moving past the age of thirty-five, not yet ready for the widely promoted menopausal hormone replacement therapy or for a postmenopausal pregnancy. However, many women who had established careers during their early thirties were now arriving at their gynecologists' offices wanting to become pregnant.

By the mid-1990s, a quarter to a third of women attempting a first pregnancy were over thirty-five.[9] These women were asking if they could take the time to try conceiving on their own. Did they need fertility treatment? Was treatment such as IVF—which disrupts one's life physically, emotionally, and financially—likely to work for them? In most cases, gynecologists had no clear answer to these questions for an individual prior to her own menopause, when her menstrual cycles were actually stopping.

Although percentages vary somewhat from study to study, depending on how the research was conducted, studies consistently demonstrate a clear reduction of fertility after the age of thirty-five. According to one 1995 report, approximately 6 percent of women under the age of twenty-five, with apparently normal reproductive systems, are unable to conceive within a year, compared to 43 percent of women between the ages of thirty-six and forty.[10] A French study of fertile women undergoing artificial insemination (because of the male's infertility) found that within one year 74 percent of women aged thirty or younger conceived, compared to 61 percent of those between the ages of thirty-one and thirty-five and 54 percent of women over thirty-five.[11] In addition, the rate of first-trimester miscarriage (i.e., before the twelfth week of a pregnancy, including very early "subclinical" miscarriages that happen before a woman is aware she has conceived) also increases as women pass through their thirties; such miscarriages often result from chromosomal abnormalities, which are more common with eggs from older women. However, for some women fertility begins dropping by the age of thirty, for others not until forty, and the drop proceeds more rapidly for some than for others. Among women whose fairly regular menstrual cycles had not changed, there was no good way to distinguish those who already have a significant fertility problem from those who may be able to conceive quite easily until they are fifty. "The most important aspect of diminished ovarian reserve and decline in reproductive potential," concluded the 1995 report, "is that its onset is highly variable."[12]

The Age Factor

By the mid-1990s, medical reports begin to incorporate more explicitly a woman's age when evaluating and recommending specific fertility treatments. At the same time, economic pressures are forcing the questions of which treatments work best—including which are most cost-effective—for patients with varying conditions and ages. Most of the reports focus on IVF—comparing it to other treatment or comparing IVF success rates with and without donor eggs.

Fallopian Tube Problems

Many women with fallopian tube abnormalities or damage must decide whether to undergo pelvic surgery and then try to conceive naturally or to bypass the problematic tubes with attempts at in vitro fertilization and embryo transfer. Acknowledging that "limited data" exist to provide useful estimates of IVF success, specialists from one IVF program have compared their cumulative pregnancy and live-birth rates (after four IVF cycles) to outcomes following tubal surgery as reported in the published medical literature (articles identified through Medline computer searches).[1] This comparison of IVF and tubal surgery highlights considerations that are important for fertility patients more generally.

First, women with fallopian tube problems are a heterogeneous group. The prognosis for surgery compared to in vitro fertilization varies, depending on the type, location, and severity of an individual's tubal abnormalities; the existence or absence of additional fertility problems in the woman or her partner; the woman's age; and the specific surgical technique. After summarizing reports on surgical repair, these specialists conclude that "young patients with mild or moderate tubal disease should be offered tubal reconstructive surgery, whereas those with severe disease, where the potential benefit of tubal reconstruction is limited, should be treated primarily with IVF."[2] Any woman who does not conceive within a year following surgery should move on to IVF.

For older women, however, this group of IVF practitioners recommends treatment that "provides the highest likelihood of success within the shortest time interval"—that is, IVF. As they note with regard to reversing tubal sterilization, "special attention should be paid to the age factor, because, with each year after age 40, fecundity drastically decreases and IVF may afford an immediate chance for conception without the potential [risks] of abdominal surgery."[3]

An advantage of successful surgical repair is that the women can attempt one or more naturally conceived pregnancies during subsequent years. The age factor complicates comparisons of IVF and surgery all the more, however, because IVF success rates drop noticeably for older women, the very ones most likely to be pushed directly toward this intervention. Doctors and patients alike face difficult trade-offs in trying not to lose valuable time before trying IVF while keeping open treatment options a woman might prefer.

In addition, comparisons and decisions must be based on success rates of the physicians and programs an individual is actually considering, not on national (or worldwide) results reported in the medical literature. Prospective patients need to interpret cumulative IVF success rates with an eye toward the number of cycles they can afford and tolerate, or the number allowed by their managed-care plan. A cumulative live-birth rate of 70 percent after four treatment cycles, as this IVF program reports, is overly optimistic for patients who will not undergo more than two IVF attempts.

Along with medical considerations, cost and insurance remain undeniable determinants of an individual's decision and outcome. Indeed, this summary of medical options for various types of tubal infertility concludes with: "In this era, in which society's increasing concern seems to be focused on cost containment, the calculated costs per live birth after tubal surgery compared with IVF is becoming a central issue. Comparisons are difficult because cost calculations do not take into account whether third-party insurance carriers will reimburse patients for either surgical or IVF expenses." After all is said and done, the overriding consideration may be that "patients are more likely to be reimbursed for surgical procedures than IVF."[4] If this country's movement toward managed care (see Chapter 8) increasingly encompasses fertility treatment, the trend may shift away from surgery, as IVF practitioners argue the cost-effectiveness of IVF, regardless of the woman's age or specific tubal condition.[5]

Multiple Pregnancies

Age became a focus for studies asking what number of embryos should be transferred during IVF treatments in order to lower risks of multiple pregnancy yet maintain acceptable success rates. For instance, one 1996 report concludes that in women younger than thirty-five, transferring four embryos, rather than three, significantly increases the risk of triplets or twins without improving overall chances for a pregnancy. In contrast, transferring four rather than three embryos does not increase multiple gestations for older women; chances for pregnancy improve with the higher number of embryos if the woman is over forty.[6] The same question became important for IVF with donor eggs when specialists observed, to their surprise, high rates of multiple gestations; the young age of egg donors was the important factor, rather than the advanced age of recipients who became pregnant.[7]

Ovarian Stimulation

Specialists are looking more explicitly at age and non-IVF treatments as well. For example, ovarian stimulation with clomiphene citrate appears to be less effective as women approach forty. Similarly, clomiphene citrate combined with intrauterine insemination seems to have an age limit. One study asks if this therapy is effective in women over the age of thirty-five; the results show a "dramatic fall" in pregnancy rates after that age. Moreover, "virtually all" pregnancies, regardless of age, occurred during the first four cycles of this treatment. The report concludes that women over thirty-five are better off with more advanced reproductive technologies than with the simpler and cheaper clomiphene-stimulated IUI, and that no one should make more than four attempts with this treatment.[8] A study of the stronger ovarian stimulant Pergonal combined with IUI also found success rates dropped for women over the age of thirty-five. (Rates also dropped if the male partner was over forty.) No pregnancies occurred in women requiring more than twenty-five ampules of Pergonal, whatever their age.[9]

---

1. Benadiva et al. 1995.
2. Benadiva et al. 1995, 1053. See also Tomaževič et al. 1996; Dubuisson et al. 1997.

3. Benadiva et al. 1995, 1054.
4. Benadiva et al. 1995, 1059.
5. Bates and Bates 1996; Penzias and DeCherney 1996.
6. Svendsen et al. 1996.
7. Sauer, Paulson, and Lobo 1995b; Wolf et al. 1997; Yaron et al. 1997.
8. Agarwal 1996.
9. Brezechffa and Buyalos 1997.

Fertility specialists did begin developing ways to test what they call "ovarian age" or "reserve"—an individual woman's remaining ability to produce adequate hormones and fertilizable eggs. The most commonly used blood test, which measures levels of follicle-stimulating hormone (FSH), was most useful in identifying women *unlikely* to become pregnant on their own because they were physiologically closer to menopause. As new tests and predictive methods appeared, some specialists began to warn their colleagues that tests were being advocated and used without adequate medical understanding of what was being measured; predicting a patient's fertility as she approached menopause, or her likely response to treatment, would require greater knowledge about the biology of fertility and aging.[13]

Nor could fertility specialists tell patients much about the likelihood of success with assisted reproductive technologies as they passed the age of forty, although researchers were gaining insights as they experimented with fertility treatments in women of varying ages. With more women undergoing assisted reproductive technologies, and their age creeping upward, the rates of success and failure were revealing. One 1995 report, for example, provides data on success rates for IVF and GIFT—also revealing is the researchers' interpretation of their results. This study asked the question: At what age can we no longer offer optimistic pregnancy rates to women seeking ART? The authors report "respectable numbers" of live-born deliveries in women aged forty to forty-three—but what they considered "respectable" was an approximately 5 percent delivery rate for IVF and 9 percent for GIFT. After the age of forty-three, the rate dropped lower, finally turning the outlook pessimistic even for these fertility specialists; not only are chances for success "extremely low," but the attempts bring "significant risks" of ovarian hyperstimulation syndrome, ectopic pregnancy, multiple gestation, miscarriage, and, if a pregnancy continues, other obstetric complications that increase with age.[14]

To get around these dismal success rates and risks, these specialists suggest egg donation for women over forty-three—a suggestion consistent with results, more generally, from other assisted reproductive technologies programs. As the numbers of women attempting assisted reproduction grew, the pattern was emerging: likelihood of success falls as a woman's age rises, *unless* she is using eggs from a young donor (preferably in her twenties). It seems a woman's uterus can function quite well, with the help of hormonal medications, even as she reaches and passes the age when her ovaries cease to produce fertile eggs. Or, as a physician from the University of Southern California group put it, "It appears that oocyte donation makes pregnancy possible in virtually any woman with a uterus."[15]

On the one hand, the accumulating evidence prompted fertility specialists to declare that the worst enemy for an infertile couple is the woman's age.[16] Even a normal result on tests of ovarian age does not bode well after the chronological age of about forty; women are likely to have some trouble conceiving, their chances diminishing with each passing year. On the other hand, this age-related fact of life was fueling development of high-tech efforts to circumvent the natural biological limit, most visibly in the postmenopausal pregnancy. The challenge for millions of women caught in the middle, between their most fertile twenties and menopause, is to benefit from information now available about age, while avoiding dangers this new emphasis brings—especially the danger of being stampeded into unnecessary medical treatment. Beyond the many questions about the wisdom of postmenopausal pregnancies is a question for any woman considering fertility treatment at a relatively "advanced reproductive age" (i.e., beyond her early thirties): How aggressive do I need to be *now* with medical intervention? For these women, overzealous application of therapies focused on age may become a worse enemy than age itself.

A Guide for Women over Thirty-Five

In the absence of accurate ways to evaluate an individual woman's fertility loss due to age—including the likelihood of pregnancy without treatment and the likelihood of successful treatment using her own eggs—one specialist offers the following checklist of positive and negative factors:[1]

Factors Suggesting Adequate Fertility

1. A history of past ability to conceive, especially in recent years.
2. Identification of a treatable condition, such as tubal blockage, that could be preventing conception, so that egg quality is less likely to be the main fertility problem.

3. Hormone tests indicating both a low follicle-stimulating hormone (FSH) and a low estrogen level in the early part of menstrual cycle—the normal pattern for women not yet showing physiological signs of approaching menopause. (Since levels vary from day to day, cycle to cycle, and between different laboratories, the physician ordering these tests should interpret the results.)

4. No change in cycle length, bleeding pattern, or other symptoms associated with menses that often signal the approach to menopause.

5. At least one ovary that responds readily with multiple follicles to low doses of fertility drugs.

Factors Suggesting Significant Loss of Fertility

1. Long-standing inability to conceive (more than three years).

2. Unexplained infertility.

3. Elevated levels of either FSH or estrogen early in the menstrual cycle—a pattern indicating the approach to menopause.

4. Shorter or irregular menstrual cycles compared to past years.

5. Ovaries that seem resistant to hormonal stimulation, requiring high doses of fertility drugs to produce only a few follicles or eggs.

---

1. Based on material from M. Martin, Northern California Resolve Conference, June 1996.

For individual women and for the field of fertility medicine, questions of age will only become more perplexing as technology provides even more types of interventions. Technically speaking, egg donation for assisted reproduction is fairly easy. More problematic for the clinics and their patients is the limited supply of available eggs. During the 1990s, fertility programs were developing their own lists (sometimes called "stables" or "pools") of donors—vendors, actually, whose eggs are available to infertile recipients for a fee. Unlike sperm, which a man can deposit by the millions on relatively short order, mature eggs are normally released from the ovary one at a time in each menstrual cycle; even hormonal superovulation yields at most about a dozen "high-quality" fertilizable eggs for one treatment cycle. Some fertility clinics offer reduced prices with a "shared donor" option; the superovulated eggs of one young donor are distributed among a number of recipients. Or a woman undergoing superovulation and egg retrieval for her own IVF gets a discount if she "donates" several of her eggs to another patient. (The Irvine clinic revelations cast an eerie shadow on this option, when that "sharing" occurred without the women's permission or knowledge.) In the mid-1990s, a new, enlarged source of "egg donors" became feasible, if not particularly appealing, as scientists announced the ability to harvest eggs from ovaries of deceased women or of aborted fetuses and then mature these eggs in the laboratory for fertilization.

Within a decade, specialists were predicting, technology would allow women to have their own eggs frozen for future use. Indeed, fertility specialists underestimated how quickly experiments on women would materialize. In December 1995, a well-known, well-advertised fertility clinic—the Genetics and IVF Institute, located in Fairfax, Virginia—sent letters to thousands of cancer specialists offering a new reproductive procedure to nearly any woman about to undergo chemotherapy or radiation who might, in the future, want to conceive and bear her own biological child.[17] In an attempt to circumvent the ovarian damage and subsequent infertility cancer treatments can cause, a surgeon would remove the woman's ovaries, then freeze and store them in liquid nitrogen—for a charge of $3,000–4,000. Portions of a woman's cryopreserved ovaries could be replaced at some later time, when (and if) she was considered free of cancer—generally a wait of at least five years.

Preserving the fertility of women facing cancer treatment is a laudable goal. This goal, however, should not divert our focus from the way this new reproductive intervention is developing. As with so many other fertility treatments, it is burdened by serious ethical questions and social concerns, both immediate and long-term. Perhaps most blatant is the questionable ethics of offering to perform this experiment on patients who are exceedingly vulnerable, of making the offer so early in the procedure's development, and of charging several thousand dollars to do it. At the time of the fertility clinic's solicitation, the technique's originator, Dr. Roger Gosden, of the University of Leeds in England, had removed ovaries from only four cancer patients (including a 3-year-old), the first before the 1994 publication of the results from his experiments with animals. Although Gosden reported success with the completed technique in sheep, resulting in the birth of live offspring, no one had yet reimplanted ovarian tissue in humans, let alone observed whether a woman could then produce fertile eggs and have a successful pregnancy. Nor could anyone predict the impact of such an attempt on her overall health. Among the most obvious questions was whether this reproductive technique, successful or not, would trigger a recurrence of cancer. Such concerns led Gosden to stop removing ovaries from cancer patients until he determined at least that the later steps of this experiment could restore fertility in women who had the initial operations. (He had also excluded women with breast cancer, due to concern about recurrence, a precaution not taken by the Virginia clinic.)

In this country, plans to begin performing the procedure took other fertility specialists by surprise. Dr. Alan DeCherney, who had just finished his term as president of the American Society for Reproductive Medicine, was "taken aback" by the "bold step." He noted, however, that reproductive technology is market driven. (See Figure 4.) In other words, this clinic was staking early claim to a potentially large market share. Since these women have no other options for preserving their fertility, DeCherney added, "Theoretically, it sounds fine."[18]

In fact, these very circumstances make the clinic's plan more troubling than exciting, both as an immediate operation for women with cancer and, in the longer run, as a reflection of decisions made at fertility medicine's cutting edge. That a woman sees this experiment as her only apparent chance for someday having a biological child, and that she faces an illness in the present that may take her life before that someday ever comes, leaves her more emotionally vulnerable than other women who are deciding about an experimental reproductive treatment. Physicians need to proceed even more cautiously, zealously ensuring that these cancer patients reach well-informed decisions, free of undue pressure and manipulated hope. A doctor's medical oath to "do no harm" can mean *not* attempting a medical intervention. Physicians and patients need to ask even more persistently if a goal of future pregnancy is narrowing too severely their focus, clouding their assessment of risks, benefits, and unknowns to the point where they lose sight of the woman's overall health and well-being.

Physicians and patients should also ask whether this reproductive procedure is the only option for women who may want to attempt conceiving a pregnancy rather than pursuing adoption (an alternative generally downplayed in fertility medicine). Are there—or might there be developed in the same five to ten years before reimplantation can proceed for today's patients—less risky interventions that would preserve cancer patients' fertility? While letters to cancer specialists were offering to remove women's ovaries, for instance, other physicians were reporting less drastic techniques that could help women receiving radiation treatment for one type of cancer, Hodgkin's disease, approximately half of whom experience premature ovarian failure following radiation and aggressive chemotherapy. [19]

At the least, to safeguard participants in this reproductive experiment, the technique of ovarian cryopreservation should develop within a framework of

Donor Egg
ICSI for Male Infertility
IVF
Sperm Aspiration
Ovary Cryopreservation

Immediate Availability

The Genetics & IVF Institute is internationally respected for pioneering infertility treatments using advanced reproductive technologies. **ICSI** (intracytoplasmic sperm injection) **donor egg**, and **IVF** services are *available now with no waiting list.* We have accomplished *over 500 ICSI pregnancies* in cases of severe male infertility, and *over 1500 pregnancies* through IVF technology. And our highly successful donor egg program has *over 100 fully screened donors immediately accessible* to patients requiring oocyte donation. Other innovative services such as *non-surgical aspiration of sperm* (an alternative to vasectomy reversal), and *ovary freezing* are also available.

GIVF is conveniently located in suburban Washington, D.C. We are deeply committed to courteous, responsive, personal service, and have effectively assisted patients from throughout the United States and the world. Joseph D. Schulman, M.D., GIVF Director and founder and Richard J. Sherins, M.D., Director of Andrology, are two of the many specialists available to respond to your inquiries.

GENETICS & IVF INSTITUTE

3020 Javier Road
Fairfax, Virginia 22031

800-552-4363, ext. 150

E-mail: givf@givf.com
WWW: http://www.givf.com

© GIVF 1997

GENETICS & IVF INSTITUTE

Figure 4. Within weeks of the announcement of a new technique for removing and freezing ovaries of cancer patients for later reimplantation, a clinic adds this procedure to its lengthening list of services advertised in newspapers, in magazines, and on the Internet.

well-planned, thoroughly reviewed scientific trials—an approach consistently lacking in fertility medicine. Researchers need to provide information about the likelihood of infertility after cancer treatment; patients need to discuss and understand these probabilities in order to decide whether to take the risks now of an experimental "preventive" surgery—including the risks that cancer may recur and that the procedure may not even work in humans. Far from proceeding cautiously, with a systematic, scientific approach, the Virginia clinic's offer constitutes a bulk mailing to drum up business by inviting cancer patients to pay for being experimental subjects.

Granted, to learn whether this technique can work in humans, it must at some point be tried on humans. But on whom should doctors experiment, under what conditions, with what risks considered acceptable, and at whose expense? These difficult questions require painstaking deliberations and scrupulous review, processes that often do not survive a free medical marketplace. Although this clinic chose cancer patients for initial human experiments, the potential market is ultimately much larger, possibly expanding to all young women. The teenage girl excited today about her first menstrual period may not have to choose between career and childbearing. She might embark on each simultaneously, during her most fertile years, *if* she chose to have pieces of her ovary removed, cryopreserved, and deposited in her egg-bank account, to be reimplanted when she reaches thirty-five, or forty, or sixty. This goal in itself requires social and ethical deliberations about the directions of reproductive medicine before the new technology slips into common practice, like others before it, as a fait accompli. A more immediate concern, however, is the use of women cancer patients as a means—the human guinea pigs—toward a much more general entrepreneurial and medical end. Attempts to justify this use may claim that cancer patients most need this operation, having no other options, or that these women have nothing to lose in trying. Yet, they may have the *most* to lose—a hard-fought, perhaps fragile recovery from cancer and their future health.

News of this reproductive experiment did not meet with unanimous approval in the medical specialty. Four months after media reports describing the Virginia clinic's plans, the American Society for Reproductive Medicine issued a highly unusual press release. Perhaps stung by ongoing revelations emanating from the Irvine clinic, the professional organization took a stand opposing a "bold" new fertility intervention. Without naming the clinic, the society's statement declared its belief that "there is insufficient scientific evidence to justify the use of cryopreservation of ovarian tissue for later replacement to restore reproductive and endocrine function." The procedure should not be offered to patients until systematic, well-designed research—with informed consent and approval from a hospital review committee—demonstrated the treatment's safety and efficacy. The press release concluded, "Exploitation of patients must be avoided. Patient welfare and the safety and effectiveness of reproductive health care are of paramount importance to [ASRM]."

Another press release came just two days later. This terse official statement following up the first official statement revealed the clinic's identity. Issued "at the request of" the Virginia clinic, the second release stated, "According to the Genetics & IVF Institute, they are in full compliance with the guidelines proposed by the ASRM in its press release . . . on cryopreservation of ovarian tissue." The society did get its own last word: "ASRM continues to emphasize that research involving human reproductive tissue should comply with the established standards for informed consent and the protection of human subjects. Promotional material should clearly distinguish between research and newly accepted procedures for the clinical care of patients." [20]

Nevertheless, these pronouncements are only guidelines—the society has no authority to monitor or restrict what member physicians do. Furthermore, this controversy remained largely in-house. There was no significant press coverage; most fertility patients—and most of the general public—learned nothing of the official statements or of the crucially important disagreements underlying them. Nor would the public read the debate in a European medical journal the following year that focused explicitly on the risk of a cancer recurrence. Researchers who experimented on mice with lymphoma (a blood cell malignancy) found that after ovarian tissue was transplanted into healthy mice, the recipients developed lymphoma. Turning to humans, these scientists explain, "The implication of our results is that ovarian tissue which contains cancer cells at the time of collection has the potential to reintroduce the cancer to the cured recipient whenever it is replaced. If there is any possibility that a patient in remission has cancer reinitiated by [reimplanting their] tissue, the risk is too high. Therefore we should not be promoting the idea of ovarian tissue banking for cancer patients." They certainly think such a possibility exists. They also think a suggestion that safe techniques for reimplanting the ovarian tissue will exist by the time these cancer patients are ready "is presumptuous and could be misleading." Contending that a "predictable, safe, and reliable" alternative is as likely to arise from changes in the cancer therapies as from experimental procedures already advertised and begun by fertility specialists in Virginia, these scientists warn that "the issue of how to deal with ovarian tissues which may contain cancer cells therefore needs to be debated now, before groups start to graft ovarian tissue back into patients."[21]

Risks Revisited

While the public learned little about the ovarian cryopreservation controversy, its attention was caught periodically by the most unusual pregnancies—in women past menopause. Discussion of risks centered on problems that might face children living with older parents (especially mothers) and older parents coping with a young child or later a teen. Risks for the pregnant women received scant attention, and all the women for whom this treatment failed received even less. Physicians critical of these postmenopausal pregnancies predict that some women will die in the process of pushing the limits further, no matter how careful the health screening. And there is certainly no guarantee that all practitioners will be all that careful. Beyond direct risks to the few women likely to attempt such pregnancies, however, are more general concerns and cautions related to age that, once again, such women dramatize.

First, risks of pregnancy are not confined to postmenopausal women. Obstetric complications such as stroke, heart failure, hemorrhage, diabetes, and hypertension increase significantly beginning at about age thirty-five. The rate of miscarriage, chromosomal abnormalities, and death in newborns (mostly stillbirths) also increases.[22] Although most threats to the pregnant woman's health are manageable, maternal "disasters" (severe, long-term damage to health, or death) do occur, their frequency rising with age. Statistics from the United Kingdom reflect the increased probabilities for older women: 5.3 deaths per 100,000 pregnant women aged twenty to twenty-four, up to 53.9 above forty years old. The rate will be higher for women over fifty.[23] No one knows how high the rate of maternal death and other complications will go. Nor is there any public dialogue regarding how high is too high.

A specialist enthusiastic about these treatments does describe pregnancy as "a major stress on women's organ systems," systems which become less sturdy and resilient with age. He is more than willing, however, to forge ahead with experiments to determine not only whether (or when) the stress becomes too great for women, but whether "there is an age beyond which a woman's organ systems are unable to adequately provide the nourishment required for normal growth and development of a fetus."[24] Dr. Bernadine Healy, a former head of the National Institutes of Health, describes this concern more graphically.

Although she supports the goal of freezing and storing women's ovaries to be used later, for their own postmenopausal pregnancies, she does worry that "a crumbling scaffold riddled with osteoporosis probably is not an ideal one to go through nine months of pregnancy."[25]

By the mid-1990s, in fact, the USC group that pioneered in postmenopausal pregnancies began to report a "surprising" and "worrisome" rate of multiple gestations and other obstetric complications in pregnant women aged fifty to fifty-nine. Medical tests required before women were accepted into post-menopausal treatment—in order to select "only those women known to be in excellent physical health"—did not predict who would experience problems (including hypertension, preeclampsia, diabetes, and preterm labor) during pregnancy. Among thirty-six women, who had seventeen live births, the doctors describe the rate of complications as "at face value . . . incredibly high."[26] Their experiments with pregnancies in postmenopausal women led additionally to conclusions about the considerable risks of multiple gestations: "As our experience expands, it is becoming increasingly more difficult to recommend that more than three embryos be transferred to women of advanced reproductive age."[27] An Italian report on sixty-one treatment cycles in thirty-four post-menopausal women also found a high number of maternal complications during the eighteen pregnancies conceived, notwithstanding pretreatment screening examinations and exclusion of women with "important diseases."[28]

The view of one California obstetrician who specializes in high-risk pregnancies: "Under the age of forty, pregnancy is not a problem; over fifty it is a problem, to the same degree as under forty is not! Between forty and fifty is a gray area." Yet he observed, "It is not 'politically correct' in the medical world to say that pregnancy for women over the age of fifty is not a good idea."[29]

In addition to risks of pregnancy, the fertility treatments themselves bring an extra burden with age, whether or not the woman succeeds in conceiving and delivering a healthy baby. For example, recent studies suggest that fertility drugs that hyperstimulate a woman's ovaries may increase her chances of later developing ovarian cancer. Use of these drugs need not be the single, direct cause of her disease; ovarian cancer appears more frequently among all women as they grow older (increasing tenfold between thirty-five and fifty-five years old, from about 4 in 100,000 to 40 in 100,000 women). Older fertility patients who undergo superovulation are thus more likely to start ovarian stimulation with premalignant or malignant conditions that the treatment may promote or accelerate. A 1994 article describing two cases of advanced ovarian cancer in fertility patients warns that "the driving concern" of patients and physicians to

achieve ovulation, fertility, and pregnancy may lead physicians to overlook earlier signs of cancer (the authors suggest "judicious use" of ultrasound during the
infertility workup to detect ovarian masses). Their conclusion, which should be
heard by patients as well as doctors, emphasizes the need to avoid "medical
blinders" and the potentially harmful effects of medical care too narrowly focused on the goal of pregnancy.[30] Whether fertility drugs can cause a woman to
develop ovarian cancer, independent of a preexisting abnormality, remains an
unresolved, hotly debated question that requires further research.

As another example, use of the medication GnRH-a to suppress a woman's
menstrual cycle can result in loss of bone density (osteoporosis). This side effect
is most pronounced and least reversible when the drug is used for six months or
more, as in the treatment of endometriosis; however, shorter treatments, as are
common as a prelude to ovarian hyperstimulation, may also cause bone loss.[31]
Because the natural incidence of osteoporosis increases as women age, accelerating markedly at menopause, older fertility patients face even greater risk with
use of GnRH-a. Moreover, these older, less fertile patients may receive treatment for a longer time. One recent study targets older women specifically. Arguing that "IVF has long needed to improve pregnancy rates and reduce costs,"
the authors suggest that long-term use of GnRH-a might improve conception
and implantation rates in women over the age of thirty-five. As in rats, giving
women GnRH-a over many months, even years, may "save sufficient [egg] follicles to last them until [their] 70s."[32] This study does not mention risks of osteoporosis and bone fractures—and certainly does not question whether such a
goal is desirable. At the least, this risk suggests doctors should first assess an individual's starting point—that is, does she have adequate bone density before
treatment?—and periodically reassess during treatment.

Finally, concern with risks to women as the age of fertility patients rises
must acknowledge the facts that, at least for now, the number of treatments
using donated eggs will also rise and that egg donors (usually younger women)
take on the risks from superovulation and egg retrieval. Use of these donors
raises basic questions about benefits of the new information and interventions
focused now on women's reproductive age. Who benefits, in what ways, at
whose risk? Individuals nearing or past menopause, who are no longer fertile
but wish to become pregnant, consider the new reproductive technologies beneficial and worth the risk. Yet, is this new type of choice—with benefits for
some women that bring risks for others—an appropriate goal of medical treatment? Does the gain in pregnancies override risks, not only to the older women
but to young egg donors? Is it appropriate to pay egg donors to assume these

medical risks? Already medical reports on severe ovarian hyperstimulation syndrome include healthy donors with no known predisposition for developing this life-threatening complication of superovulation.[33] Donors face other well-documented complications, including ovarian injury, infection, infertility, and vaginal laceration as well as possible increase in the risk of ovarian cancer. And there are other unknowns, leading Dr. Florence Haseltine, then director of the Center for Population Research at the National Institutes of Health, to argue, "There is no excuse for young girls to be getting drugs to donate eggs. These are young kids. There's often a $2,000–$3,000 inducement. . . . How do you know their fertility won't be impaired? We're sticking their ovaries with needles. . . . Will they have early menopause?"[34]

Tellingly, the same USC research group that began reporting postmenopausal pregnancies during the early 1990s commented, by 1995: "As the debate over the ethics of achieving pregnancy in postmenopausal women continues, a *modicum of fact* is necessary to fully inform older patients of their chances for success" (emphasis added).[35] Unfortunately, this call for a modicum of fact appeared long after the fact of promotion and proliferation of treatment to older patients (in this 1995 study, egg donation to women aged forty-three to fifty-nine). Ethical debate unfolded within the profession as the therapy became an established technique. In 1994, 163 egg donor programs were already reporting over 3,000 treatment cycles to a voluntary ART registry.[36] A new group of women, paid egg donors, was already established, if not yet in numbers sufficient to supply the increasing demand—demand fueled in large part by fertility specialists.

Also telling are the views of Dr. Mark Sauer, who shaped and directed the USC program and helped establish other egg donation programs throughout the country. Despite his enthusiasm just a few years earlier—postmenopausal pregnancies were "a natural extension of what I do"—in 1996 he was wondering what had gone wrong. He expressed his revised outlook, not on national public television, but in a European medical journal. While he once felt "puzzled" by arguments against egg donation, he now revealed to fellow specialists alarm regarding "serious controversies." Of particular concern were escalating fees that "may certainly be considered an enticement" to attract young egg donors and the escalating age of recipients.[37]

Ten years earlier, Sauer recalls, the idea of young, unmarried women who had never been pregnant—usually students—undergoing ovarian hyperstimulation and egg retrieval, for instance as part of a research project, was "unthinkable." With risks of these invasive procedures far outweighing any benefit to donors, no ethics committee would have approved such a proposal. "Labeling the practice 'standard' or 'conventional,'" he comments, "seems to have justified it." Ten years earlier, he notes, egg donors received $250 per cycle, a payment that has increased more than tenfold. Claiming surprise at the technique's success ("I don't believe any of us expected oocyte donation to establish itself so quickly nor did we anticipate how well it would ultimately work"), he seems also bewildered at how the technique's initial patients—women with premature ovarian failure or a genetically inheritable disease—"were followed by" women nearing and past 'menopause, as if his group and the specialty itself played no role in enlarging upon the original use.

In a field "where failure is more commonly the norm," Sauer worries that the "infusion of hope" marked by treatments using donor eggs will soon be "overshadowed by the increasingly questionable practices taking hold of oocyte donation." Already he can point to "tasteless advertisements" of egg brokers and fertility clinics (e.g., "We pay top dollar") trying to increase supply for the increased demand. Impressed by "almost unanimous criticism leveled at American practitioners by colleagues abroad with respect to payment of donors" (e.g., "pimping for patients in need of eggs"), he now warns, "It is time to guard against moneyed and special interests profiting from the desperation of our patients and exploiting the goodwill of most donors."[38]

If perhaps less naive, no longer oblivious to the controversies, Sauer clings tenuously to the hope that "strong condemnation by professional peers may still have some impact," that fertility specialists can "police ourselves," maintaining freedom to "choose the way they wish to practice medicine." Yet it was the USC egg donation program—the very program he built up during the eight preceding years—that in April 1997 announced a baby born to a 63-year-old woman, "the oldest woman to deliver a child by this technology in the world."[39] The woman's USC physician professed innocence in public statements regarding the patient's age, explaining that "she lied to us."[40] He quickly acknowledges, however, that clinic age limits for egg donation are both arbitrary and flexible (USC's was fifty-five), characteristics obvious to interested women. Given this patient's outcome, he even feels somewhat glad she lied. Of course, he does not discuss patients whose outcomes were less gratifying, the failed treatment attempts and, perhaps, harm that led to this public "success." As he explains it, doctors do not know whether risks from pregnancy are greater for women in their sixties than in their forties or fifties. However, the real question is not *whether,* for risks will surely rise with age. The question is *when* will risks—including maternal deaths—have risen beyond what is considered acceptable?

And should limits be defined only by reaching the point where fertility specialists declare, "We went too far"?

Indeed, the findings reported in the journal article presenting this "unusual case of successful pregnancy achieved by oocyte donation" become a statement against establishing limits. The medical report's conclusions about reproduction in postmenopausal women are, first, that "the uterus is capable of supporting [implantation] and subsequent gestation for many years beyond natural menopause," and, second, the consequence of attempting to regulate the age of recipients is that "human beings whose age falls outside of these limits become motivated to deceive the providers of those services.[41] Both findings about humans, though probably valid, are but a partial explanation. The fact is, once a treatment exists, some doctors will offer it and some patients will want to try. With fertility interventions, individual doctors and patients are making up the rules as they go along; medical directions remain unexamined until the new developments are irrevocably on their way.

"Now Available in Your Community"

The newspaper advertisement leads with "Egg Donation: Is It for You?" For couples struggling with infertility, the message continues, this exciting new technique may be the answer. The ad provides a toll-free number to register for an informational evening, presented at a local hotel by a local medical group. A man's taped voice answers that number, sounding rather like an airline—"Physician Referral, Class, and Seminar Scheduling Line. We apologize for the short wait. All our counselors are busy right now . . . " Soft music plays until a live voice breaks in, a woman's voice with a smooth but distant Southern drawl. "Center for Reproductive Medicine. Can I help you?" She enters the prospective patient's name, address, and phone number into a computer. She will not tell just where she is, only that she is in some other state. Space at the evening seminar is confirmed, and a reminder call comes on the day before it takes place.

The presentation is free. A young, well-dressed, smiling woman greets people approaching the conference room. She checks off names from her list—women and men arriving in couples, more women alone or in twos or threes. The women range in age, with some appearing to be close to or even past menopause. Some couples have a manner of having been through much already. Most of the women and men are white; most look middle-class, except for a few of the youngest, dressed in scruffy jeans and T-shirts—potential egg donors

perhaps. At the entrance is a table displaying written handouts about egg donation and stacks of business cards for the three physicians, the IVF nurse and egg
donation coordinator, and an administrator skilled in complexities of health insurance coverage—just part of the medical team offering their services. Inside,
another table offers a pleasing array of refreshments.

The physicians speak first, over the glow and hum of the slide projector:
charts, percentages, procedures, a cartoon for brief comic relief. "Our pregnancy rate is above the [national] average," one physician reports enthusiastically. "People come from all over the United States, the world in fact, to our
program." As for the admittedly dismal in vitro success rates for women over
forty, using their own eggs, "Egg donation is a phenomenal technique for older
women." He also reports the remarkable success of this program, compared to
others, with the freezing (cryopreservation) of embryos, particularly with
donors who produce twelve to thirty good-quality, viable eggs. He cannot pin-
point reasons for these happy results, but it means their patients have more opportunities for attempting a pregnancy. (These doctors generally suggest no
more than four embryos transferred per cycle, to lessen the occurrence of multiple pregnancies, though this decision is "up to you.") If the first try is not successful, thawed embryos can be used for later attempts—a much less expensive
procedure (and, though he doesn't mention it, generally less successful) than
the initial superovulation, retrieval of eggs, and transfer of fresh embryos. It also
means that, during that initial cycle, "the more eggs the better . . . whether
from a donor or your own ovaries."

Embryos are the province of another team member, the program's IVF laboratory director, a lanky woman with large, expressive hands and easy smile. An
embryologist, she supervises the realm in which sperm and eggs actually meet.
Her job is to coax these microscopic cells—through some mix of scientific for-
mula and magic touch—to fertilize and divide into embryos a doctor can take
from the laboratory, remove from the dish, and place into the uterus or fallopian tubes of the recipient lying on a table in another room. "We are always
happy to talk with you, which patients really like," this scientist tells the audience warmly. "You can tour the lab, ask any questions you may have. . . . And
we go down to talk with the donor each time she has eggs retrieved. She wants
to know how many eggs the doctor could get, what their quality is."

And the recipient wants to know about that donor. Indeed, to a striking degree, the evening's presentation centers, not on medical information about diagnostic and treatment procedures, but on an obviously ticklish relationship between egg donors and recipients. The egg donation coordinator describes a

service that, she says, most assisted reproduction programs do not provide—an ongoing pool of egg donors from whom patients can choose. They solicit applicants for their "highly selective" pool through newspaper advertisements, colleges, day care centers, and other community agencies where fertile young women congregate, and increasingly through word of mouth—donors telling their friends, who then apply to join the pool. Along with interviews and past employment checks, potential donors must complete a 29-page questionnaire. A woman's answers help screen for the mandatory requirements—good health, fertility, emotional maturity, stability, responsibility in complying with the regimen of hormone stimulation and egg retrieval, in following through on commitments. The answers also let recipients know as much as possible about an array of additional characteristics they may desire in the egg donor they will choose and (although the coordinator does not say it) in their child. She explains that you can look over these answers, as well as photographs, compiled in a donor book. You may change your mind about what you thought were crucial characteristics—blond hair, blue eyes (she says this, though the audience is not all white), Phi Beta Kappa, a great skier. You may, like other patients, feel so anxious that you run out of the room the first time you face their collection of donor books. Once you choose a donor, the type of relationship established with her is your choice—you may want to meet or definitely not meet, exchange letters only, talk on the telephone. Of course, you can go outside the program's pool to find an egg donor. There are donor brokers, if none in the existing pool work for you. Some patients come with a sister or friend lined up. However you find a donor, the coordinator concludes, "it's an exciting process."

Whoever the donor may be, both she and the recipient will require preparation involving more than hormones and pain medications. Both will have emotional concerns, the psychological domain of two therapists who speak next. These concerns may be as concrete as the fear of an unintended waiting-room encounter between the recipient and the woman whose egg may become her child. Yet all concerns eventually become more diffuse—concerns that range from philosophical to biological to legal. What motivates the ideal donor? Not financial gain alone, the therapist says, which could lead to unpredictable psychological reactions. Beyond this stated certainty, all is vague. How can physicians be sure that women on both sides of the transfer are proceeding of their own free will, under no duress from partners or from other life circumstances? Can financial need ever enter an equation with "altruism" in defining an ideal donor, and how would anyone determine the balance? How should women and men handle new connections forged by new reproductive technologies? What does it mean to be a parent?

While a psychological minefield may await those who go ahead, the evening's final speakers give barely a hint. Two satisfied former clients laud the enjoyment of parenthood, whatever the hesitations about a donated egg. A nine-time donor conveys her contentment with the role she has played. The picture of stability, she has two treasured children of her own. She likes helping people and happily shares whatever she can, in this case fertile eggs. She jokes about days of feeling sick and bloated from superovulation drugs while dragging herself to college classes; she is not the type to change her mind at the last minute, to back out on a promise. Then, allowing a brief flash of tension to break through, she warns, "Beware of freelance donors." Voicing in an almost offhand way the most dreaded peril underlying previous talk of donor screening and emotional stability and responsibility, she advises the audience, "Be sure to find someone who won't come after [you] saying 'I want my child.' "

Questions from the audience follow. What this audience has just experienced is a sales pitch. It did receive information about egg donation, well selected to promote the medical team's recruitment message for women near or past the age of forty. Women and men listening to this message want badly to have a baby. Here now is another possibility, another hope. The evening ends with clusters of prospective patients surrounding a doctor or nurse, therapist or donor, posing their more personal concerns. Once the technology exists, who is to say these individuals shouldn't use it?

If one steps back, however, the most prominent aspects of the presentation make difficult any efforts to wrestle with such questions. To begin with, certain information was conspicuously absent. There was no mention of complexities or controversy in the way IVF success rates are tallied and reported; the doctor did not explain that the percentages displayed on the screen, reflecting their program's pregnancy rates, were calculated in the most favorable light. A physician quickly bypassed one slide, allowing only a fleeting glimpse of its title, "Limitations of success with ART," and arrows pointing to more complicated procedures for assisted fertilization, such as micromanipulation of eggs and sperm. This slide might suggest how long and expensive the venture could become for patients who, as the doctor put it (to a murmur of audience recognition), come to him with medical histories "measured by inches rather than pages." By whatever calculation, all of those women and men who do sign on for treatment will go through difficult times, and most will not succeed.

The audience did not hear about risks of treatment that use egg donation, other than multiple births, most often twins (an outcome not terribly forbidding to people who fear they can never have a child); there was no discussion of obstetric problems for older women and for any multiple pregnancy, or of fetal reduction, newborn deaths, or lifelong health problems among babies born very prematurely—particularly in multiple pregnancies. Asked about increased rates of ovarian cancer among women who used fertility drugs, one of the doctors gave a cursory response, commenting only that a recently published study "has been criticized" for a number of reasons he then quickly listed.

The presentation did not mention that in-house or affiliated therapists might not provide the objectivity needed by prospective egg recipients and donors alike. Rather it reflected the pressures from fertility medicine to keep trying. Psychologists emphasize the importance of helping infertile couples end their quest for a pregnancy when success remains elusive or biology provides undeniable closure.[42] Now there may be no clear end, even at menopause. Younger women—in their thirties, with or without partners—feel their fertility is slipping away. This new focus on age may well pressure them into treatment they do not need or push those even younger into early childbearing, unsupported by adequate child care or flexible career patterns.

For some in this audience, egg donation *is* presently their only hope for pregnancy. A 25-year-old may be seeking medical treatment for premature menopause. In what should be the most fertile of her reproductive years, her ovaries are unable to produce mature eggs. Sitting next to her is a woman three decades older and several years past her natural menopause. She may want to become pregnant for various reasons—perhaps she recently married a younger man who wants children or recently lost a teen-aged only child, as was the case for a 62-year-old Italian woman who gave birth in 1994; or perhaps her children are grown and she enjoys having babies. The medical team will welcome both women, if they meet this particular program's evaluation criteria—and if they can pay.

The presentation emphasized individual choice. Unlike previous generations of doctors, today's ob-gyns may avoid the charge of paternalism, of making decisions that should be their patients'. They may also avoid making professional judgments about whether a treatment should be offered, given its balance of potential benefit and risk. "Leaving the decision up to you," rather than restricting the number of embryos transferred or the age at which women receive certain fertility treatments, may be a selling point for prospective patients as they shop for a fertility clinic. "Choice" may, however, be too glibly portrayed.

How good is the choice between potentially harmful options with very little chance for success, with inadequate information about possible outcomes, a choice made by patients whom doctors describe as "desperate to become pregnant," patients who "never say no," who believe a long-shot intervention "will work for me," statistics notwithstanding? Who is defining acceptable developments in fertility medicine? And once a medical technology exists, who should ultimately decide it is worth a try?

Patient Choice, Physician Choices

Physicians may emphasize patient choice and insist that society define which reproductive interventions are acceptable, even as they proceed with new variations and extensions. Physicians also decide every day who will and will not use new reproductive technologies, establishing limits that they often base on nonmedical considerations. In fertility research and clinical practice, medical and nonmedical criteria may blur. The selection of social characteristics is especially prominent with a new technique, when physicians are determining which kinds of patients will be eligible.

For example, a major report on postmenopausal pregnancies demonstrates how doctors' decisions can reach beyond their medical expertise. In the list of eleven factors discovered during pretreatment evaluations that led the clinician-researchers to exclude women from the study were some significant health problems, such as diabetes, prolapsed uterus, and abdominal mass, as well as other physical or mental health characteristics such as smoking and psychological concerns. Also listed is a rather different affliction: "No husband." As described in the report's "Subjects and Methods" section, based on their medical, reproductive, and psychological screening to identify "suitable candidates" for treatment, these physicians selected only those women who "satisfied the following criteria: good physical and psychological health; nonobese; *married;* no preexisting major medical illnesses; nonsmoking; and no family history of significant cardiovascular, metabolic, renal, or hypertensive disorders" (emphasis added).[1] While concluding that "each case should be evaluated on the strength of its own merits, without discriminating against the chronologic age of the patient," the doctors were discriminating on another basis—marital status (and, secondarily, sexual orientation)—in limiting treatment to married, heterosexual couples.

An editorial accompanying this report implies definitions that extend even further. Dr. Martin Quigly, a former president of the American Society for Reproductive Medicine's group on assisted reproduction, elaborates on the study's definition of "suitable candidates" for the revolutionary new reproductive technology. He presents a stark contrast between this "special group" of married, heterosexual, healthy, nonsmoking, nonobese older middle-class women and another category of patients, portrayed as "the 'typical' prenatal population in whom some centers have reported an incidence of cocaine use as high as 50 percent. Certainly," Quigly continues, "even a 55-year-old woman who is able to pass the study group's screening criteria would be far more likely to have a successful pregnancy outcome than a poorly nourished, cocaine-addicted woman with limited prenatal care. This latter woman may be chronologically in her early 20s, but is far more likely to have a complicated pregnancy with a poor neonatal outcome."[2] The defining lines are clearly drawn as are, by implication, the type of people deserving of medical resources. Not the poor, urban, addicted young women who, some observers might have concluded, need food, drug treatment, and prenatal care more than other women need postmenopausal pregnancies.

Thus, as new reproductive technologies evolve, doctors are defining the dimensions for fertility treatments by their answers to questions that are medical, nonmedical, and in between. Their answers vary on some questions—for example, will there be age limits for assisted reproduction, and if so, what will they be? Some fertility specialists refuse to treat women after the age of about forty-three, using their own eggs, because chances of success are too low. With egg donation, some specialists see no upper limit to the possibilities; others have decided to limit fertility treatment to women's natural reproductive life (i.e., they will not provide treatment to allow postmenopausal pregnancies). Individual doctors reach different decisions about the physical and psychological requirements an egg donor must meet, especially whether to use women who have never previously been pregnant and had a child. Doctors differ about providing advanced technologies—particularly those requiring egg donation—to women who already have children. On other questions, doctors generally agree—for example, that patients must be able to pay out of pocket for medical procedures their health insurance does not cover.

---

1. Sauer, Paulson, and Lobo 1992, 1276. Indeed, having "no husband" was equivalent on their list with having a husband with no sperm.
2. Quigly 1992.

Seeing Our Future Now

No woman has ever been able to prevent the loss of fertility that comes with growing older. For the baby-boom generation and all who follow, however, the once clear-cut, unavoidable relationship between menopause and the ability to bear a child is forever altered. The current attention to older women provides some insights that can help individuals of any age respond to profound changes already realized and those soon to come. Emerging statistical and biological information about the impact of age on fertility can contribute to decisions individuals make about having a child, helping some women avoid the most serious problems of delayed childbearing. It is important to think ahead—if possible before feeling biological time pressures—about the age at which one would like to have children if life circumstances cooperate. Younger women can give themselves more time to conceive without seeking medical advice (at least one year) than can women past their mid-thirties. Women should not assume they will conceive immediately and should be aware that most women will take longer to become pregnant in their thirties than in their twenties; statistically, age-related problems become more likely after the age of thirty-seven, even more so after forty. (But one should never assume that conception *won't* happen quickly either; don't start trying before feeling prepared to care for a child.)

Women who suspect they may have a fertility problem should consult an experienced gynecologist about whether to begin a diagnostic evaluation. Those nearing or past the age of forty should ask a fertility specialist about current testing procedures that can predict individual chances of conceiving with and without treatment and what the results may suggest about whether, when, and how to intervene. Deciding when to begin such an evaluation can be a first step in an individual timeline, worked out in consultation with the physician. Timeline decisions cannot be set in any precise, definitive way, but can provide a framework for and limits to the efforts pursued. The diagnostic process itself may span several months. As part of this process, doctor and patient should discuss the chances for conceiving without medical treatment. Then, depending on the woman's age and the couple's fertility condition—and the chances for a spontaneous pregnancy—doctor and patient need to allow an appropriate amount of time for natural conception before starting the least invasive recommended intervention.

No treatment should be repeated indefinitely. In most cases, specialists now think, a treatment is most likely to succeed during the first three or four attempts; if it does not result in conception, patients need to be ready to move on: to choose the next, more aggressive treatment, reassess whether to end fertility treatment, seek a second opinion, find another physician, consider adoption, or decide not have a child. Similarly, nonmedical alternative therapies (e.g., herbal treatments, acupuncture) should not be continued indefinitely as a substitute for medical evaluation and appropriate treatment. Although these approaches may contribute to an individual's general health and well-being, no systematic research has evaluated their benefits for demonstrated fertility problems.

It is important, once again, to remember that treatments arising initially as tentative and limited experiments, usually at university research centers, do filter out into the community, where gynecologists begin using them more widely, often without giving enough attention to limits of usefulness or the potential for complications. Treatments take on a life of their own in a world of their own, a world where doctors, support staff, and patients are highly motivated to act in the single-minded pursuit of pregnancy. Patients will need to take the initiative in seeking reasons for each recommended procedure in their particular case and in obtaining information about its side effects and success rates.

Meanwhile, information about women's age and fertility is creating its own subindustry, a competitive business that requires and seeks customers. In the United States, egg "donation" might more accurately be called egg vending or marketing. If initially women provided eggs for a relative or friend without payment, the treatment has now generated brokers and agencies that mediate the flow of services; in the mid-1990s, young women generally received at least $2,500 for each cycle of ovarian hyperstimulation and egg retrieval, with fees continuing to creep higher. (Other countries severely restrict payment for sperm or eggs in order to limit commercialism and its potential for creating coercive financial inducements; see Chapter 8.) Doctors offer fertility programs that will attract patients, and patients comparison shop. Yet which treatment program to choose is a different question from whether to choose any. Within this insular marketplace, boundaries are unclear between consumer information and customer solicitation, between educating potential patients and trying to convince them to undergo treatment. And, as the Irvine clinic revelations dramatized in 1995, doctors do at times cross a line between doing all they can to attain a pregnancy and taking unethical medical liberties.

Help Wanted: Women

For decades, college campuses—particularly prestigious, selective ones—have been a source of sperm "donations," a quick and easy way for young, healthy men to earn spending money. By the mid-1990s, college newspaper want ads had gone coed. Young, healthy women would garner more than spending money for their fertile eggs. While a sperm deposit earned up to $50 in 1997, the going price for eggs had reached $3,000—more for special characteristics or hard-to-come-by ethnicities. For instance, clustered alongside the usual employment notices (e.g., for bartenders or, more related, baby-sitters), the student newspaper at the University of California at Berkeley has run on a daily basis a dozen or so classified advertisements that include

Egg Donors Desperately Wanted by infertile, hopeful parents . . .

Give the Gift of Life to a loving couple longing for a child . . .

When Your Heart is Open to helping an infertile couple build their family . . . We need women with blond or brunette hair with green or blue eyes . . .

East Indian, Chinese, Japanese and Korean Egg Donors Needed A.S.A.P. . . .

High IQ Women Needed . . . Infertile couple needs your altruistic help . . . preferably 5'5" or over, nonsmoker, athletic, avg. wgt., N. European heritage . . . $4,000 paid . . .

Seeking German/Irish/Scotch ethnic mix. Liberal arts major with creative writing skills . . .

The disparity in compensation for sperm and egg—and the actual amount offered for egg donors—highlights troubling features of this new fertility development, whether the provider of eggs is college educated or not.

To begin with, egg donation is not quick, easy, or risk-free; besides the immediate side effects attending superovulation and egg retrieval, today's donation could mean increased health risks or fertility problems when the egg provider is older. Although advocates of this reproductive technique justify the payment as fair compensation for a donor's time and trouble (rather than a "fee," which sounds too much like the selling and buying of eggs), the considerable amount offered suggests that the trouble, including potential risks, is too great to be justifiable.

In addition, unlike the millions of sperm in a single semen deposit, egg donation may seem less anonymous, random, and unconnected—resulting in greater focus on desirable physical and social characteristics. While some sperm banks recruit "high IQ" (even Nobel Prize–winning) men and provide donor profiles to potential customers, the active and immediate participation of the donor may make it easier to imagine the child as developed from a particular woman's egg— a woman who, in fact, becomes a patient undergoing medical procedures with the same doctors; whose menstrual cycle becomes synchronized to the recipient's; whose egg retrievals occur as the recipient begins her wait, through the hours after those eggs meet her partner's sperm in vitro, for the moment when the fertilized eggs are transferred to her body.

Unlike sperm, moreover, fertile eggs are in short supply. The supply-and-demand dynamics of this medical marketplace contribute to a sense of "desperation" among infertile patients who want these treatments. Doctors eager, or desperate, to accommodate their patients and attract new ones, employ questionable if not outright unethical methods to obtain eggs, including loose donor-recruitment policies; aggressive, high-yield superovulation regimens; and, in one known instance, taking eggs or embryos from other patients without their consent when no donor was available.

Finally, individual doctors and brokers are defining their own requirements for egg providers. The limits and protections—for donors and recipients—are completely arbitrary and highly variable. For example, some doctors will use donors as young as eighteen, others set a minimum age of twenty-one; some require the woman to already have had a child (both to prove her fertility and to avoid unpredictable psychological reaction), others state "no prior pregnancy necessary." Egg donors have become subjects of study, to determine who enters a program's donor pool or whom a prospective recipient should choose.[1] However, complex questions about the well-being of these young women and of reproductive medicine itself are too important to be left to the medical profession. In addition to the question of the physical and psychological impact on women who "donate" eggs during their late teens and twenties, questions arise about the pressure that comes with financial need—a pressure not compatible with informed, coercion-free consent—and about creating an underclass of women who provide eggs, at some personal risk, to women of a higher socioeconomic class.

---

1. For example, one study finds that donors with previous pregnancies are more likely to provide eggs that result in successful pregnancies than are donors who have never been pregnant (Darder et al. 1996). Another study included analysis of the impact of donor's age on success rates, finding the ideal age—associated with the best outcomes—to be twenty to twenty-three (Stolwijk et al. 1997). The very asking of such clinical questions can only contribute to categorizing fertile donors and their eggs as commodities with greater and lesser sales appeal to those selecting and purchasing.

There is surely much to say for patient choice and for a doctor recommending treatment on a case-by-case basis. However, with new fertility interventions, particularly those that can dramatically change women's natural reproductive lives, this focus on each individual desiring a baby loses sight of broader questions about medical progress, the fair and wise use of medical resources, and limits that will protect individuals from harm. Medicine and technology have reached the point where an admission that "there is nothing we can do" needs increasingly to be replaced with a question: "Should we do all that is scientifically and technically possible?" Entering the 1990s, fertility medicine was creating what one well-known specialist, Ricardo Asch, described, with almost literary foreshadowing, as reproductive anarchy—the same Dr. Asch who later became the major character in the field's most glaring public scandal. By the mid-1990s, concerns about the way fertility medicine was unfolding led some physicians, as well as the American Society for Reproductive Medicine, to suggest creating forums for public debate about the specialty's many social and ethical dilemmas.[43] Even as case-by-case interventions were accumulating, "let society decide" was a slogan more frequently heard about new reproductive technologies. However, both the slogans and the public forums remained empty.

As with other areas of medicine, resources and information flow overwhelmingly toward treatment, not prevention. While the decline in women's fertility that comes with age is not preventable, women and men can take steps to moderate the impact on their individual chances for a successful pregnancy. (See Appendix 4.) However, as information about women's age and fertility accumulates, the focus on fertility treatment also neglects another approach, less individual in some respects, yet ultimately promoting greater individual choice. This approach requires that women, early in their reproductive lives, *not* assume their only choice is a medical fallback of invasive, expensive, highly technological fertility treatment. Beyond individual efforts (as well as government health policy) to prevent problems that can exacerbate the fertility loss that comes with age, preventing delays in childbearing for those who do want to have children sooner rather than later can be a societal goal. Attaining this goal would require social, economic, and educational changes, rather than medical answers. The focus would shift to seeing individuals as potential parents, rather than potential patients. First, information about fertility, contraceptive choices, pelvic inflammatory disease (PID), and prevention and treatment of sexually transmitted disease would be widely available to teenagers as well as adults. Women and men in their twenties and early thirties would have employment and educational choices that include flexible schedules, job sharing, part-time work, generous maternal and paternal leaves, and work-at-home options (especially with widespread use of personal computer networks); high-quality child care at or near work sites; affordable health care that emphasizes prevention of infertility—and that provides health care for children. Such changes could help reduce the pressure on young women to choose between children and career, reducing also the number of potential patients who, for reasons of physiology, truly need to rely on fertility treatment as their only hope for pregnancy.

6 Of Mice and Men and, Especially, Women

Learning from Research Past, Present, and Future

Straddling a prominent urban hill that commands panoramic views of skyline, park, and ocean sits one of the country's leading medical centers, the University of California, San Francisco. Buffeted most days by cool Pacific winds, its sidewalks buzz with a continuous flow of doctors, medical students, hospital staff, visitors, and patients going to and from a multitude of specialty clinics. Occasionally, an ambulance wails. Less visible are the research scientists, surrounded by laboratory equipment, never seeing a patient. They work in spaces less presentable than areas the public generally sees—off hallways lined with file cabinets, locked refrigerators, bicycles; behind doors plastered with "biohazard" warnings; amid jumbles of beakers and jars, centrifuges, computers, a microscope, bowls of food pellets for laboratory mice. Their goal is to find answers to basic research questions, independent of practical application to medical problems.

Tucked into the thirteenth floor of one of the center's massive buildings, Dr. Gerald Cunha and dozen or so developmental biologists conduct experiments with a chemical substance well known to fertility patients—clomiphene citrate. The scientists in Cunha's lab are not pursuing treatments for infertility, nor are they all that interested in clomiphene per se; their passion is to determine how the human organism develops from the earliest stage of conception. The narrow piece of the scientific puzzle that is the focus of this group's work is the reproductive tract. More particularly, they want to know how physiological signals influence development of the right kind of cells, tissue, and organ systems from a single fertilized egg to what we all recognize as a newborn girl or boy. This focus leads them to experiments with clomiphene and other hormonal substances, such as diethylstilbestrol; for much of their research they use ingeniously bred mice to model growth processes they cannot observe directly in the developing human fetus. A by-product of their experiments, however, is concern about use of clomiphene in humans, across the street and beyond.[1] Cunha thinks clomiphene is probably relatively safe when taken before ovulation—compared, for instance, to taking DES during pregnancy. But, he says, "You are rolling the dice." He wonders about repetitive use with increased dosages (as Clomid has for years been prescribed) or inadvertent exposures after a woman conceives. He and other scientists wonder how close people want to get to a threshold beyond which a fertility medication can be harmful.

Though unseen and unheard within the doctor's office, the work of these scientists connects in vital ways to the discussion going on there. In fact, there is a world of scientific inquiry with which fertility patients should at least be acquainted. In addition to animal models and other laboratory research, epidemiological studies trace what actually happens in human populations, at times providing preliminary evidence of harm from a medical or environmental exposure. A striking feature of fertility medicine is how little the insights of scientists inform actual deliberations by patients and doctors, particularly when it comes to considering risks. Patients are mostly unaware of the scientists and their work. Physicians may be aware, if only vaguely, but seem generally to ignore hints provided by related scientific research.

As the previous chapters have described, from conventional therapies to the now routine IVF to more technologically sophisticated manipulations of eggs and sperm, fertility medicine has tended toward jumping in too soon, with too little previously established scientific groundwork, too little regard for potential harm, and too little effort to demonstrate significant benefits. Thousands of articles on highly invasive and technological interventions have filled volume after volume of obstetric-gynecologic journals during the last two decades; among their most notable features is the extent of experimentation, especially on women, despite substantial gaps in knowledge about the biological processes underlying these fertility interventions. These experiments are uncontrolled, in far more than the scientific sense, as individual doctors try out treatments on individual patients on a daily basis, with no evaluation or documentation of outcomes.

In this chapter readers can step back to view this broader world of research. The discussion returns to an example introduced at the book's outset—the synthetic hormone diethylstilbestrol (DES), used for more than three decades to treat or prevent pregnancy problems—because this large-scale human experiment so persistently illustrates concerns that continue to be paramount in fertility medicine.

If the biologists in Cunha's lab have little contact with doctors and patients sharing the same buildings, they do communicate with other scientists engaged in related research. Over periodic pizza lunches they discuss experimental techniques and findings with a group of researchers across San Francisco Bay, even further removed from patients receiving medical treatments. On the University of California's Berkeley campus, Dr. Howard Bern has devoted a long research career to studying the role of hormones in the development of cancer. In the process, he established closer connections than most research scientists—closer than he might wish—to the world of clinical medicine. His research with DES in mice pushed him across the divide, as he attempted to alert physicians about potential dangers of this estrogenic substance. Findings in his zoological laboratory raised a red flag about risks for humans. Beginning in the 1960s, he wrote letters to medical and scientific journals warning that use of DES during pregnancy might lead to cancer or other reproductive tract abnormalities in human offspring exposed to this medication before birth. In 1971, the value of animal models for predicting human outcomes gained unhappy verification when Dr. Arthur Herbst, an obstetrician-gynecologist working with epidemiologists, helped trace a rare vaginal cancer in young women to their prenatal DES exposure.[2]

Though officially retired, Bern remains a patriarch—or perhaps an irrepressible mother hen—to a far-flung network of former students who, in turn, join other scientists studying estrogens, progesterones, androgens, and other hormones. Research continues to identify previously unknown hormonal effects on a range of physiological systems. By now, several decades of research with animal models and biochemical experiments have suggested risks for humans from reproductive therapies that employ such substances. These scientists seem far more chary than are fertility specialists of altering intricate endocrine and immunologic interactions in humans.[3] When doctors hear these warnings, their response frequently sounds some variation of the theme "mice are not people." While direct extrapolation from animal experiments to humans is not always possible, animal models often provide the only hints we have about potential harm from reproductive interventions, short of experimenting on people or waiting for epidemiological evidence to materialize. DES is a prime example, not only of these scientific hints, but of the danger of ignoring them. Yet similar experiments—which may, for example, result in hormone levels that differ from those usually circulating in the body early in a pregnancy—are common today, every day, in doctors' offices, fertility clinics, and major medical centers throughout the world, as the large number of current reports on assisted reproduction, ovarian stimulation, gamete micromanipulation, and immunotherapy attest.

Doctors might even be accused of wanting to eat their cake and still have it. Though cattle are not people either, many current and upcoming reproductive technologies were pioneered in the world of livestock breeding, as well as in experiments with smaller creatures. Potential harm is not the only link between fertility patients and research using nonhuman animals. Animal studies point to prospects, as well as problems, for fertility medicine. On both scores, the fact that mice are not people can only magnify the question left to us: When and how should people intervene *intentionally* in human reproduction? It is a question for women and men as individuals and, on a broader level, for the direction of future medical endeavors. Thinking about this question does not require immersion in the more sophisticated scientific content, but rather a grasp of the basics—the three Rs, if you will—of fertility treatment: research, risk, and resources.

The Question of Research

Basic scientists have it easy when it comes to designing controlled experiments. Within their laboratories, they can systematically manipulate what they wish to study, observe outcomes among varying comparison groups (animals, tissue, or cells that receive experimental treatments and control groups that do not), and reach verifiable conclusions about the effects of their experimental manipulations. For physicians and their patients, approaching an ideal of systematic scientific research is much more difficult. In the practice of medicine, furthermore, decisions reached by individual doctors and their patients can never be a pure, consistently rigorous science: these decisions inevitably involve judgment calls and hope-filled trial and error. However, the complexity of humans, their health and well-being make it all the more important to consider carefully the choice to experiment with medical manipulations.

There has been some shift in emphasis toward more systematic clinical research (studies that, in contrast to basic science, are concerned with applications to medical diagnoses and treatments) in the 1990s. Rising medical costs and the threat of health care reform—or of insurance plans refusing to pay for experimental or unproven procedures—focused fertility specialists' attention on trying to determine what interventions *are* effective, especially cost-effective. Indeed, when one of this country's most prestigious medical journals, the *New England Journal of Medicine,* published two special articles on fertility medicine in July 1994, their topic was the high overall costs of reproductive technologies.[4] An accompanying editorial concluded: "It is customary, of course, to call for further research, but with respect to persistent infertility, research is central to the problem, because there are few conditions that are so prevalent yet lack a defined causal mechanism and a specific, effective treatment."[5]

Current Efforts—and Shortcomings

Couples who face decisions today about fertility treatments can benefit from the recent shift, in some clinical research, toward measuring efficacy, simplifying techniques, and reducing harmful and costly side effects. This research will provide more solid information upon which to base decisions about diagnoses and treatments. However, many questions are late in coming. The focus of recent studies involving commonly used treatments demonstrates just how significant these questions and their answers are to doctors' recommendations and patients' decisions. Seeking answers *before* treatments became widespread could have saved many women physical, emotional, and financial hardship. Examples include recent attempts to

Evaluate the varying, widely used ovarian-stimulation regimens, to compare success and complication rates for differing drug combinations and dosages.[6]

Identify patient subgroups (especially by the woman's age and by the woman's and man's diagnoses) with differing likelihoods of success and complications from particular fertility treatments; this information will help doctors provide a recommendation and prognosis to individual patients, and help patients decide whether a treatment is worth trying. Recent clinical research is attempting to determine who can successfully undergo assisted reproduction during the natural menstrual cycle, or with minimal medication, rather than with the aggressive superovulation that has become routine; which individuals are likely to need the expensive and inconvenient injections of GnRH-a before fertility drugs during superovulation; which women should receive few transferred embryos, based on their chances for conceiving large multiple pregnancies; and which women are likely to experience a third or fourth miscarriage, including after IVF, and so are more likely to benefit from trying experimental, potentially harmful immunologic treatments.[7]

Compare through randomized clinical trials, whenever possible, assisted reproductive technologies. For example, a 1993 study found standard in vitro fertilization and embryo transfer to the uterus to be as effective as the more complex, invasive, and expensive variation called ZIFT, in which embryos are transferred to the fallopian tube; an accompanying editorial cites use of ZIFT as "just one more example of how preliminary results may inappropriately influence clinical practice."[8] Specific components of assisted reproduction, such as the timing of various widely used medications, also came under closer scrutiny.[9]

Modify common procedures to lower risks and expense of treatment while maintaining acceptable success rates (e.g., lower drug dosage and/or alter drug administration schedule to avoid hyperstimulation syndrome and multiple pregnancies; transfer fewer embryos during IVF to lower the rate of ectopic and large multiple pregnancies; refine technique for placement of embryos in uterus to lower the rate of ectopic pregnancies).[10]

Determine a maximum number of failed attempts after which continuing a particular treatment is likely to be futile.[11]

Two studies from the mid-1990s demonstrate how basic are the biological questions still needing better answers. The first asks in its title, "How often should infertile men have intercourse to achieve conception?" The answer challenges years of doctors' advice that subfertile couples limit frequency of sexual intercourse at the time of ovulation (e.g., to once every 48 hours). This advice may, in fact, have limited their chances for a spontaneous pregnancy. According to the study's authors, a previously unquestioned "myth"—that ejaculation affects sperm production similarly in subfertile and normally fertile men— does not hold. To the contrary: men with low numbers of sperm or sperm that move sluggishly "may increase their fertility potential . . . by having intercourse every day or even twice a day, at the time of ovulation." If this new conclusion holds up under further scrutiny, some couples may be able to avoid medical treatment altogether. Additional recent research suggests, moreover, that physicians' long-standing advice to fertile and subfertile couples may have inaccurately delineated the days of a woman's menstrual cycle when she is most likely to conceive, perhaps lowering her chances for pregnancy.[12]

The second report, on ovarian stimulation using human menopausal gonadotropin (hMG, brand name Pergonal) in women who do not ovulate on their own compared with women who do, shows how physicians ignore critical biological differences among women when prescribing this drug. The result: a treatment that benefits a small group of patients brings no benefit (though, as always, risk) to a much larger number of women who also receive that treatment. Women who do not ovulate or menstruate for one fairly distinct physiological reason (traced to the hypothalamus, a region of the brain intricately involved with hormone production and regulation) responded very well to ovarian stimulation. However, for women diagnosed with other ovulatory problems, "hMG therapy may be unsuccessful at correcting the underlying defect and restoring normal fertility. Although hMG therapy is considered one of the treatments of choice for these . . . disorders, the prognosis for conception appears limited."[13] Yet doctors prescribe this therapy broadly to women with diverse fertility problems, despite the authors' caution against attempting to superimpose hormonal therapy on a woman's own menstrual cycle.

Doctors' widespread use of ovarian stimulants in general lacks the biological underpinnings that should guide such hormonal intervention. Nearly a decade after warning about the "use and abuse" of clomiphene citrate (Clomid), Dr. Melvin Taymor goes back, in a sense, to square one, reviewing for clinicians what scientists know about the natural maturation and release of a single egg during a woman's menstrual cycle. Improved care of patients, he argues, is possible only if doctors vary fertility drug regimens according to the particular medical goal (e.g., ovulation of one egg in a cycle for women who do not ovulate on their own; maturation of many eggs for assisted reproduction) and to a woman's physiological characteristics (e.g., age, hormonal responsiveness, her particular fertility problem). Although he does grant that women can benefit from ovarian stimulation, the dosage is often too high and the timing poorly adjusted to the endocrine cycle. After all these years, even the extremely common Clomid prescription may not hit the days or dosage most effective for the individual woman. Whatever the medication, Taymor concludes, with a comment surprising only in its obviousness, "Rather than using one protocol for all conditions of ovulation induction, the choice of protocol should be based upon the specific clinical problem."[14]

What direct impact might the focus and quality of existing research have on actual care for individual fertility patients? For example, suppose a laparoscopy reveals signs of endometriosis. This condition can be very painful in its more severe forms, particularly as tissue swells in response to a woman's monthly hormone cycle, and some women seek treatment to alleviate this pain. Other women, however, may not experience pain or any other symptoms. Although endometriosis is linked in some undetermined way to fertility, the relationship is most uncertain for the milder stages; indeed, recent research suggests that mild endometriosis may be a common condition that has no symptoms and does not affect fertility.[15] Yet, since the advent of laparoscopy, doctors are diagnosing many more women during infertility workups as having mild or moderate endometriosis. They then treat the endometriosis as a cause of infertility.

Over the years, various treatments, including hormonal medications, surgeries, and, more recently, assisted reproduction, have gained and sometimes lost popularity among physicians, while studies of the treatments have been poorly designed. Explanations have, in the words of one review article, been "glib" and treatment results disappointing.[16] Not only is the relationship of endometriosis to fertility a mystery; physicians do not know whether certain fertility treatments may worsen the endometriosis or cause other health problems in women with this condition. A discussion of one treatment, intrauterine insemination following superovulation, demonstrates the depth of uncertainty: "Whether minimal or mild endometriosis in infertile women is the cause of, or the result of their infertility remains uncertain. . . . As in the case with unexplained infertility, expectant management [i.e., no treatment] . . . offers acceptable pregnancy rates. IVF and GIFT have been proposed as a successful and established treatment of women with endometriosis. . . . [Other] preliminary studies suggest that superovulation alone . . . may improve [fertility]. . . . *The risks, if any, that hMG stimulation . . . has on the natural history of endometriosis are uncertain*" (emphasis added).[17]

The succession of treatments for endometriosis now includes Lupron, a medication that suppresses the production of hormones leading to ovulation and menstruation. Physicians think the monthly rise in hormonal activity aggravates endometriosis. Aside from the question of whether this therapy ultimately improves a woman's fertility, critics cite the risk from Lupron of developing osteoporosis. One Stanford University physician cautions that without adequate monitoring for loss of bone mass, this treatment "may needlessly [put women] at risk for osteoporosis later in life."[18] Some physicians are now experimenting with the addition of estrogen, clomiphene, or other drugs to counter this worrisome side effect.

Although proponents acknowledge that women receiving Lupron (or other types of GnRH-a) should be monitored for signs of bone density loss, most clinicians are unlikely to provide the needed tests and may keep women on this therapy beyond a point where potential benefit outweighs risk. Physicians also may not adequately assess who should and should not be taking Lupron in the first place. This assessment requires more than a baseline measurement. Not surprisingly, the danger of osteoporosis may be heightened as women approach their forties, when natural bone loss accelerates and time is short for reversing loss caused by treatment. But risks may also be high for young women who have not yet reached their peak in bone density (which is generally achieved during a woman's mid-twenties).[19] Indeed, the risk for fertility patients is a double bind. On the one hand, more women now undergo fertility treatment, including use of Lupron, when they are older, facing greater risk from bone loss. On the other hand, given fertility medicine's increasing focus on women's age, doctors may also treat endometriosis aggressively with Lupron in younger patients, women in their early twenties, so they can attempt pregnancy before they hit their thirties; with a natural peak in bone density thus undermined, these women, too, may ultimately be facing greater risk of osteoporosis.

Questions remain about other side effects of Lupron. For example, a preliminary study published in 1996 suggests that "memory disruption may be a more common side effect of GnRH-a treatment than currently is recognized," caused by the rapid drop in estrogen this drug brings.[20] Clearly, there have not been enough well-designed clinical studies or basic biological research to provide a good sense of the benefits and risks in treating endometriosis. If physicians understood the reason women develop this condition and what its relationship to fertility really is, they could perhaps develop better treatment, more directly targeted to a cause, instead of broad, scattershot therapies that may compromise a woman's fertility or her more general health. How significant is mild or even moderate endometriosis in lowering fertility? Is the endometriosis a cause of infertility that treatment will help, or is this abnormally located tissue a symptom of some other underlying condition—perhaps hormonal and/or immunologic—that interferes with pregnancy? Women might also avoid a different extreme in treatment: one doctor advised a patient she would never conceive and recommended hysterectomy to relieve the pain of her endometriosis; the woman gave birth to two healthy babies following in vitro fertilization.[21]

A diagnosis of endometriosis is usually followed by fertility treatments, often IVF and GIFT (although a 1994 study showed less success with GIFT in women with endometriosis).[22] If these treatments are not successful, a new term may surface in the doctor's office—IVF failures (a label all the more difficult for patients in hinting that the failure lies with them rather than with the procedure). Physicians may be learning from this phenomenon just how complex the reproductive process is, and perhaps formulating new ideas for overcoming problems that arise, but patients need to question the way fertility medicine progresses.

Could research have laid a better groundwork so that a proportion of IVF failures might have been avoided? Could sperm that do not fertilize eggs be less of a surprise, repeated early miscarriage better predicted? Nearly two decades after the first in vitro success, for example, with hundreds of clinics performing hundreds of thousands of assisted reproductive treatments worldwide, fertility specialists cannot answer this basic question: Why does IVF so often fail? They stimulate women's ovaries, watch egg follicles enlarge on the ultrasound screen, measure the rise and fall of hormone levels in blood samples. They extract and fertilize the eggs. They transfer multiple embryos into the uterus—then wait, knowing implantation is where this process often ends in failure. For all the ultrasound scans and hormone assays, such fundamentals as monitoring a treatment cycle's progress—deciding when an attempt should proceed or whether to cancel—are not based on solid understanding of the biological processes being watched and measured. Among these processes, the significance of the amount of estrogen circulating in a woman's bloodstream is poorly understood. This hormone's function is to prepare the uterine lining (the endometrium) to accept and nourish an embryo—but what hormone levels are most desirable? Doctors may cancel a patient's treatment cycle after ovarian stimulation based, at least in part, on low hormone levels measured in blood samples; yet the endometrium may be just fine. Or doctors and patients cheer a steep estrogen rise that may actually be impairing conditions necessary for successful implantation. Doctors may, in other words, be stimulating undesirable outcomes and accumulating the wrong measurements. "As obvious as this conclusion may seem," comments a 1996 review of the role of hormones in assisted reproduction, "the goal of effective treatment and monitoring strategies" should focus elsewhere—at the site where the embryo must implant.[23]

A Case Report

The medical literature not only demonstrates the need for greater biological understanding before experimentation on women; these journals also provide reminders of how profoundly individual lives are affected by fertility medicine's usual approach. Through the cold clinical jargon of one case report comes a glimpse of what one woman has been through in her attempt to become pregnant. The report's authors, fertility specialists, present this case as a short journal article to alert colleagues that a procedure intended to prevent severe ovarian hyperstimulation syndrome—administering albumin intravenously at the time of egg retrieval—does not always work.[1] Their patient is "a 30-year-old gravida two, para zero with regular menses"—meaning she has been pregnant twice, but never delivered a baby, and her menstrual cycle is normal. "Past gynecological history is significant for an episode of pelvic inflammatory disease at the age of 17. Her two pregnancies resulted in two ectopic gestations, which necessitated a left salpingostomy [removal of the affected fallopian tube] in 1988 followed by a right salpingostomy in 1993." The report outlines this patient's fertility treatment, including several blood tests for hormone levels, ultrasound of the ovaries, suppression of her natural pituitary hormones using GnRH-a (Lupron), followed by two weeks of ovarian stimulants (injections totaling 27 ampules) and a shot of hCG (human chorionic gonadotropin) to trigger the final maturation of eggs.

> Thirty-six hours later, 22 oocytes were collected transvaginally. At retrieval, 50 g of human albumin . . . was administered. The patient was discharged home and underwent a day 3 ET [embryo transfer] with four embryos. She continued on 50 mg P [progesterone injections] in oil daily for luteal support. On day 12 after ET the patient complained of bloating, abdominal pain, nausea, and vomiting. Her vital signs were stable without evidence of hypotension [low blood pressure] or tachycardia [rapid heartbeats]. Decreased breath sounds were revealed by auscultation [listening with stethoscope] and dullness was elicited with percussion in the base of the right posterior lung field, demonstrating a right pleural effusion [fluid collecting in lung]. Abdominal exam showed a "double bubble" sign with the contour of the enlarged ovary and displaced intestines apparent on visual inspection. Her abdomen was tense but not significantly tender. Significant labial edema [swelling caused by fluid accumulation] was present. . . . Ultrasound revealed . . . the right ovary measuring 8 x 9 cm and the left ovary measuring 7 x 9 cm. . . . The diagnosis of severe ovarian hyperstimulation was made and the patient was admitted for supportive therapy. One hundred milliliters of

The process through which doctors recognized—and are learning from—IVF failures presents a classic case of rapidly proliferating interventions that are, in fact, experiments on women. As one journal editor commented a decade after the first in vitro birth: "There are now so many possible [IVF] techniques and approaches to be used that controls will be next to impossible to design, and any true comparison will be difficult to make. . . . Whether any of the alphabetical techniques are an improvement is . . . [a] completely unsolved matter."[24] During the 1990s, the acronyms multiply while matters of comparison remain unsolved. One overview, finding few comparative studies and serious methodological problems with those that exist, argues, "In recent times it would be almost unheard of to unleash drugs or devices into medicine without long and exhaustive research evaluations, yet many new techniques, including assisted reproductive techniques, are clinically adopted before such assessments are completed."[25] The latest phenomenon—injecting all manner of sperm into an egg (ICSI)—is expanding freely, in the absence of systematic controlled studies that could establish benefits (for example, which couples require this procedure, rather than a less invasive one, in order to have a baby and how much are their chances improved) and risks (including to offspring). This clinical rush to ICSI ignores questions about causes of male infertility, questions that must be answered before preventive measures or less invasive treatments can develop.[26] Immunologic treatments, too, are spreading, pushed by some physicians beyond careful attempts to piece together this fertility puzzle. More generally, another editor reminds his colleagues, "We continue to forget that if we do not follow the rules of clinical trials before determination of therapy, we will end up in disaster. Unfortunately, toward the end of the 20th century, we embark on new therapies and new medications without having rigorous tests of their worth. We join the bandwagon touting new modalities without informing our patients that some of these procedures really should be viewed as investigational."[27]

At some point, of course, solving complex matters of fertility and its treatment must include experimental or investigational attempts with humans, but this process needs to be done rigorously, before a treatment falls into common use. As one physician admonishes, "Once the genie escapes from the bottle, it is extremely difficult, and usually impossible, to put him back in."[28] What is the more rigorous approach then: the clinical trials longed for by critics? And how do patients fit in?

Randomized Controlled Trials

Though medical journals fill monthly with reports on fertility treatments in humans, few take the form of controlled studies, the type of clinical research that provides the most useful results about a treatment's effects—both desired and unintended. Patients seeing doctors affiliated with a medical school are most likely to be offered the option of entering a randomized clinical trial. The couple with unexplained infertility, for instance, arrives at their appointment to discuss the specialist's opinion about what to do next. He suggests they participate in a scientifically controlled study, testing whether a new hormonal medication, given to a woman for one week after ovulation, improves pregnancy rates in couples with unexplained infertility.

What do patients need to know about such a study? The paramount ethical requirement involves efficacy and safety; a medical institution's ethics (or "human subjects") committee normally reviews all study proposals for adherence to legal and professional standards. First, physicians must truly not know whether the treatment being tested is better than existing alternatives (or better than no treatment, if no proven treatment presently exists). That is, patients may be just as well off *not* receiving the new, unproven treatment. Second, there must be no evidence, from in vitro, animal, or preliminary human studies, that possible harm to this patient is likely to outweigh benefits of participating in the study. That is, the physician-researchers must adhere to the medical precept "First, do no harm."

In a formal randomized controlled trial, researchers need patients who are similar to one another, so that the differing interventions that make up the study are, to the extent possible, isolated as the factors responsible for differing outcomes. Patients are randomly assigned to receive an experimental treatment, an alternative treatment, or no treatment, depending on particulars of the study. The goal of randomized groupings is to avoid biases of choosing and to distribute unknown differences across all of the groups. In addition, neither the patients nor medical personnel know who is receiving what treatment (or none). The goal of this "double-blinding" is to avoid a "placebo effect," biasing the results through subtle differences in the way doctors or nurses behave toward patients they know are receiving the new treatment, who in turn respond positively, or through the possible psychological-physiological effects in patients who know what treatment they are receiving.

For the hormonal medication study, the doctor explains, this couple's diagnostic test results, length of time trying to conceive, and their age make them eligible to participate. If the woman agrees, she will sign a lengthy consent form that delineates the procedures and lists possible benefits and possible risks for study participants. After she signs on the dotted line, indicating her "informed consent" to participate, a computer will transpose her name into an identification number, then randomly assign that number to one of three groups. Group 1 receives the new medication; Group 2, a commonly used fertility drug; Group 3, a sugar-pill placebo, without medicinal substance. Since the new treatment may be no more effective than existing medications or than recommending the couple wait six months while continuing to have intercourse on the woman's most fertile days, the researchers have no ethical qualms about relying on the luck of the draw. A pharmacist will place the designated pills into a small envelope marked only with the identification number. A nurse with the list of numbers distributes these envelopes to the women. All pills look exactly alike. No one knows what pills each patient is taking until the study is completed, the pregnancy rates for the three groups calculated, and the identification code broken. The nurse will also instruct every couple on how to determine the most fertile days of their monthly cycle—information that was significantly revised in 1995 (see Chapter 4)—so that they will all be timing intercourse in the same way.

Why are randomized blinded studies of fertility treatments—including comparisons with no treatment—so rarely done? One reason, say many physicians, is that patients will not agree to participate. They want the new treatment, or at least some type of treatment, even though the least invasive and safer alternative—no treatment—may be equally effective. They do not want their options left to chance. Enrolling enough participants with similar fertility characteristics becomes difficult, often requiring a study to include several doctors and their patients, which adds logistical and methodological complications and expense. Physicians themselves also undermine the research process by claiming that unproven therapies work. Too often, fertility treatments become popular with physicians in the absence of systematic evaluation. Once a treatment becomes established, or physicians believe a treatment works, medical ethics argue against assigning patients randomly to what the doctor—or professional consensus— now regards as lesser care. And there are other obstacles to randomized controlled trials. Funding for research on fertility treatment is hard to come by. Carrying out a study properly is itself fraught with difficulties, none more challenging than avoiding the placebo effect.

None of these obstacles is unique to fertility medicine. Carrying out well-designed, scientifically controlled, ethically acceptable trials of treatment for cancer or heart disease is not easy. However, fertility patients differ from patients with cancer or heart disease in a crucial respect. They are essentially healthy women and men for whom treatment is not aimed at saving or prolonging life or at relieving physical pain. Many might reach their goal of pregnancy without medical treatment (though who these individuals are is not always clear, nor is actually attaining that goal ever guaranteed). Since harm to the woman or offspring from a treatment may not be immediately apparent, doctors and patients may be more inclined to "take a chance"—the chance that the treatment may cause health problems now or in the future. Yet, the very uncertainty of benefit for patients who start out healthy—patients pressured in various ways to try a medical treatment in spite of potential for harm—compels a close look, first at this prominent question of minimizing harm and then at the wider question of risk.

Doing No Harm

No one knows better the basic medical requirement to "do no harm" than some of the women who have been fertility patients during the past three decades. Cathy, who is now approaching fifty, has had problems from the time she was a teenager. She was the last of her friends to menstruate, and then her periods were always irregular. At her first pelvic examination, the gynecologist saw strange-looking tissue lining her vagina; her cervix looked as if it wore a hood. Her Pap tests usually show results that are unusual. After years of trying to conceive came the preterm delivery of her only child, who lives with brain and lung damage resulting from prematurity.

Cathy seemed to have every reason to expect an easy, problem-free reproductive life. Her older sister had no difficulties. Her mother never had fertility or pregnancy problems. She was a strong, healthy graduate student at the University of Chicago when Cathy was born. As a patient at the university's clinic during that pregnancy, however, she participated in a randomized study testing whether the synthetic hormone diethylstilbestrol prevented miscarriages. Though her first pregnancy had been normal, Cathy's mother was assigned, by chance, to receive the hormone; the other group took sugar pills.

This scientifically controlled study in humans, published in 1953, finally demonstrated that DES did not prevent miscarriage.[29] The findings contradicted testimonials of prominent doctors as well as drug company advertisements in medical journals that promoted DES not only for problem pregnancies but also to "make normal pregnancies more normal." This important knowledge came at a high cost, however. As study participants, hundreds of healthy women with normal pregnancies—and their babies, among them Cathy—were exposed to a medication they would not otherwise have received. With use of DES already widespread, this trial could be seen as coming too late. Seen another way, however, any time was too soon. The systematic clinical research proceeded in spite of hundreds of studies in scientific laboratories that indicated the potential for harm from DES, clear evidence that experiments on women and their prenatally exposed offspring—whether in clinical trials or in daily obstetric practice—should not proceed at all.

Women like Cathy are living examples of the result.[30] And she is not alone. Even as systematic studies of fertility treatments begin to accumulate, prodded by economic pressures, the ugly reality of unjustified human experimentation persists. Unfortunately, fertility patients must understand that this danger is not an aberration, an incidental aspect of gynecology. During the earliest years of the specialty in the United States, in the mid-nineteenth century, doctors developed new techniques through surgical experiments on slaves, with permission of their owners. "Physicians are taught to emulate [such innovation]," writes Dr. David Richardson in a 1994 essay on gynecologic ethics; far from being unusual, the profession "teaches and promulgates" this behavior. Though experimental interventions often take a nonsurgical form when applied to infertility today, his words resonate just the same: "Whether one talks about nonstandard therapies, therapeutic research, clinical investigation, nonvalidated practice, innovation, or experimentation, the semantic distinctions should not obscure the fact that . . . unscientific . . . innovation is wrong."[31]

Egregious examples of experimentation on humans continue to surface—on a scale more systematic and widespread than people once imagined. Poor Southern black men were victims of the infamous Tuskegee syphilis studies begun in the 1930s, in which physicians withheld a known effective treatment from unknowing participants in order to observe the "natural" course of this ravaging disease. The exposé of this study was one spur toward developing informed consent requirements in this country. More recently the public learned of decades-long human studies on the effects of exposure to radiation and toxic biological agents. Frequently, such vulnerable populations as the mentally ill or retarded, prison inmates, and the terminally ill have been used as research subjects; in some instances, a geographic area (e.g., downwind of a toxic release) defined who became the unwitting participants in these government-supported studies. And in 1995, this sorry history reached into the present, with the public accusation of unethical conduct by physicians at the Irvine fertility clinic. Along with the most disturbing charges of misappropriating eggs and embryos of women undergoing assisted reproduction, doctors conducted laboratory and other research, all without the women's knowledge or consent.

Unlike the earlier examples, the Irvine clinic "research" was not officially sanctioned by oversight agencies. The university maintained the required human subjects committee, established to review and monitor all medical research, but the researchers did not follow the existing approval process; the oversight system was clearly inadequate to restrain doctors and protect patients. At a higher level, the federal government's refusal, since the Reagan administration, to touch assisted reproduction has left this field open to a frenzy of unregulated, uncontrolled experimentation and, in some cases, patient mistreatment. This particular clinic was a scandal waiting to happen—and then waiting to be uncovered. As Dr. Arthur Caplan, director of biomedical ethics at the University of Pennsylvania, observed: "These [fertility specialists] aren't on the fringe. . . . It's not like this was done at a new clinic or a seat-of-the-pants operation. . . . It's basically a market free-for-all with very little oversight over who offers services, what they do, how much they charge." In the absence of oversight, assisted reproduction had developed into "an ethical cesspool." The director of another fertility center also commented: "Things are done in this field that would never, ever be done in any other field of medicine without review or without big studies that look at efficacy or safety."[32] Indeed, as Dr. Caplan pointed out, interventions in human fertility are less regulated than is animal-breeding.

Perhaps as shocking as charges that doctors wantonly disregarded medical ethics is another conclusion reached by outside investigators once the public alarm did sound—that the doctors involved seemed not to comprehend how serious the accusations were or to understand distinctions between standard medical practice and experimentation. A different reaction among outsiders is chilling as well—a reaction less of shock or surprise than of wondering just how common such reprehensible medical behaviors are.[33] Perhaps most unsettling in the long run about this publicized scandal is that it affirms the need to ask: What *is* going on in the day-to-day of fertility medicine? How *can* patients be protected? Fertility patients are a vulnerable population in their eagerness to conceive and to believe claims of doctors who hold out so much hope. Patients and physicians are swept along by the momentum of the pursuit and of the competitive fertility industry that has grown around assisted reproduction. Although many physicians do agonize over ethics of their practice, many patients lack the good fortune—material and otherwise—to obtain care from those who have the greatest knowledge, skill, or, in some instances, ethical scruples.

In the wake of ethical violations at the Irvine clinic, the director of the Office for Protection from Research Risks of the National Institutes of Health summarized informed consent requirements in the specialty journal *Fertility and Sterility*.[34] Before agreeing to participate in research—whether a randomized controlled trial or any other type of study—fertility patients (and others) should be sure the physician provides "basic elements of informed consent"; all research should be approved by an independent review panel (see Appendix 3). Although the director states his "fervent hope" that none of this summary is news to journal readers who conduct reproductive research involving humans, he acknowledges that recent reports from major research institutions reveal "startling ignorance or underappreciation" of review and consent requirements. And with embryo research receiving only private funding, government protections do not apply.

The Question of Risk

Women who face the prospect of fertility treatment learn—or should learn—of various side effects that treatment may bring. They must then decide whether possible benefits are worth the risk of these undesirable outcomes. Of all potential risks, cancer looms for patients and doctors alike as the most feared, the life-threatening risk around which their hesitations dance. In 1993, the cancer risk gained concrete dimensions: an epidemiological study suggested a possible link between women's use of fertility drugs and increased risk of ovarian cancer. (See Appendix 2 on types of studies.) Based on comparisons between women who were diagnosed with the disease and similar women who were not, this "case-control," or retrospective, study reported on a broad range of characteristics that may affect women's chances for developing ovarian cancer.[35] The findings include an increased risk (nearly threefold) for developing invasive epithelial ovarian cancer among Caucasian women who used fertility drugs, compared to women with no history of infertility; the risk was higher among a subgroup of fertility drug users who never became pregnant.

Considering how widely prescribed fertility drugs had become during the previous decade, an unusual mustering of professional response was, perhaps, not surprising. Within days of publication, in January 1993, the American Society for Reproductive Medicine issued a press release criticizing this particular study. Acknowledging that the research was "carried out by reputable investigators," the professional organization went on to list deficiencies in the study's methods and conclusions. An international federation of fertility societies published a more extensive critique, emphasizing the inability to say that fertility drugs cause ovarian cancer based on the available information. Their advice to physicians: "Continue to reassure patients who receive drug treatment for their infertility."[36] Clearly, the study hit a sensitive nerve. Already, widespread use of fertility drugs was gathering criticism focused on the known dangers of multiple gestations for both the pregnant women and the desired babies. The physician organizations seemed intent on discrediting the ovarian cancer study and on reassuring fertility patients as well as their doctors.

The report's lead author, Dr. Alice Whittemore of Stanford University, was the first to point out limitations of this study. In the researchers' own press release at the time of publication, she stated that the fertility drug finding "is by no means certain. It is based on very small numbers and is really very tenuous." Though only a single report, with definite limitations, this episode—the publication of epidemiological findings on ovarian cancer risk and the response of fertility specialists—captures issues central to decisions that patients and doctors are making every day about fertility treatment. Observing patterns of human disease through epidemiological studies is one tool for probing the ever-present question of potential risks from medical treatment, as well as from environmental or other sources. In conjunction with animal models and laboratory experiments, epidemiological research provides hints about medical risks that need to be pursued through larger, more comprehensive studies. In fact, however, most decisions about complex medical interventions must rely on small pieces of knowledge gleaned from several studies; at best, patients and doctors reach conclusions based on the current accumulation of evidence.

Several pieces of evidence about fertility drugs and cancer currently suggest a disturbing, albeit preliminary, picture. A 1993 *Lancet* report describes twelve patients with a different type of ovarian cancer (granulosa-cell tumors) detected after ovarian stimulation using clomiphene citrate and/or hMG. During earlier years, in the United States and Europe, isolated case reports of women developing ovarian cancer after using fertility drugs dotted the medical literature.[37] In 1994 the *New England Journal of Medicine* published a study finding increased risk of ovarian cancer in women who used clomiphene citrate for one year or more.[38] This study might be considered the other shoe dropping, though it provoked less public attention than Whittemore's report. Large numbers of women have taken or presently take clomiphene. As of 1988, one survey estimated that of the nearly 2 million women who had taken medications to stimulate ovulation, perhaps two-thirds used clomiphene.[39] This study avoids certain problems inherent in the Whittemore analysis. First, it followed women over time (prospectively, rather than retrospectively); these women had a known fertility diagnosis and were known to have taken the specific drug. The increased risk was found in women with and without ovulation problems and in women who did and did not become pregnant; therefore, the risk cannot be attributed solely to an ovulatory problem or to an intractable fertility problem that thwarts any pregnancy, as critics of the Whittemore study suggested. In response to the clomiphene study, specialists commonly said that women should not use this medication for as long as a year in any case; if unsuccessful after three or four months, they should move on to other treatment. However, this view has not always prevailed among physicians. In the past many women took clomiphene for at least twelve months, and some still do today. And because women typically move on from Clomid to stronger ovarian stimulants, their cumulative exposure to some type of fertility drug can easily exceed one year.

Two other brief reports, also published in 1994, suggest a link between fertility drugs and increased risk of breast cancer. One study reported on sixteen women—out of 950 patients who had undergone ovarian stimulation at an Israeli clinic—who were diagnosed with breast cancer between the ages of thirty-one and forty-seven. The authors question whether excessive levels of estrogen and progesterone resulting from ovarian stimulation may mean hazardous stimulation for breast tissue; this risk might be highest for women who have never completed a full-term pregnancy, a characteristic that itself raises chances for developing breast cancer and that is common among fertility patients.[40] The second report described a woman with a family history of breast cancer diagnosed with this disease following ovarian stimulation.[41] These authors suggest that the hormonal stimulation from fertility drugs may speed the growth of existing, undetected malignancies in women with a genetic predisposition. Though relatively few women fit this particular profile, the suggestion could certainly be important to them; furthermore, now that certain genes for breast cancer have been identified, a screening test may become available, allowing more women to know whether they have an inherited increase in risk before deciding whether to add a possible risk from fertility drugs. (Other risk factors an individual may have, such as no pregnancy or late age at first pregnancy, must also be part of this equation.)

The drug hMG (Pergonal) was the focus of a 1996 report on epithelial ovarian cancer, showing a threefold increase among women who took this drug compared to women who did not; women who used hMG were at even greater risk for developing ovarian tumors described as borderline (may or may not develop into invasive cancer). Noting that most of the women used clomiphene citrate for three to six cycles before switching to hMG, these researchers suggest that prolonged treatment (again, for more than one year) with ovarian stimulants in general, rather than the particular type of drug, may be the more important factor contributing to an increased cancer risk. They recommend that "until more data are collected, women who use fertility drugs be under regular gynecologic surveillance."[42] A study published the following year found no statistically significant increase in risk from fertility drugs (never being pregnant did increase a woman's risk); however, the results did raise similar questions about hMG and borderline tumors, as well as about risks from prolonged treatment with various stimulants.[43]

Current biological theories about causes of ovarian cancer support the plausibility of increased risk after use of fertility drugs, although each possibility is certainly open to dispute.[44] Among the most prominent theories are, first, that an excessive number of ovulations and/or egg retrieval punctures, each a small trauma to the ovary, contributes to a cancer-producing physiological response; second, that the exceedingly high levels of hormones needed to hyperstimulate the ovary in order to mature many eggs during a treatment cycle contribute to development of malignancies; and third, that the fertility drugs themselves have a direct carcinogenic effect on ovarian tissue.

A Surprising Piece of Evidence

One study of breast and ovarian cancer in 10,000 women who were patients at an Australian IVF clinic highlights the need both for long-term follow-up of fertility patients and for greater understanding of the biology of cancer development.[1] In this prospective study, approximately half of the women received ovarian stimulation and half did not (they either had natural cycle IVF or ended up not receiving treatment). The two groups did not differ in rates of breast cancer; and this study found no statistically significant increase in ovarian cancer among the women who had taken fertility drugs, although the authors emphasize that the number of women is too small (i.e., given the rarity of ovarian cancer) and time span too short (i.e., to cover the latency period during which cancer might develop) to provide reliable data. More intriguing—and in need of further study—are two other findings of a statistically significant increase in cancer risk, even with the short follow-up time. Whether they took fertility drugs or not, the fertility clinic patients overall had higher rates of uterine cancer than the general population. And women with unexplained infertility—whether they took fertility drugs or not—were more likely to develop ovarian and uterine cancer than women with known causes of infertility. These findings, if confirmed in future studies, would certainly be important considerations when counseling differing subgroups of fertility patients about their risks and benefits from fertility treatments.

1. Venn et al. 1995.

These theories, the recent studies that suggest an association, and existing case reports from the United States and Europe of ovarian tumors in women who took fertility drugs have prompted researchers at the National Institutes of Health to take this possible connection seriously—more so, apparently, than do the professional fertility societies.[45] The NIH intends to fund expanded studies of long-term health risks for women who take fertility drugs. Among the questions needing answers is whether further research confirms the suggested increase in rates of cancer among women who have used fertility drugs. If yes, do specific medications increase the risk? What dosage and duration of use? Do certain subgroups of women have a greater risk than others, depending on the fertility problem or other medical history? What other long-term health effects are associated with use of fertility drugs? (For example, some researchers suggest the possibility of earlier menopause, an outcome that could shorten the time available to women who can conceive spontaneously.) Further research also needs to clarify benefits of using fertility drugs, so that patients and doctors can weigh them against potential, as well as known, risks. Most important, for which groups of fertility patients do fertility drugs improve chances of successful pregnancy, and how much are their chances raised compared to not taking these medications?

The study of ovarian cancer is a complex area of scientific inquiry into what causes or contributes to development of this disease. The possible impact of fertility drugs is only one of many factors needing additional epidemiological and biological investigation. The focus by many fertility specialists on whether recent studies prove that fertility drugs cause ovarian cancer ignores other important questions about how these drugs may promote development of malignancies in some women.[46] An interesting case-control study of ovarian cancer published in 1997 found that women who developed this disease had both a high number of lifetime ovulations (i.e., ovulatory menstrual cycles between the ages of twelve and fifty) and alteration of a gene involved in suppressing tumor growth.[47] Determining whether these associations shed any light on effects of ovarian stimulation by fertility drugs would require careful research among fertility patients who have and have not undergone such treatments.

Preliminary hints of risk from ovarian stimulation did compel gynecologists to acknowledge this most dreaded of potential long-term side effects. Though quick to point out weaknesses in the Whittemore study and others, fertility specialists are now more likely to admit there is a legitimate concern, to advise moderation in use of ovarian stimulants, and—for patients' health and doctors' legal protection—to specify this risk as part of the informed consent process. (At the same time, they more frequently call attention to research on alternative treatments that could eliminate the need for fertility drugs in some cases.)[48]

Until more is known about the drugs' relationship to ovarian cancer, patients and doctors can take precautionary steps, beginning with a careful assessment of a woman's individual risks, as well as benefits, in taking fertility drugs. (For example, have related family members experienced ovarian, breast, or other cancers?) In addition to a routine pelvic examination of the ovaries, an ultrasound or other imaging scan before and during treatment may detect an existing malignant or premalignant ovarian abnormality that could greatly increase the potential cancer risks of ovarian stimulants. If a woman decides to take fertility drugs, individualized treatment—rather than a blanket regimen prescribed for all patients—can minimize exposure to the medications. For example, dosage during an initial cycle should be calibrated to a woman's age and weight (women of younger age and/or lower weight generally need less medication); for subsequent cycles, dosage can be based on her previous response to the treatment. Additional precautions include use of natural-cycle IVF or low-dose ovarian stimulation, if possible; more potent ovarian stimulation alternated with less; and a limited number of total fertility drug cycles. Finally, doctors and patients can keep thorough records of all fertility drugs taken, with doctors maintaining addresses and phone numbers of patients, for future health surveys and for providing further information regarding risks.

Unfortunately, this last suggestion—and critiques of the research methods used in the recent studies—highlights the very limited types of follow-up possible for fertility drug use or any other reproductive treatment. This country lacks systematic, ongoing record keeping for the most basic of data on treatments, outcomes, complications, and long-term health of fertility patients and their offspring.[49] On use of fertility drugs with assisted reproductive technologies alone, two specialists, writing in the *Journal of the American Medical Association,* comment that "unfortunately," whatever data fertility clinics do keep "defy analysis" because of their haphazard and incomplete nature.[50] Indeed, a frequent criticism of the Whittemore study—that its data are incomplete regarding the specific type and dosage of drugs, and the women's specific fertility diagnosis— is disingenuous, since it is the physicians who are responsible for keeping such records. Aside from estimates based on limited pharmaceutical industry marketing information, there are no records even to document how many women have taken which medications. In contrast, several European countries maintain registries that not only record medical treatments of fertility patients but that also link reproductive outcomes in the general population to men and women's occupational exposures to reproductive hazards.

Cancer is surely not the only unproven risk attached to fertility treatments. Various medical interventions now in use could jeopardize a woman's existing good health or actually lower fertility among women who can become pregnant without treatment. And—as the DES story has shown, in particular—children exposed in utero to fertility treatments must be considered. Aside from potential long-term effects on a fetus from medications given to the woman (e.g., immunosuppressive drugs, GnRH-a, clomiphene citrate), new questions shadow new therapies that more directly manipulate sperm and eggs. Are sperm requiring assistance to fertilize an egg more likely to carry defects apparent only later in offspring? Do micromanipulative procedures themselves carry risks for the child who is born?

Fertility patients have a right to know potential risks—explained as such— based on whatever preliminary hints there are. People differ in their personal desires about having a baby and in their willingness to take even minimal risks—and, of course, in their particular medical characteristics. To a woman whose mother died of ovarian cancer or who has a family history of breast cancer, preliminary information may tip the balance against taking fertility drugs. Some women who ovulate normally may not want to take any risk with drugs whose only certain benefit is to stimulate ovulation. To a young woman considering her prospects, financial or psychological gains of donating eggs to be implanted in an older woman may not be worth a possible increase in risk of later developing cancer.

Women taking on risks of a fertility treatment should gain a reasonable likelihood of benefit. That is, for an individual patient with a particular fertility problem, is there adequate evidence that fertility drugs increase the likelihood of having a healthy baby? Along with fertility specialists, epidemiologists like Whittemore cite the benefits of pregnancy as an important consideration when deciding whether to take fertility medications—benefits that include lowered rates of breast and ovarian cancer. However, this consideration assumes appropriate prescribing of the ovarian stimulants to women who can benefit from taking them, which is too often not the case.

In a sense women must now choose their risks as they reach individual decisions about a medical intervention. Questions of cancer risk seem more complicated with every new study. For example, a case-control study of cervical cancer suggests that women with fertility problems who used clomiphene citrate had less chance of developing this disease than did similar women who never used the medication. Noting that this finding "was unexpected and must be interpreted cautiously," the researchers speculate that the anti-estrogenic effect of clomiphene on cervical mucus could reduce the occurrence of cancerous cervical changes.[51] If such findings are confirmed through further research, women will need not only to compare the magnitude of increase and decrease, but also to consider the possibilities for doing anything about the various risks from this medication. Unlike ovarian cancer, however, cervical cancer can be detected easily and treated effectively, and cervical changes that result from sexually transmitted viruses can be avoided through preventive measures. Therefore, cervical protection that might come with taking clomiphene citrate may not outweigh the possible increased chance of developing ovarian cancer. Another quandary is that many other characteristics of a woman's reproductive life (e.g., age at first menstruation, first full-term pregnancy, menopause, use of oral contraceptives) increase her risk for certain cancers even as some of them reduce risks or protect against other diseases, including other cancers. The challenge is to resist becoming overwhelmed by these multiple considerations, choosing to just not think about them at all.

When physicians think about their patients' view of risk—for instance, ovarian cancer—they often contend that women will choose treatment anyway; they never say no. Even if an increased risk of cancer from fertility drugs is confirmed, women will take the chance, as they do with known dangers of assisted reproduction such as ovarian hyperstimulation syndrome, large multiple pregnancies, and infection. Doubtless many will. However, a decision to proceed with fertility treatment despite risks—those hinted and confirmed—should be based on the best available information. Patients may think a treatment improves their likelihood of pregnancy when it does not; that is, the treatment has never been proven effective or their doctor did not prescribe it appropriately. Patients may not know the extent of improvement treatment offers compared to their chances without treatment, information needed for weighing benefits against risks. Nor does a woman's intense desire to conceive, to take any chance against all odds and risks, mean physicians have no professional judgments to make about a treatment's merits. Indeed, the intensity of a patient's desire and inclination to throw caution to the wind requires doctors to exercise caution all the more. For many fertility patients facing difficult decisions, a doctor's recommendation that a treatment is inappropriate or too risky or that only a limited number of cycles should be tried will at the least be an important consideration.

Finally, some physicians assert more generally that progress often requires the taking of risks. Forging ahead also allows for the serendipitous, the fortuitous finding that not only helps the individual patient but points the way to new and improved fertility treatments. Many patients who have tried standard fertility drugs, surgery, and/or in vitro procedures without success indeed agree to try a newly emerging treatment or an existing therapy used in an unusual way, even if the doctor acknowledges explicitly, "We don't quite know what to do in a case like yours. . . . We don't know if this will help." Before trying something new, however, patients need to recognize that what they are being offered is an experiment, at best an educated guess by an experienced, knowledgeable clinician, applying plausible biological principles in this particular case. A trial-and-error attempt may succeed; perhaps this small experiment will blossom into a treatment that helps other patients. But patients need first to consider—with their doctors and others they may consult—whether the rationale is plausible enough in their case and what prior research underlies the proposed treatment. They need to hear the advice of one fertility specialist to his colleagues: "View the results of new treatment[s] with caution . . . [and] consider 'making haste slowly' before going to overly aggressive, heroic, stressful, and expensive measures to achieve pregnancies in a population that stands a reasonable chance of conceiving with relatively little intervention, or even none at all."[52] And they need to be aware that many such efforts lead nowhere. Often, treatment merely escalates to no avail, interventions added on to counteract problems with the previous intervention—the errors of the original trial.

In the early 1980s, a diagnosis of inadequate or "hostile" cervical mucus led physicians to prescribe estrogen as a way of improving mucus production at the time of ovulation. Unfortunately, this estrogen could interfere with ovulation itself; the more estrogen taken, the more problematic the side effect. To counter this interference, doctors tried using the increasingly popular medication for stimulating a woman's ovaries, hMG (Pergonal). However, the estrogen interfered with monitoring the dosage of hMG; patients on this regimen faced even higher risks than others of not ovulating at all or of ovarian hyperstimulation syndrome and multiple births.[1] Doctors could better control that problem when they began using ultrasound to monitor egg development during cervical mucus treatment. Although the intervention was ballooning in complexity and cost, there was no evidence the original estrogen supplementation improved cervical factor infertility—which in itself was a diagnosis of questionable validity in the first place.

As scientists learned more about the menstrual cycle, a substance was developed (GnRH-a) that could shut down hormonal signals leading to ovulation. Though initially considered promising for contraception, GnRH-a soon found a prominent role in fertility treatments. First, clinicians tried this substance on women who did not respond well to ovarian stimulation medications; GnRH-a could eliminate their natural menstrual cycle, leaving a clean slate upon which to begin ovarian hyperstimulation. Before long, fertility specialists were expanding use of this regimen beyond "poor responders," making it a routine treatment for most women undergoing assisted reproduction.[2] Greater control over a woman's hormonal cycle reduced the number of treatment cancellations before egg retrieval and facilitated timing of the egg retrieval procedure. The next several years produced no cumulative data on success rates, though reports of scheduling benefits did appear (for instance, use of GnRH-a meant doctors could avoid performing egg retrievals on weekends or could even limit this procedure to three days a week).[3] Unfortunately, use of GnRH-a requires larger doses of the drugs used to stimulate the ovaries (hMG), resulting in increased risk of ovarian hyperstimulation syndrome and large multiple pregnancies. Recent studies of ovarian stimulation suggest, moreover, that higher doses of hMG result in lower pregnancy rates.[4] Now some researchers are questioning the trend toward using increased amounts of this drug. They question also the routine use of GnRH-a during fertility treatment, which is not only expensive but also then requires higher doses of ovarian stimulation drugs. A recent study suggests "selective use" of GnRH-a, based on a woman's response to hormonal pretesting; that is, identify first those women whose endocrine profile suggests the GnRH-a regimen will be helpful. Another study suggests a "minidose" of this expensive drug, only in certain women with a poor hormonal response during previous attempts. Use of GnRH-a, furthermore, may include the risk of prenatal exposure to the drug, since this component of fertility treatment is sometimes started before a pregnancy can be detected.[5]

1. Check 1984.

2. Chetkowski, Kruse, and Nass 1989.

3. Tan et al. 1994 (Cumulative conception).

4. Brzechffa and Buyalos 1997 report no pregnancies for women needing more than twenty-five ampules of hMG for egg maturation. See also Manzi et al. 1994; Stadtmauer et al. 1994. The Stadtmauer study not only suggests that hMG dosage not be increased if a woman's response is poor, but concludes: "Further investigation is needed to determine whether patients requiring high doses of hMG for adequate ovarian stimulation would benefit from alternative approaches to [in vitro fertilization–embryo transfer]" (p. 1063). As with studies of endometriosis that relied on observing visible reduction of normal tissue rather than pregnancy rates, once researchers looked at pregnancy rates following superovulation, they found that neither high estrogen levels, large number of mature eggs, nor improved cancellation rates translated into increased fertility.

5. Feldberg et al. 1994; Manzi et al. 1995; Wilshire et al. 1993; Young, Snabes, and Poindexter 1993. An earlier report (Diamond, Tarlatzis, and DeCherney 1987) describes the first published case of superovulation in a fertility patient with an undetected pregnancy. Although this report focuses on the "interesting" physiology of ovarian hyperstimulation during early stages of embryo development, with birth of an apparently normal infant (i.e., no observable birth defects), it does cite a "practical lesson"—in women with open fallopian tubes who are undergoing in vitro fertilization, there is a "potential for pregnancy." The report does not cite the additional lessons of possibly unnecessary fertility treatment *and* inadvertent prenatal exposure to potent hormonal medications.

Bulb Baster Does the Trick

When medical science cannot provide the answer: "A surrogate mother eager to provide a child . . . used a turkey baster to inseminate herself and stood on her head for 30 minutes after each treatment. . . . After failing to get pregnant using more scientific means, Janet Johnson sterilized a $2.95 kitchen baster. . . . 'We were kind of fed up with the doctors.' " (Associated Press, April 21, 1993)

The Question of Resources

It all takes money: basic science to answer biological questions; scientifically controlled clinical research to evaluate diagnostic tests and treatments; epidemiological studies of long-term health consequences for women who received fertility treatment and for their offspring. Registries that keep track of former patients and their daughters and sons are costly as well. However, only by establishing and maintaining records of who receives what medications and undergoes what procedures, as some European countries and Australian states do, can follow-up studies document the health impact of fertility treatments. Increased occurrence of cancers in treated women, for example, may not be detectable for several years or even decades; and, as DES demonstrated so definitively, health problems or other abnormalities in offspring may not take the form of immediately observable birth defects.

If well-funded, well-designed studies were to proceed, the woman and man visiting their doctor in coming years might undergo fewer diagnostic and treatment procedures that are futile or harmful. However, still missing from this picture is prevention. If resources flowed toward studying what reduces fertility and developing programs to prevent those processes, how many of these patients would never need to see a doctor in the first place? With fertility treatments growing ever more technological, invasive, and costly, attention to preventing the problem remains sorely neglected. Galvanizing this attention will certainly require government support. Although individuals can take some preventive measures to protect their fertility (see Appendix 4), other measures are beyond the power of individual actions to control, except as they pressure government officials and agencies that could be taking needed steps. One such step that pulls together research, risks, and need for resources aimed at prevention is to study carefully evidence that certain chemicals used in agriculture and industry may be disrupting normal reproductive processes in animals, including humans. Here the DES example recurs, but on a global scale. Failure to pay attention to available evidence—from basic science, epidemiology, wildlife studies, and from the use of DES on a previous generation of pregnant women—may jeopardize the reproductive health of women and men attempting to have children today and in the future.

Chemical Soup and Chemical Cocktails

Many chemicals used in agriculture and industry appear to affect complex hormonal messages and pathways of the endocrine system; they exert physiological actions that in some instances mimic, in others interfere with, the animal's natural estrogenic and other hormones. Unlike DES, which doctors prescribed as a medical therapy, these chemicals are all around us, in rivers and lakes, on crops, in paper processing and plastics, in the food we eat. They seep into water, food, and our bodies from pesticides, weed killers, food wrappings, hair colorings. Wildlife experts worry that recently observed reproductive abnormalities in fish, birds, and mammals may be caused by exposure to pollutants they call endocrine disrupters. The abnormalities, which include lowered fertility, could mean that some species "are on a fast track to extinction," says Dr. Theo Colborn, a zoologist with the World Wildlife Fund.[1] Scientists are now wondering, what of the human species? Even at low doses, these chemicals accumulate and their residues linger in human tissue. Of particular concern is the possibility that exposures during pregnancy could be disrupting normal fetal development—with effects that become apparent only years after the initial prenatal exposure occurs.

In 1991 Colborn organized a conference of researchers from various scientific fields to analyze and discuss existing studies of estrogenic chemicals and of dangers they may pose.[2] Among the participants were scientists who have studied DES in animal models and biochemical experiments, including Howard Bern, Gerald Cunha, and Dr. John McLachlan, then director of research at the National Institute of Environmental Health Sciences. Based on numerous studies of mice and of molecules, and given our present knowledge from the past human experiment with DES during pregnancy, these scientists worry about the wider implications regarding present estrogenic exposures—for both males and females.

Meanwhile, other diverse studies were revealing birth defects, reproductive tract abnormalities, lowered fertility, and eggs that won't hatch in birds, fish, turtles, and alligators exposed in the wild to chemicals that disrupt normal endocrine processes. And then, in the early 1990s, came initial reports from European researchers that during the past thirty to fifty years, decades that saw the development and widespread use of agricultural and industrial chemicals, testicular cancer and other reproductive disorders have approximately doubled, while sperm counts have dropped by about one-half, among men in industrialized countries. These scientists, and subsequent investigators, suggest that environmental exposures—particularly during critical weeks of fetal development—may be responsible for this disturbing trend.[3] With such suggestions, endocrine disrupters became a hot topic, focusing attention at scientific meetings worldwide, in popular national magazines, in the local health food store newsletter, and on television news.[4] There are scientists who dispute the hypothesis that environmental estrogens and other endocrine disrupters can explain observed reproductive disorders, and some question how real the decline of sperm is in the human species.[5] However, it does appear that the century's end brings not only increased recognition among physicians of male infertility, but evidence that this problem may be increasing from causes humans not only created but could prevent.

The complexity of developing measures to reverse the pattern and protect human fertility became evident in 1996 when a team of scientists led by

McLachlan (now directing the Tulane-Xavier Center for Bioenvironmental Research) reported a fascinating next step in research. They combined pesticide chemicals that, tested alone, show only weak, apparently insignificant estrogenic effects; tested as combined pairs, these effects were 500 to 1,000 times more potent.[6] As McLachlan explained, "Instead of one plus one equaling two, we found in some cases that one plus one equals a thousand." If this dramatic synergistic effect is confirmed through additional research in various animal species, current testing of individual pesticide and industrial chemicals is missing the mark; so too are present government policies intended to protect the public's health.

1. Stevens 1994.

2. Data, discussion, and conference conclusions are summarized in Colborn and Clement 1992.

3. Sharpe and Skakkebaek 1993. See also Auger et al. 1995; Bahadur, King, and Katz 1996; Ginsburg et al. 1994; James 1997; Joffe, 1996. The Augur study, by a group of skeptical French researchers, set out to disprove previous reports; to the investigators' surprise, their own findings confirmed a decline in sperm counts. Indeed, when DES effects in women exposed before birth became apparent, McLachlan noted, "If there are no effects on the men exposed prenatally to DES, we are the only species I know of where only one sex is affected by a reproductive toxin" (personal communication). In January 1995 Denmark's Environmental Protection Agency and its Ministry of Environment and Energy sponsored an international conference that noted increasing evidence of changes in male reproductive health that may be linked to estrogenic environmental compounds, particularly from exposure during fetal development; see *Lancet* 1995.

4. Pinchbeck 1996; Wright1996. It seems fitting that *Esquire's* first issue of 1996 covered the sperm decline story. In addition to popular magazines and newspapers focusing on the sperm angle, a science newsletter, *Endocrine/Estrogen News*, now reports conferences and research worldwide investigating the broader substantive concerns. The work of Colborn and others provides the basis of a well-publicized book published in 1996, with a foreword written by Vice President Al Gore (Colborn, Dumanoski, and Myers 1996).

5. See Olsen et al. 1995; the first four of five coauthors of this reanalysis of sperm data are scientists employed by chemical corporations (including Dow and Shell Oil); the last author is a urologist. One contentious question is whether the decline is global or varies in different geographic areas—a question that does need an answer but should not lessen the concern. The May 1996 issue of *Fertility and Sterility* included four articles questioning an overall decline in sperm counts: Fisch and Goluboff 1996; Fisch et al. 1996; Lipshultz 1996; Paulsen, Berman, and Wang 1996. See also Becker and Berhane 1997. Another question is whether decreased sperm count, if confirmed, is resulting in decreased fertility—or could if current trends are not reversed.

6. Arnold et al. 1996.

Although the connections between environmental chemicals and fertility are far from certain, with cause and effect relationships extremely difficult, if not impossible, to confirm, it is clear that estrogenic and other hormone-like chemicals are far more complex than physicians and scientists previously assumed, with a potential impact on human fertility only recently imagined. Existing safety requirements apply to a relatively small proportion of chemicals in contemporary use; rates of cancer, death, or visible birth defects may be monitored, but reproductive, endocrine, and immunologic abnormalities are not. Current testing procedures, based on acute high doses, cannot measure the impact of low-level or accumulated exposures, particularly as they affect the developing fetus; scientists and regulatory agencies may be seriously underestimating hazards posed by combined chemicals which, tested by themselves, may appear relatively innocuous. If in fact some part of the mysterious unexplained or immunologic infertility or of an increased incidence of endometriosis results from environmental toxins, then surely this country's research and treatment priorities need to be altered.[53] The usual medical response to a couple's infertility—attempting a highly technological solution that superovulates the woman, micromanipulates egg and sperm in a laboratory dish, and transfers embryos to her uterus—is dangerously short-sighted to the extent that significant resources are not committed to identifying and attempting to undo environmental harm that modern societies have accomplished. Louis Guillette, a professor of zoology at the University of Florida, captures the irony of where the usual approach many be heading. He wonders about the potential threat to human fertility, given the severe endocrine abnormalities he observes in Everglade alligators. Speaking at a 1995 meeting of scientists and citizens concerned about contamination of their local rivers and reservoirs, he posed this question to the audience: "Will we all need reproductive technologies in years to come?"[54]

Making Progress: Good News and Bad

The ongoing story of fertility medicine remains ambiguous, even as it alters the course of patients' lives. A mid-1990s assessment of male infertility published in *Lancet,* citing new treatments such as IVF and micromanipulation of eggs and sperm, could well be describing more generally interventions offered patients past and present. "Recent research has brought good news for infertile couples. . . . The bad news, however, is that this progress is restricted mainly to treatment of symptoms; there has been little gain in prevention and clarification of the underlying causes."[55]

Even improvements in technique can have a darker side. For example, devising ways to lower risk of serious harm from ovarian hyperstimulation is good news. With the most inhibiting threat removed, however, the bad news is that more doctors are likely to give more fertility drugs to hyperstimulate more women, in many cases unnecessarily. Mincing no words about the threat to a woman's health from standard methods of superovulation, members of a group of assisted reproduction practitioners describe a modified fertility drug protocol intended to avert the "life-endangering complications" of severe ovarian hyperstimulation syndrome, without having to cancel the treatment cycle. Many physicians, they comment, have avoided use of the most potent fertility drugs because of those complications. "If our results, based on patients undergoing IVF-ET, prove applicable to the non-IVF patient, they could lead to safer administration of [the more potent drugs], with obvious advantage for many infertile couples."[56] However, these drugs will likely also be administered to women whose condition does not require or cannot be improved by this treatment.

The news yet to come is whether fertility medicine, prodded finally by economics, will maintain a long-delayed focus on identifying what interventions can benefit what patients, with what risks—as well as what measures can help avoid such interventions. Already concern with costs is leading some specialists to suggest that the "true patient pool" needing active medical care for fertility problems may be approximately one-third lower than commonly claimed during the past two decades.[57] Will cost concerns restrain inappropriate treatments, the trial-and-error experiments that have flourished all too freely? Will more attention focus on preventing conditions that lead to a need for expensive therapies? That would be good news indeed. The same economic pressures, however, can also bring bad news. As cost dominates medical decisions and as patients are squeezed increasingly into corporate managed-care health plans, will doctors economize on tests or procedures that can more thoroughly diagnose an individual's condition and individualize care? Will economics dictate wholesale application of treatments to any patient who walks through the managed care door? Will patients be able to choose the doctor best able to handle their particular case or the treatment determined by their particular problem rather than by its cost or insurance coverage? Already the rapid expansion of ICSI for patients who can pay threatens to divert attention and resources from research on causes, diagnostic techniques, prevention, and less invasive (and less expensive) treatments for male fertility problems.[58]

As this story unfolds, patients are waiting in their doctor's office. The tendency of doctors to favor medical intervention and the motivation of patients to try anything remains a potentially risky combination; and the shared responsibility for assessing chances of success and of harm is no simple matter. Subfertile patients—and their doctors—need to pull back from the push to precipitous intervention. For many couples, a recommended treatment is not the only option, let alone their only hope for pregnancy. As eager as doctor and patients are to see the woman pregnant—and as difficult as it feels to *not* "do something"—doing nothing, except sexual intercourse on the most fertile days of her menstrual cycle, may be the wisest choice. Wanting a pregnancy badly— whatever that desire's source—surely weights the risk patients are willing to tolerate. The essential question, however, is not how badly a couple wants a pregnancy, but how badly they need treatment.

The questions of research, risks, and resources reach beyond the individual patient and doctor. Does the decision to plunge ahead with a medical intervention remain always with the patient, no matter how overwhelming the likelihood of failure or how threatening the risks? Is there a point of diminishing medical returns beyond which physicians should refuse to supply a requested service? To increase those medical returns, at what point are experiments and scientifically controlled trials using women and men justified and necessary? Are there qualitative boundaries of human reproductive nature beyond which researchers should not follow a new treatment path? And who defines these points and boundaries, on what basis, with what power to enforce?

7 How Is Consent Informed?

For everyone who enters the world of fertility medicine, undergoes basic diagnostic tests, and reads books and brochures about infertility, the moment comes when the doctor recommends a medical treatment, and the patient must decide yes or no. Whether the recommendation is an experimental reproductive technology or a more conventional approach, whatever the particular diagnosis and whatever a woman's age, whether as part of a research study or not, the patient must—by law and the ethics of medicine—give consent. And that consent must be "informed." This fundamental legal and ethical requirement that doctors inform patients about a medical procedure is but one aspect of a patient's decision process.[1] This chapter considers information and consent in a broader sense, as occurs when patients choose a course of action. Beyond the legal consent form, with its sometimes overwhelming list of risks and benefits, what is the information patients receive on which to base a yes or a no?

Patients considering a doctor's recommendation often ask themselves, *How informed is my consent?* That is, how much information did I obtain, and was it enough? This chapter suggests a different question: *How is my consent informed?* The alteration seems slight, yet it opens up a range of considerations crucial to making a decision about treatment. This question examines the origins of information, the influences shaping both it and the choices that a patient makes. This chapter asks, first, what are the main sources of information and—equally important—what are *their* sources?

Doctors

For most fertility patients, the main source of information is their doctor. To greater or lesser degrees, the doctor explains a diagnosis and possible medical treatments. A doctor may provide brochures to read; a nurse may be available to answer questions. Established assisted reproduction programs typically distribute written informational (and promotional) materials to prospective patients; some programs include audiotapes. Information about fertility clinics and the treatments they offer now appears on home computer screens through E-mail and Internet web sites. Some infertility specialists organize "seminars," advertised to the public; others hold orientation meetings only after women and men decide to become patients, to avoid "enticing" them into treatment they might not otherwise pursue.

Doctors develop expertise and skills needed to overcome certain fertility problems. After medical school, obstetrician-gynecologists and urologists complete residency training in their specialty (usually four years); the subspecialty that actually concentrates on infertility—reproductive endocrinology—requires two additional years. Throughout their careers, doctors must obtain a minimum number of continuing education credits; they can attend additional classes, seminars, and conferences. There is also a never-ending parade of medical journals to help them keep up with the latest information. Within these publications—this world literature of medicine—doctors can read reports of recent research, as well as editorials commenting on a particular study or a topic of more general concern.

One limit on information doctors can convey to patients, as Chapter 6 indicated, is that the lack of systematic follow-up studies and other well-designed research means that some important information remains inaccessible to doctors as well as to their patients. A University of Toronto medical ethicist addresses this concern with the example of ovarian hyperstimulation syndrome. Writing of a reported death caused by this side effect of superovulation, she notes that the case was presented as "the first reported death from associated stroke worldwide." To the contrary, other women had died previously from strokes brought on by ovarian hyperstimulation; without follow-up studies and other means for recording complications, however, "inadequate information about risks leads clinicians to present treatment options in an undeservedly positive light, and patients may agree to treatments that they would reject if given more accurate outcome probabilities." With only the occasional anecdotal report of complications, "long-term effects can remain undetected until multiple case-reports suggest a pattern several years later. . . . The failure by clinical researchers to undertake structured follow-up studies or to ensure that they are done by others is an abdication of their responsibilities. . . . In the absence of conclusive studies confirming safety and efficacy, clinicians talking to patients must be explicit about what is unknown." [2]

Even when information is available, doctors differ in the extent to which they attempt to keep up to date. Those who do read medical journals know of one persistent concern expressed within those pages, a concern that might surprise patients: doctors are not adequately evaluating the articles filling these journals, nor do they apply new data appropriately to patients they see. Rather than provide needed expertise, funneling useful information into a patient's decision process, doctors too often become a weak link. In this country, patients' choice of physician is increasingly limited, primarily by finances; however, a broader view of doctors' expertise can help in seeking the best available doctor or, at least, avoiding the weakest. What are the most prominent flaws in the ways some doctors are informing their patients?

First, for all their medical training, many doctors receive little formal education in statistics and scientific research methods, knowledge essential to analyzing research findings, choosing and interpreting diagnostic tests, and incorporating data appropriately into care for individual patients. Evaluating and applying research findings can be complicated. Medical studies vary in methods and types of patients included. One study may contradict the study published just a month before. Research varies in quality of design and execution as well. In recent years, increased economic pressure on doctors to demonstrate the usefulness and cost-effectiveness of tests and treatments they recommend has forced greater attention to evaluating new, as well as established, medical procedures. Journal articles that review "the basics" of research design, randomized controlled trials, and statistical tests provide doctors with helpful remedial lessons, but also underscore the fact that such a need exists. "It is only by translating good evidence into good clinical decisions that we can be sure that we do more good than harm for our patients," explains one review of research methods. Only then can doctors reach decisions based on more than "hope or authority."[3] (Many of the basic definitions and concepts summarized for physicians—aimed at improving their ability to evaluate medical journal articles—can be helpful for patients as well; see Appendix 2.)

Second, doctors, like many people, tend to stick with what is familiar, in this case, their preferred diagnostic and treatment methods; they may resist, or even creatively misinterpret, scientific findings that indicate a favored method is ineffective or less useful than another approach. Fertility tests for men are a prime example. As one urologist notes about the sperm analyses on which physicians commonly base treatments, "It will be difficult to change the mindset [doctors have] perpetuated for many decades" about diagnostic tests now shown to be inadequate.[4]

When Does Consent Become Informed?

"While everyone at the IVF clinic was caring and informative, there were some things no one ever mentioned to us," says a woman who underwent ovarian stimulation and embryo transfer that resulted in multiple conceptions. Joy over the pregnancy dissolved quickly into agony over what to do next. In such cases, recognizing that nearly all such pregnancies end prematurely, with a considerable chance that no infant will survive in good health, obstetricians may offer another medical intervention: they can attempt to reduce the pregnancy to twins by terminating two, three, or more fetuses. This woman's doctor advised reducing the number of fetuses from four to two. "It was the single most horrible experience of my life thus far," she recalls. "No one ever told me that there was a possibility of this happening."[1]

Two medical reports on fetal reduction demonstrate jarring differences in the way doctors provide information to patients in this situation—and in when they provide it. One group of Belgian obstetricians performs the procedure two or three weeks after the pregnancies are confirmed; in addition to medical considerations, the concern is that the patient have time to become informed and to consider the options.[2] A report on 200 cases performed by specialists in New

---

York describes a different experience: "All of the procedures were done . . . after a counseling session by the operator [i.e., the obstetrician performing the procedure] that lasted an average of 1 hour. . . . All patients were counseled about the risks and possible benefits of multifetal pregnancy reduction at least *1 day before the procedure,* to allow them some time to consider the issues that were discussed" (emphasis added).[3]

It is important to note that in both reports, patients receive information on multifetal reduction only *after* they have conceived a large multiple pregnancy. They have a day or two, or a few weeks at most, in which to decide. Yet giving patients information about this potential outcome *before* they attempt to conceive would seem essential to fully informed decisions, not only about fetal reduction, but about the initial treatment that can lead to such difficult choices. Understanding that she may face this dilemma might help a woman discuss with her doctor the risks of transferring many embryos compared to the increase in chances for pregnancy. A woman who could not agree to fetal reduction might decide not to undergo in vitro fertilization, for instance, or could choose to transfer fewer embryos than a woman willing to undergo fetal reduction if she did conceive triplets or more.

At whatever time a physician presents this option, his own preferences will shape the information he conveys. That preference may be primarily technical, reflecting his own skills and success rates with different procedures. Physicians with a good record of healthy newborns following fetal reduction, compared to their record of healthy live births following pregnancies with triplets or quadruplets (or more) will likely recommend the reduction procedure. If cryopreservation (freezing extra embryos) is not available, the doctor may suggest transferring more embryos, with fetal reduction the backup plan. Fertility clinics connected to hospitals with exemplary newborn intensive care units may have better success with triplets than with fetal reduction. The preference may reflect a doctor's ethical views on abortion. In order to be adequately informed, the patient needs to have the physician's preferences—and the reasons for them—made explicit. She also needs the kinds of information and comparisons most helpful to her individual decision. In considering fetal reduction, for example, she needs to know the rates of success and of complications (including loss of the entire pregnancy) at her hospital, performed by her physicians, not rates based on someone else's published study; she needs to know risks of prematurity with and without reduction, and the outcomes for babies treated in that hospital's newborn intensive care unit. And she needs this information at a time when she can best hear and comprehend it.

1. Robin 1993.
2. Bollen et al. 1993. See also Frederiksen, Keith, and Sabbagha 1992.
3. Berkowitz et al. 1993, 18.

While patients may assume a doctor's recommendation reflects solid numbers and scientific evidence, less obvious nonmedical influences also help determine the treatment he recommends and information he provides. To better understand how doctors inform patients, let us turn the tables and ask about doctor, not patient, characteristics contributing to the treatment options offered. Patients may want to consider the following questions when seeking a physician skilled not only in performing medical techniques but in evaluating and communicating medical knowledge—whether as their primary doctor or for a second (or third) opinion about a difficult medical decision.[5]

Where did this doctor receive medical training? When checking the diploma on a doctor's wall, think beyond the prestige and ranking of medical schools and residency programs. Different schools and programs emphasize different treatment approaches (e.g., surgery or endocrinology), as well as more general philosophies about medical intervention (e.g., more or less aggressive)—all of which shape what a doctor trained there is likely to do. Patients may want to ask doctors directly about the type of training they received and their general approach to diagnosis and treatment. What do they consider to be a thorough fertility evaluation? What evidence do they need before recommending a medical treatment?[6] If a diagnosis or treatment is controversial, patients can seek opinions from physicians with a differing background and orientation.

How long ago did the doctor receive medical training? The treatment a doctor recommends may be influenced by the number of years since residency training (sometimes, though not always, reflected in the doctor's age). A study of hysterectomy rates showed that doctors trained more recently (who, in this study, were younger) performed fewer hysterectomies; they were also more open to patients' preferences about whether to have elective surgery.[7] Applied more generally, fertility patients need to consider whether a doctor has a thorough understanding of recent developments in reproductive endocrinology and assisted reproduction. More experienced physicians, however, may have the advantage of knowledge gained from treating more patients. They may also have developed a more tempered perspective on reproductive interventions and a keener appreciation of the futility and harm that are too often the legacy of highly touted medical breakthroughs.

Is the doctor working in an academic, research-oriented setting or in private practice in the community? Specialists at a university medical center may base their recommendations on a more sophisticated understanding of statistics and current research than the average community physician. They may also be less influenced by personal financial returns. However, recommendations from these research-oriented physicians can bring other shadings. Researchers may become true believers, adherents of a particular "camp" of physicians advocating a treatment on which they have staked their academic career. Their devotion to a particular theory may go beyond the existing evidence. In the extreme, specialists at the "cutting edge" of research and treatment may establish medical fiefdoms, often with the encouragement and material support of their institution; the ego-enhancing payoffs they enjoy as benevolent (or not!) dictators may distort the advice and interventions they provide.

Where is this doctor practicing medicine? Surgery rates vary by geographic area, as doctors coalesce within regional medical communities of shared beliefs. Less concretely, different regions of the country become identified with differing medical approaches and preferences, as do different countries.[8] A recent study of surgery rates and costs, reported in 1996, reveals even greater regional variation than did previous studies. Although fertility treatments were not among the specific procedures included, its general conclusions are worth noting. First of all, a doctor's treatment recommendation depends more on medical philosophy and interpretations than on straightforward, demonstrable facts. Physicians cluster in like-minded groups, most often near the medical school where they trained—reinforcing and perpetuating the prevailing viewpoint in that locale. Doctors who move to a new area tend to adopt that region's medical philosophy and practices. Commenting on this study, Uwe Reinhardt, a Princeton University health economist, explains that medical care "is driven by fads, and the fads are regional. . . . We don't call it fads—we call it 'professional norms.' "[9] Second, the greater the number of doctors clustered in a region, the more medical procedures are performed. In a reversal of usual economic dynamics, the *demand* for medical services responds to the *supply*. Third, variation by geography is most striking with conditions for which a best treatment remains uncertain. Finally, and in a sense the bottom line, people living in regions with more frequent or costly medical procedures are no healthier than people living elsewhere.

Fertility medicine displays this geographic divide when a California woman consults by phone a specialist at an East Coast medical school; he disagrees with her doctor's treatment recommendation, which is based on results of a hysteroscopy (viewing inside the uterus through a narrow telescopic instrument), explaining, "They do a lot of that on the West Coast." And a West Coast specialist, asked about intrauterine insemination with ovarian hyperstimulation, says, "It's very popular back East."

In addition to geographic variation in procedures and philosophies, patients also need to remember that doctors do form an intangible medical community in which a quiet, informal knowledge circulates about other members of that community. Though physicians shy from discussing colleagues publicly, an insider's view (off the record, from a doctor friend perhaps—with all due awareness of the dynamics of envy, competition, and just plain gossip) can provide patients with an appraisal they would not otherwise hear of how a local doctor treats patients, particularly at the extremes of good and bad.

Has the doctor or the hospital with which he is affiliated purchased a laparoscope, a laser machine, or an IVF laboratory? Having the equipment pulls physicians, and their patients, toward treatment that uses that equipment, in order to make the purchase financially worthwhile. Short courses gynecologists take to learn a new procedure also have the effect of encouraging use of that procedure. As one example, a continuing education announcement arrives in the mail inviting doctors to learn "the easy way" to perform all manner of laparoscopic treatment— including for infertility—"all in two days . . . and at a fee of $875!"[10]

Are you seeing this doctor as part of a managed-care insurance plan (e.g., a health maintenance organization, or HMO)? In this country, costs and insurance reimbursement shape the type of treatment doctors offer patients. The move toward managed care means patients must be all the more vigilant when evaluating medical information. With a goal of keeping costs down, some doctors may neglect to mention certain options to patients. Or a doctor may push a treatment that is less appropriate for the individual patient because insurance will cover it. For example, the high cost of fertility medications—not usually covered by insurance— may lead a doctor to convey overly optimistic information about surgical procedures that are reimbursed. The expense of in vitro–related treatments—with limited insurance coverage, if any—encourages some doctors and patients to go for a quicker success, by maturing more eggs, transferring more embryos, and taking greater risks (including reliance on fetal reduction if necessary). Specialists may exaggerate the necessity of a specialized treatment, in hopes of attracting referrals from managed-care plans unable to provide that treatment.

Fertility patients may feel other effects of recent health insurance trends. Earlier models of managed care generally paid doctors straight salaries, but by the mid-1990s the income of physicians increasingly reflected, in part, how well they furthered the profits of a managed-care organization. A capitation system (paying doctors and hospitals a set fee per patient, often monthly, regardless of services provided) motivates doctors to limit both time spent with patients and procedures performed. In addition, many managed-care plans give doctors bonuses based on success in reducing services and increasing enrollment of patients who will not need much medical care. Some plans penalize doctors for using too many services—for instance, docking pay for each diagnostic procedure a doctor orders beyond a set limit. A *New England Journal of Medicine* editorial warns against physician behaviors that "shun the sick or withhold information to benefit ourselves. This system pressures doctors to exploit patients' trust for financial gain. . . . The ways we are paid often distort our clinical and moral judgment and seldom improve it."[11] Distortion is most possible and likely when diagnostic and/or treatment decisions are uncertain—a situation exceedingly common for fertility patients. (Chapter 8 discusses more specifically the types of distortion fertility patients may face.)

In addition, many doctors are forbidden to discuss these circumstances with patients, leaving patients unaware of ways their health insurance plan may affect their health care. In December 1995 *New York Times* reporter Robert Pear interviewed physicians around the country about restrictions written into their contracts with HMOs, including "gag clauses" that prohibit doctors from telling patients about those very restrictions. According to these doctors, health maintenance organizations "routinely limit their ability to talk freely with patients about treatment options and HMO payment policies, including financial bonuses for doctors who save money by withholding care." Among the most common restrictions are limitations on access to certain tests and treatments and requirements that doctors obtain permission from the HMO before offering a medical procedure. According to the executive director of the Medical Society of New Jersey, the gag clauses, in particular, "intimidate physicians and discourage them from talking openly to patients about the need for specialty care and the role of managed-care companies in limiting tests and treatments. . . . It's more like managed silence than managed care."[12]

Not telling patients all appropriate diagnostic and treatment options is bad enough, but these informational distortions can bring serious medical consequences as well. An example: an HMO member, trying to become pregnant, begins taking a more powerful ovarian stimulant after a year of taking Clomid. Her physician never tells her about an alternative, the GnRH ovulation pump, nor does he order diagnostic tests that would indicate whether she could benefit from this treatment. Although safer and more effective than Clomid (which is relatively inexpensive) or Pergonal for some women, use of the pump requires physician time and expertise; it is not included in her health plan. If she does conceive while taking Pergonal, she faces an increased chance of a large multiple gestation with all its particular risks. Or suppose she wakes in the middle of the night feeling sharp pain that shoots up to her shoulder. She calls the number listed for her doctor, explains her symptoms to the voice that answers, then waits for a return call. Hours pass before a message is conveyed that she should come to the office in the morning if she still feels discomfort. With the pain worsening, she and her husband decide instead to go to the emergency room—where a doctor must remove an ectopic pregnancy. The couple may then face long-drawn-out appeals trying to force their health plan to pay for this emergency visit—but, as a nurse told the woman in the hospital's recovery room, she should be thankful to be alive.

The excessive cost of fertility drugs points to a final flaw in relying on the ways physicians inform patients: drug manufacturers exert a direct and powerful impact on what doctors tell patients because the makers of medicines are a major source of doctors' knowledge about medicines. While the manner and degree of influence on individual doctors vary, the pharmaceutical industry's role is nonetheless pervasive; patients need to recognize the diverse forms and overall impact of this source on what they are learning about fertility treatments.

Drug Companies

Nearly all fertility patients will, at some point, leave their doctor's office with a prescription and some explanation of why they should take this medication. (Indeed, in nearly two-thirds of all visits to the doctor in this country, the patient leaves with a prescription.) How does the pharmaceutical industry feed into this seemingly simple interaction between a doctor and patients, and how might its involvement distort information the patient is now digesting? Consider, as an example, a drug that became a routine component of various fertility treatments in the early 1990s—Lupron, the brand name for GnRH-agonist, a hormone-related chemical used to suppress a woman's menstrual cycle. Doctors were prescribing daily injections to increasing numbers of women diagnosed with endometriosis and women undergoing ovarian hyperstimulation before an assisted reproductive treatment. The doctor's explanation of this new hormone regimen probably sounded enthusiastic and knowledgeable. But where were doctors obtaining their knowledge? How did they arrive at this recommendation? As it turns out, drug manufacturers pursue well-orchestrated strategies aimed at getting doctors to write prescriptions, making use of medical journals, sales representatives, and educational activities.

No one denies that drug manufacturers produce medications for which people are grateful—products that save lives, ease pain, allow some infertile couples to have a baby. At the same time, drug companies, like other corporations, seek to make a profit. Pursuit of profitable business is not always compatible with individual patients' needs, however. Often medications are overpromoted and end up prescribed to many patients who do not need them, people who may in fact be harmed.

The most obvious and straightforward displays of pharmaceutical persuasion are advertisements through which a reader must wade to find articles in a medical journal. The busy physician, with time only to skim through a recently arrived journal, finds his attention inescapably drawn to the colorful visual magnets of commercial messages. Advertisements are, of course, designed not to provide balanced assessment of medical pros and cons, but to increase sales of a product. Too often, this goal can result in advertisements that are false or misleading, in violation of Food and Drug Administration regulations.

And Now This Brief Commercial Message

That drug manufacturers are a major force shaping health care is no longer news. The collapse of health care reform in the 1990s—victim in no small measure of lobbying by the pharmaceutical industry and large health insurers—removed any public camouflage over the high stakes and extensive reach of this industry. Nor is an inordinate influence of drug companies on doctors' prescribing habits a recent phenomenon. During the mid-1970s, a few critics within the medical profession were documenting and protesting a long-standing, unhealthy relationship between the pharmaceutical industry and physicians.[1] A 1992 study focused on drug company journal advertisements. Researchers asked physicians and pharmacists involved in physician education to analyze advertisements from leading medical journals, including *Obstetrics and Gynecology.* (Tellingly, an initial requirement for physicians who would review the advertisements—that they had not accepted more than $300 from the pharmaceutical industry during the previous two years—had to be dropped for lack of eligible physicians.)

Beyond finding most of the advertisements to be "of little or no educational value," the reviewers noted that many were misleading and neglected facts about dangerous side effects. "The large proportion of advertisements (62 percent) that the reviewers judged to need major revisions before publication or that they would have rejected outright should arouse concern." With 92 percent of the advertisements potentially violating at least one FDA regulation, the study concluded that existing regulations defining standards of honesty, accuracy, and balance "appear to go unheeded."[2]

---

1. Lee and Silverman 1974. The coauthor of this prominent early critique, titled *Pills, Profits, and Politics,* Dr. Philip Lee, became President Clinton's assistant secretary for health and human services two decades later.

2. Wilkes, Doblin, and Shapiro 1992.

A more personal approach is through sales representatives—known as "detail men"—who visit doctors' offices and hospitals, bearing advice and small gifts. They leave behind friendly reminders—prescription pads and pens decorated with company insignia or, more pointedly, with the name of a specific drug to be prescribed from that pad. They leave free samples of medications, introductory offers that help establish brand-name identification and loyalty. Brochures announcing uses of a company's drug advise doctors, in prominent print, to avoid generic versions (less expensive and probably made by other companies) and to circumvent policies intended to make the least expensive drugs available to patients: "Protect your prescription by specifying 'no substitutions.' You must not only specify brand name, but take additional steps needed in your state to prevent substitutions."

An estimated 45,000 detail persons (one for every twelve to fifteen doctors) circulate throughout the country; a quarter of every prescription dollar flows into promoting drugs and providing trinkets directly to physicians.[13] A typical doctor's office averages two or three visits per week from different representatives covering that territory for their company. Although they are generally unseen by the public, patients may catch a glimpse of a man passing through the waiting room, dressed in suit and tie and polished shoes, carrying a large briefcase, looking like the traveling salesman he is; or the company may send a woman, well dressed, attaché case in hand.

Presence—and Presents

Doctors become familiar with the practices of pharmaceutical manufacturers long before they have an office for a detail man to visit. A medical student's first stethoscope or reflex hammer arrives during orientation week, courtesy of one or another drug company. Workbooks embossed with a company name help students study for exams. Sales representatives host periodic "donut rounds" where they meet with hospital residents. Medical interns enjoy a free ski trip, if only they attend a brief seminar about a new drug. It hardly seems unusual, then, to be offered fancier dinners and additional gifts after one becomes a physician with an established practice. Some egregious gifts (for example, luring doctors with frequent flyer mileage or with bogus continuing education credit for every prescription they write) have provoked investigations in some states, causing the company to desist. Some hospitals now restrict contact between detail men and doctors; some professional medical societies have established voluntary, though unenforceable, guidelines. Yet the influence persists. Dr. Alan DeCherney, no radical critic of the medical establishment, says of the profligate use of ovarian stimulants and the resultant multiple gestations and fetal reductions: "The pharmaceutical industry is responsible to a great degree for this predicament because for years they've been telling physicians that they can use ovulation induction agents without any special training."[1]

The pharmaceutical industry is, of course, international in its reach. A *Lancet* editorial comments on the British medical scene: "Doctors are becoming so accustomed to [drug company] sponsored postgraduate education that it is difficult to attract them to meetings where they have to pay for their own registration and refreshments. Postgraduate education is thus tending to become the responsibility of the drug industry rather than of postgraduate deans, clinical tutors, and the profession itself. This trend should be a cause of major concern to us all, because of the potential for distorting postgraduate medical education away from the needs of patients and the health service, towards the requirements of the industry."[2]

---

1. Penzias and DeCherney 1996, 1223.
2. Rawlins 1984.

Pharmaceutical companies pour money into promoting their drugs to doctors—an estimated $5,000 per physician per year at the start of the 1990s—because the marketing strategies work.[14] Doctors draw a surprising proportion of their pharmacological knowledge from advertisements and sales pitches. Prescription numbers, as well as brand loyalty, rise with the number of interactions a doctor has with a drug's manufacturer. So too do requests by physicians to add a drug to a hospital's list of authorized medications—a particularly lucrative payoff for the manufacturer, since all doctors using the hospital must choose from this list (the "formulary") when prescribing drugs for hospital patients.[15] One study commissioned by five pharmaceutical companies concluded that "manufacturers can have confidence that . . . when sales messages are communicated through journal advertising market shares of new prescriptions will increase."[16] Even when doctors think they pay little attention to advertisements and sales representatives, their actual beliefs about specific drugs reflect commercial messages rather than scientific sources such as peer-reviewed published studies and review articles that offer contradictory information.[17]

Patients should be aware of comments by critics who have an inside view. A physician in the Department of Pharmacology at the University of Massachusetts states: "I can see no role whatsoever for drug advertising. . . . I can see that it is reasonable for the telephone company to try to persuade us to use the telephone more. I cannot see that it is appropriate for a drug company to get us to prescribe a drug we would not otherwise prescribe. The party line, of course, is that the advertising provides education. If you were buying a used car, would you get your information from Sam, the friendly used-car salesman? . . . Time and again, our Pharmacy and Therapeutics Committee is asked to add a drug to the formulary, and it is quite clear that the motivating force is the arrival of some detail man. The drug industry's advertising budget appears to be well spent."[18]

His counterpart at a British university's Department of Pharmacology observes, "Few doctors accept that they themselves have been corrupted. Most doctors believe . . . that they are uninfluenced by the promotional propaganda they receive; that they can enjoy a company's 'generosity' in the form of gifts and hospitality without prescribing its products. The degree to which the profession . . . can practise such self-deceit is quite extraordinary. No drug company gives away its shareholders' money in an act of disinterested generosity. . . . The harsh truth is that not one of us is impervious to the promotional activities of the industry, and that the industry uses its various sales techniques because they are effective."[19] And a former executive with two major pharmaceutical manufacturers testified at Senate Labor and Human Resources Committee hearings in 1990 about drug company promotional practices that "the companies entice doctors into prescribing drugs that are of no use to the patient" and that their strategies are intentional—for example, providing researchers with funding for studies that are "purely devices the companies use to get patients on their drugs." [20]

With advertisements and detail persons, at least, the commercial goal is explicit. Another avenue for influencing doctors passes into a pharmaceutical netherworld where sales tactics intersect with educational endeavors, where lines blur between promoting increased sales and increasing medical knowledge. This more direct involvement with doctors' ongoing education brings even greater potential for distorting information patients ultimately receive. One example is editorials actually written by drug company ghostwriters. Many physicians draw upon opinions and comments published in journals when determining how to handle specific medical problems of their patients. Like many physicians, Dr. Troyen Brennan, of the Harvard School of Public Health, assumed medical editors invite well-informed experts to share their opinions about new research or controversies involving current treatments. He was surprised to learn firsthand of a rather different process, which he describes as "buying editorials":

> I . . . receive[d] a call from . . . a public relations firm in New York, asking whether I would be interested in writing an editorial for a medical journal. . . . The caller said that I would not really have to do much

work on this project. I would discuss the matter with them, and they would then have a professional writer compose the editorial, which I could modify as I saw fit. I would earn $2,500 for what was estimated to be several hours of work. . . . The caller stated that the entire project would be funded by a pharmaceutical manufacturer; her firm was merely the intermediary.[21]

Brennan goes on to describe a "glossy brochure" sent by the caller, which outlined ways the public relations firm solves problems of bad pharmaceutical publicity. In addition to journal advertisements and commissioned articles, the firm's services include special medical symposia, management of the press, and public appearances by leading medical experts. Realizing that the proposed editorial was part of a deliberate industry strategy to change the medical opinion of readers, this prospective author declined. "Of course," he concludes, "if I were to state that I was paid $2,500 to help a public relations firm write an editorial, my opinion might carry less weight with readers. That is the point."

Other "educational activities" occur at medical conventions. Gynecologists who began prescribing Lupron to fertility patients might have first learned of this drug at such a meeting—the American College of Obstetricians and Gynecologists or the American Society for Reproductive Medicine—held each year at one or another large hotel in one or another convention city. At the 1989 convention of ASRM, physicians browsed through floors of displays mounted by one pharmaceutical company after another, alongside makers of medical equipment, publishers of medical texts, and providers of laboratory services. Although the convention program listed display booths as "technical exhibits," the men and women accompanying these booths looked and acted very much like detail persons, offering not only free samples, trinkets, and tickets to an evening of food, drink, and entertainment, but informational videos, brochures for doctors and for doctors to distribute to patients, conveniently reprinted medical journal articles—with interpretive comments—reporting their product's favorable results. The theme of Booth #700: "Innovations in GnRH-Agonist Research," the display of TAP Pharmaceuticals, Inc., manufacturer of Lupron. With information and free samples in hand, doctors returned home to prescribe this innovative treatment.

So what is the problem? Why shouldn't doctors, and their patients, rely on this source in deciding to embark on a newly developing fertility treatment? One hint surfaced in a small conference room upstairs at that ASRM meeting where three physicians held a press briefing on ethical issues raised by assisted reproduction. Asked about risks to women taking fertility drugs, a past president of this professional society cited Food and Drug Administration requirements that medications be proven safe and effective before they are approved for sale in this country. Reminded by the questioner that doctors can prescribe an FDA-approved drug for any use—even if it was never tested for that purpose—he paused, then angrily described a certain manufacturer's display announcing "potential" uses of its drug for an array of fertility problems. "It's approved for one thing," he exclaimed, "—treatment of prostate cancer. . . . I'm really offended."

What offended this physician was Lupron's manufacturer urging doctors to prescribe their product for uses that were neither tested nor approved by the FDA, at best straddling a regulatory line that separates the commercial from the educational. Drug manufacturers know well the gaping loophole through which they can bypass FDA regulations intended to protect patients from useless and harmful medications. A drug must withstand only one approval process, as treatment for one condition, before it is on the market; then doctors can prescribe it for whatever they wish. Drug makers often suggest "potential"—i.e., unapproved—uses for their product; promoting such use (a commercial activity) is illegal, but exchanging scientific information (an educational activity) is allowed. Inspired by the suggestion of a pharmaceutical display or sales representative, doctors can and do prescribe medications for conditions far beyond what existing research has demonstrated to be safe and effective. Lupron, approved to treat cancer of the prostate, becomes a treatment for women's infertility and endometriosis. At first it is tried on women who do not respond well to fertility drugs commonly used for ovarian stimulation; the next suggestion is to incorporate this medication routinely for nearly all women undergoing assisted reproduction.

Unapproved use tends to be inadequately tested use. This prostate cancer drug may not be safe and effective for women, for women with endometriosis, for women undergoing fertility treatment. Furthermore, even if it is helpful for some patients, the medication will be prescribed far more widely by doctors who do not understand it well. Which women need to take it? What complications may arise, and how should they be handled? Can complications be avoided? Using GnRH-a to treat endometriosis may at least temporarily improve symptoms, but it brings the risk of irreversible bone loss. Using GnRH-a before ovarian stimulation may result in more eggs but may also contribute to more severe hyperstimulation syndrome and fewer successful pregnancies, to the expense and personal demands of fertility treatment, to the specialty's reliance on superovulating women as the means of increasing pregnancy rates. Although this regimen is shorter than that for treating endometriosis, it may still affect bone density adversely in some women.[22] In fact, by the mid-1990s, doctors were pulling back some, looking at "selective" rather than routine use of Lupron before ovarian stimulation.

And there is another problem, one that clouds the search for scientific evidence itself. The fine print of a medical journal article reprinted and distributed freely to doctors at a convention or by a detail person visiting the office reveals that funding for the study showing a drug's success was provided by the drug's manufacturer. Fertility specialists who conduct research may be less vulnerable than a general ob-gyn to direct pharmaceutical "education" about medications they prescribe, but they are far from immune to industry influence wielded through research grants. Government funding is increasingly hard to come by. Other than charging patients for experimental trials of a therapy—which carries its own ethical problems—researchers see no alternative. They need money for research, not only to answer medical questions, but to advance professionally. The design of a study may be limited by what manufacturers will accept. For example, they may refuse to support a study of drug effectiveness if a competitor's medication is included. A drug's manufacturer may be less likely to fund a study that could uncover a new, problematic side effect—for instance, investigating complaints of memory loss among women who are taking Lupron.[23] "Is it a conflict?" asks one researcher who has received such funding. He shrugs and nods. The past president of the American Society for Reproductive Medicine puts it more forcefully: "It is a tremendous conflict of commitment" for a doctor to conduct research funded by a drug company.

The entanglement of drug manufacturers with medical researchers reaches to the very roots of knowledge about medical treatments. Before unapproved use of a drug ever becomes a problem, the drug must gain FDA approval, and that process relies heavily on studies conducted or funded by the drug's manufacturer. The role of drug companies in evaluating their own products grows ever larger as government resources for independent evaluations shrink—and this role has historically been fraught with inadequate, and at times dishonest, testing and reporting, in some instances with fatal consequences (to name a few—DES, the arthritis drug Oroflex, the antidepressant Prozac, the heart arrhythmia drug Tambacor).[24]

Once a drug gains approval, industry-funded studies become published articles doctors see not only at a convention display or in a visit from a detail person, but also in medical journals. In addition, physicians with connections to a drug's manufacturer become speakers (with travel expenses paid) at annual meetings and at smaller continuing education programs, many sponsored by pharmaceutical companies and repeated region by region throughout the country. For even wider dissemination, proceedings of such programs may be published as a special supplement to a major medical journal (with costs paid by the sponsoring company). With the supplement's format identical to the journal's main volume, a reader may not realize that a pharmaceutical company is providing this specialized information or that these articles have not undergone the journal's usual review process.[25] With research, drug approval, journal articles and supplements, continuing education programs, and "technical exhibits," the pharmaceutical industry completes the circle, tying up all ends of an educational process that emerges ultimately as prescriptions and information given to patients.

New and Unimproved

Many new products pharmaceutical companies develop and promote *are* "me-too" drugs—not significantly better, but often significantly more expensive than medications already available. A letter to the editor in the *Journal of the American Medical Association* reports, in wry medical form, how these new medications become widely used. A physician and pharmacist describe a "Food-Borne Outbreak of Expensive Antibiotic Use" in their teaching hospital. Routine review of drugs prescribed by doctors at this hospital, aimed at assuring cost-effective use of medications, has identified "a prescribing outbreak as well as its probable source." The patient is a 32-year-old man who arrives at the emergency room with fever and a red, swollen insect bite. "Therapy with a new, expensive, broad-spectrum antibiotic was initiated. When asked about his antibiotic choice, the admitting intern noted at morning report that he had planned on giving penicillin or nafcillin, but had been overruled by the supervising resident who insisted on a 'more modern choice for a severely ill patient.'" The investigators find that use of the new antibiotic "abruptly increased [following] an extravagant dinner party . . . held for incoming and current house staff. . . . The sponsor of this dinner was the manufacturer of the antibiotic. The increase in use of this agent bore a striking temporal association with this dinner. Furthermore, the prescribing resident had attended the dinner and had directed the admitting intern to use the drug instead of nafcillin. . . . Although this agent is not contraindicated . . . it is much more expensive ($183.20 per day) than other effective drugs such as nafcillin ($84 per day). . . . We do not know if the resident's attendance at the dinner caused his therapeutic choice. However, the striking epidemiological association between resident attendance at this drug company–sponsored event and the subsequent

Drug manufacturers also pitch educational activities more directly at patients, albeit often with doctors' assistance. A stack of brochures about in vitro fertilization written for patients sits in the doctor's waiting room, but patients would be wise to ask what may be the real message. For example, one brochure written by the educational arm of Serono Laboraboies, a major producer of fertility drugs used during in vitro fertilization, describes this treatment in glowing terms. The patient is a "candidate" being "considered" or "selected" and, the literature implies, she should feel fortunate to be chosen for such treatment—a very different attitude than questioning whether she should choose it.

Well aware that doctors are not the only source of information for today's patients, Serono Labs and other fertility drug makers extend their educational activities into alternative channels. Resolve, the national consumer organization focusing on infertility, depends on pharmaceutical company resources to support many of its activities. Just as Serono, the maker of Pergonal and other fertility drugs, underwrites the American Society for Reproductive Medicine's newsletter sent to physician members, it also finances Resolve's informational materials. It also funds and helps organize Resolve conferences—planning programs and identifying doctors who will speak. A Serono representative sits on Resolve's national board of directors. The dilemma is clear, as is the conflict of interest. Without the contributions of drug companies, the consumer organization might not be able to provide information and emotional support to women and men struggling with infertility. Yet how might the involvement of drug companies—which profit from patients undergoing treatment, successful or not—influence the content and tone of information patients receive? How strong will be the pull toward medical treatment, how compelling the lure of medical miracles and progress fueling a single-minded drive toward a pregnancy at all costs? How often will patients be encouraged to stop, reassess, and keep always in mind that defining medical edict to do no harm? As with doctors who wish to conduct research, the organization's very real need for resources—and its members' very real need for information—is what makes its pharmaceutical sponsor both irresistible and problematic.

The public has another source of information about fertility treatments, one that is hard to avoid. A front-page newspaper headline proclaims: "It Worked—Baby's Due in February." The photograph shows a smiling woman, hands resting on a slightly rounded belly; her doctor sits nearby. The short, snappy paragraphs describe a happy and grateful couple who have finally conceived after three and a half years of marriage, "thanks to a team of researchers . . . who for the first time took a single sperm cell from [the husband] and injected it under the microscope directly into the center of a single egg cell from his wife."[26] Their problem, explains the article, was the man's low sperm count, a problem "shared by about 40 percent of the couples who each year cope with the inability to have children."

A true story, with real people. But how informative is this news account? Certainly, the public learns of a new medical technique, called intracytoplasmic sperm injection (ICSI). Yet, as is common in media coverage, this enthusiastic medical report glosses over certain facts, to a point that could mislead its audience. True, in approximately 40 percent of infertile couples, the problem can be traced primarily to the man. However, this considerable number includes not just "low sperm count" but a range of other conditions that are poorly understood (see Chapter 4). Although the reporter ties news of this pregnancy to "thousands of [other couples] who fear permanent infertility," he neglects to mention that this fear is usually not the reality. Many such couples will conceive without fertility treatment, or with far less invasive and expensive interventions than intracytoplasmic sperm injection. The newly developing technique might be appropriate for only a small fraction of couples with male fertility problems, for men with the most severe sperm deficits. The report does not say how long this couple actually attempted to conceive. Nor does it even hint at the uncertainties and cautions expressed among fertility specialists about this experimental treatment and about diagnosing male infertility. Citing 100 births worldwide following ICSI, the article states that the rate of birth defects is "the same as in all normal pregnancies"; this statement does not begin to explain how very preliminary these results are, how vast the unknowns about actual success rates and about abnormalities that may not appear immediately in offspring as observable birth defects.

This account is a prime example of "gee-whiz" science reporting. Reporters dwell on the wonders of science and medicine, sounding too much like advocates and too little like analysts, let alone skeptics, of new developments. Frequently, journalists are reporting from only a press release or from a conference or "staged news event" whose organizers have a definite interest in gaining public attention and support—a drug manufacturer, the American Cancer Society, the American Heart Association, the National Cancer Institute. Unlike obvious advertisements, such medical news may arouse less skepticism in the public as well.

Injection of a sperm into an egg, continues this article, "promises a real revolution in the treatment of male factor infertility," stemming from "an ingenious succession of experimental efforts under [infertility experts'] microscopes to help the reluctant sperm." Not explained is that these experts are concentrating now on direct injection because of discouragingly low success rates and the technical difficulty of those ingenious experiments; nor would readers learn of limits on potential applications of this new experiment even if systematic evaluation should confirm greater success in achieving pregnancies for certain fertility problems.

The media do not generally cover extended follow-up studies to tell us when a revolutionary breakthrough fails to live up to its initial promise. Bad news stories that do appear later usually tell of individuals failed or harmed by a popular medical treatment. In vitro fertilization success stories, for instance, eventually gave way to a few IVF horror stories. In place of happy couples were victims—women suffering side effects of powerful fertility drugs during cycle after disappointing cycle; couples spending years in pursuit of a pregnancy, left with neither a baby nor a bank account. Among doctors, the media spotlights the scandalous—a charlatan finally revealed and prosecuted for using his own sperm to inseminate at least fifty women;[27] the world-renowned specialist at the UC Irvine fertility clinic transferring eggs and embryos, without consent, from one woman to another.

Most infertility news stories portray in black and white a terrain that is filled with shades of gray. Neglect of complexities in media reports is perhaps not surprising, given the tyranny of deadlines, limits of space and sound bites, the need for positive audience response. Members of the audience, however, should recognize two important additional characteristics of this information and their own responses to it.

First is the power of anecdotes. Stories of individuals grab us; a real-life example feels accessible, easy to grasp and relate to, and it sticks in memory as statistics and clinical information do not. However, "hearing about a woman who . . . " is not the best way to understand likelihoods and probabilities—dimensions that give fertility medicine some structure. When deciding whether to undergo a medical intervention the questions should be: Was that woman the one success out of a hundred cases of women who are similar to me? One out of two? One in a million? How *does* her experience apply to me? Doctors too are swayed by the anecdotal. They may remember well the happy patient who finally had a baby while forty similar cases that failed grow dim. And along with stories heard in the hospital cafeteria, many medical journal articles are but formalized versions of anecdotes, ranging from a single case report to accumulated experiences with a series of patients. These stories have value in revealing variations and nuances not captured by more rigorous scientific method. Individual patients do not always match population statistics, computer models, or overall study results. However, medical judgments do require a basis in fact—in both biology and numbers.

Stories of success commonly hold greater sway than instances of failure or harm. The understanding of statistical chances can be slippery. Considering success, patients often think "that one in a thousand could be me." Or a fertility specialist tells a group of prospective patients: "We had a 46-year-old woman who came to us for IVF. We told her honestly that her chance of conceiving using her own eggs was 1 percent. She insisted on trying, she got pregnant and had her baby." As for risks, many people tend to believe "it won't happen to me." For the patient who ends up with a baby, and for her doctor, success is 100 percent; patients and doctors tend not to count so absolutely the failures. And certainly, statistics are subject to individual conclusions and wishes. "We tell a woman her chance of pregnancy is only 3 percent," relates one fertility specialist, "and she says that means it's not zero."[28]

The media also help shape and fuel patient demand. Within the medical community exists a phenomenon laypeople may not perceive—consumer demand for diagnostic tests and treatments. Physicians tell of patients who march into their office requesting, or insisting on, a specific medicine or procedure. Their friends are having intrauterine inseminations, so they want to try that too. Or they want to increase their fertility drug dosage beyond what the doctor recommends. Or attempt yet another assisted reproduction cycle after too many failures—patients known in the trade as "IVF junkies." Most often, doctors blame a recent media report for creating pressure to supply the demanded service, particularly if it is something new. Most problematic, medical interventions that make news are usually not yet proven safe and effective. Some physicians try to explain why the latest discovery may *not* be the answer, seeking to correct misimpressions and to apply the newly reported information to a patient's individual case. Others follow a path of less resistance, arguing that if they don't accommodate the patient, someone else will surely give her the treatment.

The dynamic of patient demand and doctor response can only become more prominent as the public gains access to information beyond newspapers, magazines, and television. Already, laypeople throughout the country are sitting at personal computers, tapping into medical databases and networks.

Whatever the information from any of these media, the immediate result is a patient going to a doctor, where the fundamental communication about fertility decisions will occur. As in the office where this chapter began, a doctor may be writing a prescription. Like any doctor, he brings to this moment a perception of patients and of how well they understand explanations he provides. Like many fertility specialists, he may claim, "We tell them the numbers, but they don't hear," or "Patients hear what they want," or "They hear, but then they're surprised," or "Patients always say yes to treatment." However, communication within a doctor's office is more complex and circular. In fact, doctors commonly provide an overly optimistic assessment, and patients (as well as news reporters) eat it up. Doctors may not hear their own way of presenting treatment options or recognize various influences upon their explanations. A doctor who views patients as "always saying yes to treatment" may not be seeing or remembering the patients who decided no at some stage in the pregnancy quest; yet his view may lead him to be less careful or thorough in explaining statistical likelihoods of success or describing potential risks. Physicians seem surprisingly weak in the face of "patient demand." Some doctors end up blaming the victim when explaining disappointing outcomes or disastrous experiences. For instance, a fertility clinic director interviewed on NPR about how the Irvine clinic scandal could happen focused on the women who seek assisted reproductive technologies and pressure doctors to do all they can; these women are "high achievers," "not used to failure," wanting a pregnancy at the time they planned, yet often "wrongly optimistic" about their chances for success.[29] Missing from his portrayal is any feel for the seductive pull of reproductive technologies held out now to patients or for the vulnerability of even the most informed and assertive patient to the technology and the fertility specialist.

"We are the most obedient and desperate of clients," writes one such woman, a journalist and self-described feminist, "willing to sign on for anything, take anything. I am a rational, educated woman who cannot stop walking down this road, even as it seems I am throwing good money after bad. And yet I am simply marking time until they let me back in, let me start up again, let me plunge ahead, mindless of the increasingly decreasing odds. . . . What fancy new procedure will they dream up when my back is turned to reseduce me with . . . again [with] no statistics, just a flurry of hope among practitioners and patients. . . . I wish sometimes that . . . the doctors would somehow agree that I was beyond their help. . . . Sometimes I wish I just had the guts to junk the quest myself."[30]

Whether the patient marches into a doctor's office to demand treatment or somewhat more tentatively asks for information and advice, doctor and patient share a need to be aware that dominant sources of information advocate medical intervention, not caution. Beyond vulnerability to advertisements, anecdotes, and the momentum of treatment, doctors and patients also share a vested interest in the optimistic outlook and a compelling desire to "do something," to be part of a success. For doctors, the desire is reinforced by a perceived consumer demand, by a view skewed toward the most tenacious patients, and by the overall thrust and competition of the medical-pharmaceutical industry. For patients, the desire is reinforced by ubiquitous social pressures and by every new hope, endlessly reignited, like trick candles, with each newly announced reproductive therapy.

Offers Too Good to Be True?

In the best of worlds, a patient's sources of information would combine to enlighten difficult medical decisions. With access to much more information than in years past, laypeople would work with medical professionals to sort through complexities of fertility diagnoses and treatments. Individuals would benefit from another trend emphasized in recent years, at least in theory—that patients should be "partners with their doctors." Unfortunately, the informational pieces do not always fall together in such a harmonious and empowering way. Chapter 5 depicted one reproductive development—the focus on women's age—as played out at a presentation by one group of fertility specialists. Consider now another free seminar conducted by a fertility center—an example of how "informing patients" about a range of fertility problems can touch, even drastically change, people's lives. This time a small group of women and men gather in a medical suite on a workday evening in early spring to attend an informational session, one of several to be repeated here in the months ahead. They have come in response to a newspaper advertisement. "Are You Trying to Have a Baby?" the bold print asks over the picture of a wide-eyed infant. A small, in-depth seminar, claims the advertisement, will help these prospective patients learn about "recent medical breakthroughs [that] offer renewed hope." Indeed, the topics listed are the specialty's hot ones, described in Chapter 4: male infertility ("virtually doubled IVF success rates"); immunology and infertility ("a newly discovered link"); and IVF with egg donation ("nearly a 50 percent chance of having a baby after only one try"). "Space is limited," the advertisement warns, "so call for reservations today."

Eleven women and five men have reserved the space tonight. The seminar coordinator hands each a folder filled with explanations of various medical procedures and financial plans, written by clinic personnel, as well as two research articles by this clinic's doctors and a news clipping about the research. Also available is a tape cassette entitled "Women Helping Women," an interview with the center's director about their egg donation program. The coordinator guides the group through a maze of waiting areas, scales, blood-pressure equipment, examination rooms, the closed doors of the doctors' inner offices to a conference room. They take seats around a large table and wait quietly, skimming through their folders, until a doctor in white coat hurries in. He introduces himself, welcomes them, and launches into the presentation, speaking easily, diagramming now and then on a flip chart. He is confident, authoritative and personable. As presented by this doctor within this conference room, the claims sound even grander. What do these women and men learn on this evening—and what do they not learn?

"Male factor infertility is finished" the audience learns first from this doctor. "A revolution in treatment during the last six months means there is no such thing anymore. Male infertility is no longer an issue at all." The breakthrough is ICSI, to obtain fertilization in vitro followed by embryo transfer. A man need have only one sperm, just the head of a single sperm, which can even be extracted from the testicle with a needle if necessary, "and you can have your own genetic child." Among babies born following ICSI, he reports, there is no increase in abnormalities. The fertilization rate with ICSI is so good at this center (around 80 percent of eggs are successfully fertilized), they will soon use the procedure for *all* of their IVF treatments, whatever the couple's fertility problem.

What the audience does not learn is that the few fertility centers performing this new procedure throughout the world can report only very preliminary results. Though other specialists consider this treatment to be the one approach that brings some success with severe cases of male infertility, they emphasize that technical problems still hamper ICSI. Methods for removing sperm from the testicle, if need be, are newly developing and not without risk.[31] As to recommending ICSI for all male infertility, let alone all IVF, one physician remarks, "At this time, that is like recommending a Caesarean section for every woman giving birth. Only a small percentage would benefit, but what about the requirement to do no harm?" Notes another, "If you employ ICSI for all IVF in a practice where most patients undergo IVF, you are adding at least $1,500 extra per treatment cycle."

The presentation does not explain that determining which patients need ICSI has barely been addressed by clinical studies, though many specialists worry already about its overuse. They worry that doctors will ignore questions of cause, bypassing diagnosis altogether. Not only will many couples be subjected to more invasive techniques than they need, with presently unknown risks to offspring, indiscriminate use of ICSI will hamper scientific efforts to improve diagnostic techniques and to develop less invasive treatments for male infertility.[32]

Certainly, it is far too early to provide information about the rate of abnormalities in offspring, who are presently few in number and young in age. Also premature is the report handed out that evening entitled "ICSI Statistics," bearing the signature of the center's executive medical director and executive laboratory director. These "results" tally the early pregnancies out of forty-seven attempts during their ICSI program's first two and a half months—before any patient can have progressed beyond the first trimester of a pregnancy (a time when miscarriages are common). Most of the reported pregnancies are "biochemical," not yet actually confirmed through ultrasound. The handout's bottom line, in bold type, is an "*anticipated* birth rate per egg retrieval" (emphasis added)—a fictive success rate reflecting a questionable estimate of what their results will eventually be. This information is a far cry from reporting a year's worth of completed treatment and outcomes—including live births, pregnancy loss, and complications.

This audience next learns that the cause of infertility or miscarriages (often occurring before a woman misses her period) for one category of patients is an immunologic problem. Some women who try for months and months to conceive feel sure they were pregnant; they feel the early signs, their period may come a day or two late. The big breakthrough is discovering that a woman's abnormal production of antibodies can disrupt embryo implantation or cause later pregnancy failure. "All are treatable," the doctor quickly reassures the audience in response to anxious questions. Research at this fertility center (as described in the journal articles and news clipping enclosed in each folder) shows success of a new preventive treatment that the center's written information describes as "benign . . . and almost risk-free." All of their patients are tested through a sensitive blood assay to measure several destructive types of antibodies. "We now know," the doctor explains, "that women who lose pregnancies early or late have increased antibody levels that kill the baby." The preventive medications (the blood thinners heparin and aspirin), along with one other therapy (intravenous gamma globulin), may even improve pregnancy rates in women who do *not* show increased antibody levels. New patients at this center will join a research study of the same treatment in women whose test results are normal.

Information, Consent, and Research

The need for carefully designed and monitored clinical research raises additional thorny questions about the way doctors provide information to patients. There are many invitations and inducements—subtle and not so subtle—aimed at gaining patients' participation in research. When do inducements to join a study become coercive, in that they are just too hard to decline?

The evening seminar. The women and men hearing about "recent breakthroughs" in fertility treatment learn briefly of ways these physicians involve patients in research. All new patients, the doctor tells them, will be part of a study to test a preventive treatment that may improve pregnancy rates. Choosing this fertility center means agreeing to join the study (a requirement not in keeping with basic elements of informed consent; a patient who does not wish to participate in research should be offered an appropriate established treatment). Some new patients—those who qualify for a special IVF payment option—can also choose to join a second study. The financing plan is attractive. For a set fee, just under the price of two basic in vitro fertilization–embryo transfer cycles, "medically eligible" couples can receive up to three basic IVF-ET cycles, plus an additional three transfers of thawed frozen embryos, within one year. This payment option is available to patients the doctors identify as meeting minimal fertility requirements (*not* the most difficult cases with low chances for success and not necessarily patients with greatest financial need). Given that a good portion of patients selected will conceive on the first cycle, fees will be more than enough to cover costs for those needing a second or third try; these quickly successful customers, with their new babies, are not likely to complain about the extra money spent. A bonus offer comes with this package: a fourth IVF-ET cycle within that year. To receive this extra chance at pregnancy, the couple need only participate in an experiment, a study of a new egg retrieval and maturation technique; the doctor will attempt to retrieve immature eggs from the woman's ovaries, to be matured in the laboratory before transfer. This "fourth" basic IVF cycle—with experimental technique—must be the couples' *first* attempt during the year. The experimental first cycle is prepaid as part of the overall financial package; women who cannot tolerate four IVF-ET cycles (and frozen embryo transfers) within one year could, unfortunately, lose their "extra" try, but the physicians and embryologists will have accomplished their experiment. For most fertility patients, the expense of treatment looms as a major concern. For many, reproductive technologies appear as a hope beyond their financial grasp. At the least, this financial pressure will bear upon patients' decisions as they consider the doctor's offer of an "extra" try, an offer made on the condition that they consent to participate in an experiment.

Soliciting in the name of research? "Infertile Women Needed for Research Study," announces a newspaper advertisement, placed by a different fertility center. Study participants will receive up to two cycles of basic IVF-ET treatment at a reduced cost of about $6,000, not including medications and pre-cycle testing (fertility centers generally exclude these two costs from stated prices for assisted reproduction). This study "is not experimenting on people," the nurse-coordinator states vaguely to inquiring women, because the procedure "has been done before." The method has been successful in another part of the country, she explains. This study is "research to see if the method is successful here too."

Fertility medicine, like other branches of medicine, does need patients willing to participate in well-designed clinical studies—especially randomized controlled trials of new procedures. However, what are the ethics of asking patients to foot the bill to be research subjects, whether it is called an experiment or not? Even a reduced bill—or, perhaps, especially a reduced bill—can be coercive. Moreover, it does seem self-serving to invite women to join a two-cycle study when many will likely want to try again if these two attempts fail—and will not likely want to start over with a different IVF clinic.

Patients need to scrutinize the possible risks, benefits, and motives of invitations to participate in research. Among questions to consider:

1. How is the study conducted? Specifically, who receives the "experimental" treatment, and who does not? Is this study randomized and blinded? What extra medical interventions do participants undergo (e.g., medications, egg retrievals, embryo transfers, surgical procedures)? What manipulations of egg, sperm, embryos? Who is supervising and accountable for what happens to study participants and to their eggs, sperm, embryos?

2. What added benefits might participants gain (medical, financial, or other)? What are the known added risks, and is there any preliminary evidence of possible additional risks?[1] In some instances, research may benefit only future patients rather than those who actually participate; if the research brings virtually no additional risk (e.g., blood tests or laboratory studies of nonviable eggs, sperm, or embryos), individuals may wish to participate in

order to increase knowledge and help others. This altruistic benefit, however, needs to be clear.

3. If a patient does not wish to join a study, will the doctor provide another appropriate, standard fertility treatment, or is the message "Take it or leave it?"

4. Who benefits most directly from the study? Patients, present or future? Doctors who need patients? (That is, does this invitation seem to be a come-on, a way to attract patients to this fertility center?) Drug manufacturers who want doctors to prescribe a medication being studied?

5. Did a reputable ethics committee—independently chosen from among physicians and scientists not connected to this group—review the study before it began, and is there regular independent monitoring of the research process? Most major American biomedical research institutions and hospitals that receive federal funds are formally pledged to comply with federal government regulations designed to protect human research participants, including review by a "human subjects committee" or "institutional review board" (IRB). Clinics not affiliated with such institutions are not subject to this commitment. Doctors can voluntarily submit a research proposal to independent evaluation (for example, to the National Advisory Board on Ethics and Reproduction), but few do.[2] In fact, with the government refusing to support research involving embryos, privately funded studies of assisted reproduction have proceeded untouched by federal requirements established to protect participants in medical experiments. The existence of government, university, or hospital regulations does not guarantee compliance, as the Irvine clinic scandal made clear. However, if the design and ethics of a clinical study did not undergo a truly independent review, and if no mechanism exists for monitoring the way a study proceeds, then fertility patients are being invited to participate in research with less regulation and oversight than is now required to protect research laboratory rats.

---

1. For example, as of 1996, information from the National Institutes of Health seeking participants for a randomized clinical trial of superovulation and artificial insemination did not mention the possible increased risk of ovarian cancer associated with fertility drugs—even though the NIH, on the basis of preliminary research findings, was supporting further study of this risk.

2. Physicians may handpick and even pay members of an ethics panel, skirting the spirit of an "independent" review. Congressional hearings in May 1977 revealed the growth of a new commercial enterprise—research review panels for hire. Even if researchers do not select their own IRB, they can shop around until they find an approving panel (Stolberg 1997).

Hands shoot up, the listeners seeking answers they haven't heard before. They are eager to learn how to get these blood tests done. They know well other fertility tests; results already pad their medical charts. But antibody measures, the "sensitive" laboratory analyses just mentioned, are one thing their current doctor has never ordered. What these women and men do not learn is that controversy and uncertainty permeate nearly every statement the doctor made so definitively about immunologic infertility. The audience is not informed that the antibody explanation is, at best, one theory in an ongoing medical debate about the possible contribution of abnormal immune reactions to infertility or repeated early miscarriage. Among the reasons a doctor may not have measured their antibody levels is that these new and very expensive blood tests are still evolving. Their value in identifying women who may need treatment remains a hotly disputed question among fertility specialists—as do the treatments themselves, which always bring risks.

Were these listeners to consult another specialist in the community—a reproductive immunologist who studies only this problem and does not run a general fertility program—they would hear cautions about immune testing unless a woman has experienced at least three miscarriages; then further cautions about intervening with treatment unless the tests show a consistent pattern of several highly abnormal results along with the miscarriages. At that point, "trying something new"—something unproven, not well understood, but hopefully of benefit—might be justified. The scientific data are too new and incomplete, he asserts, to rely on an "abnormal" test result or "subclinical" (i.e., no symptoms) autoimmunity; certainly, women with "normal" immunologic test results should not undergo unproven immunologic treatment.

Participants in this seminar are also not hearing the opinion of other doctors in the community: that immunologic infertility "is a confused field. . . . No one really knows what they are doing"; that the recommended drugs "have great potential for harm" and are "to be avoided" unless a specific and reliable medical reason exists. They are not learning that the combination of heparin and aspirin may heighten the risk of bleeding problems because at least two clotting mechanisms are suppressed, that this effect cannot be immediately reversed, as can the effect of heparin alone, by injection of an antidote (although this medication also brings other risks), and that current tests to monitor levels of these drugs may not adequately reflect the mechanisms affected when a woman is taking both. Prospective patients will not receive reprints of studies that conflict with this doctor's explanation about preventive benefits of the immunotherapy for infertile women. They will not read a medical journal editorial—the same journal that published the doctors' research article—warning strongly against too quickly and indiscriminately applying the experimental treatment on the basis of preliminary research findings, the very danger here gathering steam.

The Ultimate Risk

There are risks no one dwells on—not the hopeful fertility patient, not the pregnant woman, her partner, or her doctor. One year after the informational seminar described in this chapter, a patient of this center—a woman just seven weeks pregnant with triplets following in vitro fertilization—experienced a headache severe enough to take her to a hospital where she died, on Mother's Day. The immediate cause of death listed on her death certificate was brainstem compression, this due to cerebral edema (swelling), due to intracerebral hemorrhage (bleeding), due to a right temporal arteriovenous malformation and aneurysm (a balloonlike abnormality). Like 1–2 percent of the general population—fertility patients and pregnant women included—she had a misconfiguration of veins and artery that was probably congenital. Most of these people are unaware of a weak spot in their brain's vital circulation network, unless it begins, unpredictably, to bleed—a slow leak or, worse yet, a "blowout."

This woman and her husband could afford fertility treatments. They consented to the treatment her doctor recommended, wanting to do everything they could to have a baby. In addition to undergoing IVF with transfer of several embryos, she was taking heparin, aspirin, and intravenous immunoglobulin (IVIG). For some women with arteriovenous malformations, changes in blood pressure that occur normally during pregnancy can trigger a leak or blowout; the result can be what obstetricians call a maternal "catastrophe" or "disaster." Sometimes the woman can be saved, if the bleeding can be stopped and the damage repaired. Doctors do not understand completely the way the medications this woman was taking affect bleeding and coagulation; current methods of monitoring to ensure "safe" dosage may miss important physiologic mechanisms. In the view of one physician who watched her die, the immunotherapy might have doomed emergency efforts to save her.

Whether or not blood-thinning medications contributed to this particular woman's death or frustrated the attempts to save her, this couple's story is a red flag. Like successes, complications are a matter of numbers and probabilities. Among any group of patients are various unknown, unpredictable disorders, of which arteriovenous malformation is one example. If a doctor gives blood thinners and IVIG to ten carefully selected patients—women with previous miscarriages and considerable abnormalities in immunologic tests—a respectable proportion may benefit. Chances are, none will suffer from arteriovenous malformation. But if treatment is extended to nearly every patient in a busy fertility practice, the proportion that can benefit will diminish. For every hundred treated unnecessarily, one or two are likely to suffer from arteriovenous malformation or another similarly rare disorder that could result in unforeseen, perhaps poorly understood, complications—including death.

While immunotherapy may someday prove effective for a small proportion of couples, "big breakthrough" overstates the uncertain knowledge and tentative abilities fertility specialists can fairly claim. True, some IVF failures involve problems with embryo implantation, some of which may relate to immunologic reactions, but there are other possible explanations as well (see Chapter 4). True, some women do experience very early miscarriages, before knowing they were pregnant; some may even feel certain they conceived during months of trying. Yet, how convenient the explanation, heard this night, that certain antibodies cause pregnancy tests never to become positive. How irresistible the thought that I was pregnant after all or that those treatment failures I went through can be prevented by these doctors the next time. Anything is "treatable," of course, but appropriately? With reasonable chances for success? With adequate attention to safety? The danger here is that a doctor's presentation of the potential success—a small possibility grounded in fact—ignores the unfavorable odds and minimizes potential harm, playing mercilessly on the longings of these women and men. In the hands of doctors with too little care for "doing no harm," physically or emotionally, patients learn to *never* give up hope, to try and then try again.

In fact, the editorial comment on this center's research mentioned above concludes that use of the suggested treatment "antedates by many years our knowledge of the ways in which the immune system plays a role in the mechanism of implantation. . . . Too often, following the initial enthusiasm associated with preliminary studies insufficient to prove benefit, treatment patterns are established only later to be proven ineffectual or even harmful. The history of the misuse of diethylstilbestrol (DES) in the treatment of threatened abortion provides a clear lesson. Given the great need and even desperation of couples entering into assisted reproduction, the potential for uncritical application of the treatments . . . prior to their more rigorous proof of effectiveness is great."[33] Regarding immunotherapy more generally, another critic argues: "Existing data . . . are meager. This has not prevented some physicians and clinics from aggressively advertising and promoting this expensive therapy to patients and other physicians. . . . More study . . . should take place only in the context of formal research protocols. The alternative is uncontrolled human experimentation, an approach both unscientific and unethical. Until randomized controlled trials establish the merit of this treatment, immunotherapy should not be used in clinical practice."[34] And a third states: "An entrepreneurial atmosphere has clouded the rational scientific evaluation of couples suffering recurrent miscarriage. The ethical duty of every physician is to be sure that the tests and procedures he or she uses are worth the money, inconvenience, and risks involved. Unfortunately, until all physicians . . . realize this, it is incumbent upon the couples themselves to heed the Latin adage *caveat emptor,* meaning 'buyer beware.'"[35]

Back at the seminar, the doctor asserts that a third group of patients who might in the past have lost hope "will have a successful pregnancy" using egg donation with IVF. These women cannot produce fertilizable eggs, usually because of a premature or natural menopause. As with male infertility, declares the doctor, ovarian failure "is a non-issue." This fertility center now has a 58-year-old woman halfway through a pregnancy, her first. With the particular hormone regimen this program uses to prepare egg recipients, he states enthusiastically, "We can synchronize things perfectly. . . . We can make a better uterine lining than a natural one," even in women past the age of fifty. Numbers flow freely—percentages, ages, months trying to conceive. The bottom line of blurred, and ultimately misleading, statistics claims that with six to eight attempts, chances for pregnancy are "close to 100 percent." Of course, egg recipients must be healthy and egg donors "as young as possible"—though over eighteen, the doctor adds.

Once again, important information is not mentioned: questions about the clinic's drug regimen during egg donation cycles, which could result in fetal exposure to unsafe hormone levels if pregnancy does occur.[36] Also not mentioned: the increased obstetric complications for older women who do conceive with donated eggs; at best, the pregnant patient and her doctor can view such pregnancies with "cautious optimism," as one specialist put it, rather than with the certainty expressed here tonight.[37] And of course not mentioned to these potential egg recipients: the physical and psychological risk to a fertility specialist's other patients, women as young as eighteen, recruited to supply the eggs.

•

They make it sound so easy. The evening is filled with "We know that . . . ," "You need . . . ," "Without doubt," and "People come from all over the world." Definitive statements describe "big breakthroughs . . . a revolution in the last six months . . . " New answers, new hope, reason to keep trying and to keep trying here. These women and men are ready to sign up, to get that test or treatment, the one thing their doctor has not done.

This free informational seminar raises far more questions than it could ever claim to answer. These prospective patients did not march into this office demanding a treatment. Nor do their stories, related briefly that night in capsule form, suggest that their considerable past experience with tests and treatments was based on the best of medical information. They are weary from the hardship and disappointment of past failures. Their attention was caught by an enticing advertisement—which suggests the first questions.

Where are the lines between education and enticement, between useful information and a strong play to people's great yearnings? Do these doctors portray fairly the state of the art or embellish a sketchy medical picture? Will the numbers tossed out tonight—or printed and bound as an official audit—illuminate or obfuscate decisions these women and men now face? Are doctors downplaying potential risks, convincing people there is no harm in trying rather than helping them understand and assess legitimate concerns? Is the audience at this and other seminars hearing professional enthusiasm and optimism or echoes of unfulfilled therapeutic claims previous generations heard?

How will these women and men evaluate what they hear tonight and what they see in the literature they carry home? A yearly audit, gladly distributed by this fertility center, confirms impressive success calculations. The printed report, duly signed by an independent accounting firm, looks official, as if it could verify medical achievements. But accountants count whatever numbers they are given, in this case given by the center. The audit can confirm *only* the calculations, not that raw numbers document accurately what occurred or that the calculations fairly represent a rate of success. Clinic reports provide no data on duration of patients' infertility before doctors begin aggressive treatment. And does the typical reader understand such nuances shading these calculations—that is, the variability tied to characteristics of the patients treated, or the superovulation regimen employed, or the number of embryos transferred? When choosing among competing fertility programs, members of this audience cannot directly judge the technical skill of a physician or an embryology laboratory; they have only the numbers and percentages, which inflate easily. A lay audience may interpret more literally than is warranted such terms as "perfected" techniques or "statistically proven" results. They receive a single medical journal reprint; yet this study and its conclusions are only one small piece in the ongoing medical exchange this audience will never read about the experimental, as yet unproven therapy. Is this fertility clinic providing patients with a journal article in order to help patients better understand a complex medical topic or to impress by the reprint's face value? When these women and men do become patients here, will the doctor be

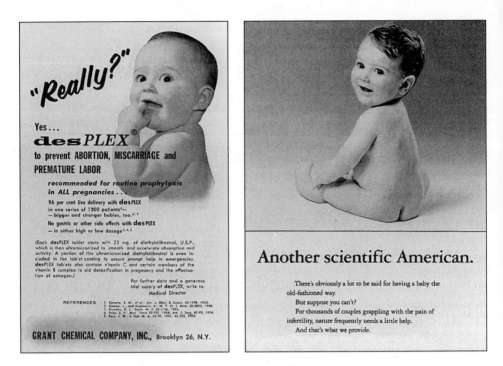

Figure 5. An ageless baby appeals to doctors and patients alike. On the left, a 1957 ad in a medical journal recommends DES for "ALL pregnancies" to prevent miscarriage—a claim that had already been disproved by clinical studies. On the right, an ad from the 1990s, which appeared in the *New York Times Magazine*, seeks patients for a New York City fertility clinic. Another of the clinic's ads gets more specific: "Thanks to techniques like [GIFT] we can now offer hope where none existed before." Today, GIFT has lost its luster for many specialists, because of high cost, questions about success rates—and perhaps because it was developed by Dr. Ricardo Asch.

---

explaining the wisdom of a medical recommendation—helping his patients understand the advice—or persuading them to buy it? In fact, the medical director of this same clinic, in a sudden change of pace from his usual exuberance, had commented a few years earlier on how willing patients are to undergo new procedures a physician might suggest: "It's the saddest thing. . . . They'll go for anything if we steer them to it."

Don't Ask, Don't Tell

"After my IVF, they did a very early pregnancy test which was positive. Just before I was scheduled to have the ultrasound [to confirm pregnancy], I started to bleed. . . . They denied it, told me I wasn't having a miscarriage. The doctors didn't even return my calls—the nurse relayed their answers, that bleeding is common, that I felt terrible just like any pregnant woman who cries when she sees the dog on a TV commercial . . . "

Aside from the uncaring manner this former fertility clinic patient experienced, what does the doctors' response, or lack of it, say about the statistics presented to future patients? Was this really a pregnancy, or only a false positive test resulting from hormones taken during treatment? And if this woman did, in fact, conceive and then miscarry, will this miscarriage ever appear in the center's reported numbers, statistics that become the basis of their audited "Estimated Birth Rate?"[1] What of other patients who get further along in a pregnancy, then have a miscarriage? This fertility center does no obstetric care; their "successfully" pregnant patients will see an obstetrician in another office, or city, or country. How many miscarriages will never be recorded? The technical description among researchers for such patients is "lost to follow-up," a group highly problematic when analyzing results and reaching conclusions. For a fertility center's purposes, the description might be, "Don't ask, don't tell."

---

1. The final accompanying note of the audit report for this clinic—notes filling three pages with definitions and explanations—reveals that the "Estimated Birth Rate" is not adjusted for losses of ongoing pregnancies. The percentage that "management believes" will occur is, compared to other fertility programs, inexplicably low.

How do matters of cost push these doctors to persuade patients? The expensive reproductive technologies are where they make their money: the more procedures, the more billable services. With these treatments paid in advance ("no later than cycle Day 2," no waiting for insurance reimbursement that might cover certain nonexperimental procedures), how many people who do not require such sophisticated and invasive fertility treatments—but can afford to pay in full—will be caught up in a broad sweep toward high-volume sales? The doctor proudly describes "pro bono" treatments this clinic provides. However, its policy requires nine new paying patients for every one receiving a free treatment. (Other clinics, by contrast, provide a set number of pro bono patients per month or per year, regardless of the number of new patients treated.)

Hidden Costs

Beyond costs added to the basic IVF fee (diagnostic tests, fertility drugs and other medications, special procedures such as ICSI or IVIG), what unmentioned costs might patients face? The expense of complications is not thrown in for free. For instance, attaining high pregnancy rates may require high numbers of embryos transferred and, therefore, selective reduction of multiple fetuses and/or intensive care for newborns—all costly measures. Hidden more deeply are costs no patient thinks to ask about. A prominent fertility center, once attached to a large, respected hospital, now stands alone; its doctors perform assisted reproductive procedures, including surgery, within its own facilities. For some medical services—for example, anesthesiology—these doctors contract with a specialty group. Especially in a practice known for its entrepreneurial edge, what impact might profit calculations have, literally, on the center's daily operations? One anesthesiologist explains why he no longer works with this center: "They went for the lowest bidder." His own group, still affiliated with the hospital, could not accept the fertility center's offer, a bottom line that did not provide for regular equipment calibration and servicing, certain backup machines, or keeping particular drugs in stock to handle a woman's unusual reaction to an antibiotic, anesthetic, or other medication. Not that monitoring equipment would be broken, just not working at its best, not checked regularly by technicians or repaired or replaced promptly. It is not that most fertility procedures require a hospital setting, but that they proceed best with a comfortable safety cushion this anesthesiologist finds lacking here.

Even as the doctor spoke to this group, other physicians in the community were asking themselves similar questions. Over the years, this fertility center was developing a reputation. Among themselves, other physicians criticized the brash commercialism, the treatment of fertility medicine primarily as a business operation. Of discount plans and free offers, local skeptics doubted costs came out of the doctors' pockets; rather, strict medical eligibility requirements would more than take care of costs. Some said that research emanating from this center was flawed (for instance, not randomized and blinded, wrong control group, questionable determinations of "abnormal" immunologic results), its conclusions far too quickly applied. Efforts to minimize pressure or coercion when enlisting patients as research participants might not be rigorous enough. Most troubling to other specialists in the community, based on what some patients related—for instance, when seeking a second opinion—these doctors seemed to overstate what was known and what individual patients would need based on unproven diagnostic methods; perhaps to ensure a brisk business, a high success rate and profit margin, they tended to employ overly aggressive, invasive, and risky treatments on patients who could do just as well with less.

In communities throughout the country, similar dynamics characterize the daily reality of doctors treating patients, for better or worse, and of doctors developing medical opinions about their colleagues. The particulars will vary, as will the degree of concern aroused. Such opinions among professional colleagues remain inside information, murmured under a collective medical breath. Granted, success rates at this fertility center were among the best, and these voices might be merely envy of the competition. Yet if professional consensus about medical practices so crucial to the lives of patients does grow to a critical mass, should patients not be aware of that too? Certainly, an audience at this center's free seminar will not be learning *this* information. And so a final question: How can these women and men—or any fertility patients seeing any physicians—know what they don't ever hear?

Ultimately, an individual's decision depends on the relationship and communication between patient and doctor. Suffusing that relationship is an ineffable mix of supportive optimism and realistic pessimism, of a doctor's advice and pressure, benevolence and manipulation. Heightening the vulnerability of many patients considering aggressive fertility treatment is the sad fact that often they are not currently receiving high-quality care. All too typical, for instance, are the doctor prescribing escalating doses of Clomid for the past eighteen months; the doctor performing tubal surgery on a woman without ever testing whether her partner is fertile; the doctor employing ineffective therapies (e.g., repeated intrauterine inseminations) when significant male infertility is discovered. A missing ingredient, from newspaper advertisements to informational meetings and materials to any doctor's office, is an effective way to protect fertility patients from the incompetent, unethical, or scandalous.

8 Protecting Patients

Work Enough for All

Midway through the last decade of the twentieth century, with reproductive medicine developing ever more sophisticated manipulations of fertility, a respected physician, an associate professor of obstetrics and gynecology and director of a highly regarded in vitro fertilization program, states, "This is an anguishing time for our specialty." The assessment sounds disheartened, even sorrowful. The physician offers this admission in the quiet of a tiny, mildly cluttered office, a refuge—if only for a few squeezed minutes each day—from the constant bustle and relentless pace of the surrounding UCSF medical center as well as from more far-reaching professional demands. Buffeted by the same Pacific winds atop the same urban hill as the research scientists studying hormones described in Chapter 6, this medical doctor feels very different pressures.

There are, first of all, patients—women lying in hospital rooms down the hall awaiting or recovering from surgery or having babies; couples pursuing rigorous monthly regimens of hormone injections, ultrasound monitoring, and blood tests, all timed as precisely as possible toward an afternoon slot the doctor reserves for their embryo-transfer procedure. Any fertility patient would do well to find a physician like this one, not only immersed in the specialty's current knowledge and practices, but obviously concerned about the well-being of individual patients. That patient would also do well to understand that the concerns reach beyond individuals this doctor actually sees to touch all fertility patients as well as their doctors:

> How can patients be protected from incompetent or unethical medical treatment?

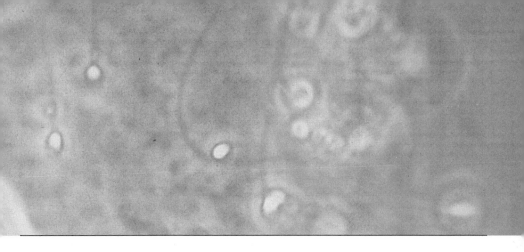

How can patients and doctors maintain trust, particularly after the 1995 revelations that a world-famous specialist had expropriated eggs and embryos from women under his care?

Is there a way to break the political logjam that has blocked needed research on assisted reproduction, research that might increase chances for successful treatment and lessen the occurrence of futile and harmful interventions?

This chapter not only asks about the role of doctors and patients in creating safeguards and building trust, but also poses a question that seems to haunt the medical profession—what is the role of government? The discussion considers the issues of professional guidelines, government regulations and health policies, research funding and oversight.

To better appreciate how profoundly these wider issues affect the well-being of fertility patients, consider the activities of this obstetrician-gynecologist whose position within fertility medicine captures so comprehensively the specialty's broader pressures: an active member of the American Society for Reproductive Medicine; past president of that society's affiliated group on assisted reproductive technologies, serving at a time when success rates and laboratory accreditation were gaining increased attention within and outside the profession; president of a regional professional society of reproductive endocrinologists (trained and certified as fertility specialists); member of local and national committees addressing the ethics of fertility research; one of three University of California faculty investigating fertility medicine's worst scandal. And now, at the age of fifty, with her career firmly established, Dr. Mary Martin has recently married. Like many of her patients, she knows well the ultimatum of a ticking biological clock. She too has reached very personal, individual (and in her case, extraordinarily informed) decisions about pregnancy—as a professional woman in her thirties, a single woman turning forty, a newlywed approaching the age of menopause, she has chosen not to pursue a pregnancy of her own.

For those now experiencing fertility problems, this chapter may seem remote, not nearly as pressing as immediate decisions about diagnosis and treatment. Yet, just as Dr. Martin finds herself "sidetracked," on a regular basis, from actual care of patients, so too must patients keep some perspective on professional, political, and economic realities beyond their consuming immediate concerns—and on the potential impact of these realities on their medical outcomes.

Regulation and Monitoring

Dr. Martin's first inkling of trouble at another University of California fertility program came in a phone call on a warm fall day of 1994. The chancellor of the Irvine campus was on the line, asking if Dr. Martin would serve on a panel of three university medical school professors looking into possible problems at the Center for Reproductive Health. The nature of the problems was left quite vague, says Martin. In fact, she hung up thinking the chancellor's concern had mainly to do with misuse of certain fertility drugs. "I naively figured I could go down there [to southern California] and assist the university by helping them clarify some misunderstanding involving the fertility clinic." Perhaps there were some disgruntled employees; apparently members of the clinic staff had filed complaints under a university "whistle-blower" policy, which had set in motion a formal investigation process.

Only later, when Martin arrived for meetings in Irvine, did she realize that she "really had no idea what it was all about." As she and the other panel members began sifting through cartons filled with patient files and clinic records, and tracing a history of letters from clinic staff to medical school administrators, the magnitude of the trouble began to hit. The faculty investigators submitted their report to the chancellor in January 1995; they confirmed the truth of at least some of the allegations about egg and embryo misappropriation, as well as wrongdoing in conducting research, handling finances, and using fertility drugs. In the spring, as the university quietly pursued legal action to close the clinic, the local newspaper received photocopies of documents from someone with access to clinic files, and the scandal hit the headlines.

Throughout that summer, further reports filtered into public view—initially through the *Orange County Register* (gaining the newspaper a Pulitzer prize for investigative journalism) and the *Los Angeles Times*—revealing more pregnancies and babies from misappropriated eggs or embryos, more unsuspecting couples, more research without patient consent. The nearly universal reaction was dismay at the absence of regulations or outside monitoring of what goes on within fertility clinics and the laboratories that handle eggs, sperm, and embryos. Previously, no one paid much attention to regulatory needs. Now came talk of big changes. Such talk remained noticeably lacking in specifics, however, and the prognosis for change seemed less than promising in that a key faction seemed not to join in the dismay.

"The best thing we can do is resist the onslaught of changes [people] want," was the reaction of Dr. Alan DeCherney, then president of the American Society for Reproductive Medicine.[1] In his view, new regulations would be an overreaction. Explaining the Irvine clinic transgressions as extremely rare, the immoral actions of one or two individual physicians, DeCherney argued that new licensing or inspection requirements for fertility medicine as a whole were unnecessary. Mechanisms already existed—legislation passed in 1992 requiring fertility clinics to report success rates to the Department of Health and Human Services, a program run by his organization and the College of American Pathology for licensing embryo laboratories. Additional efforts to regulate the hundreds of fertility clinics in this country would merely result in additional expense that would be passed on to patients. Not mentioned by DeCherney was that the legislation he cited never received the funding necessary for implementation, that the licensing program was completely voluntary (the Irvine clinic was one of many that do not participate), and that the nationwide organization of fertility patients, Resolve, fully supported new protective regulations.

That DeCherney, a longtime vocal foe of government regulation or monitoring, reigned as the professional society's president while the Irvine scandal broke is fitting coincidence. This official spokesman was voicing sentiments maintained by members of this specialty throughout two decades of phenomenal growth. While he might claim credit for his organization's cooperation in developing existing (though unfunded) legislation and licensing mechanisms, the fact is fertility specialists and their society fought even such minimal measures at every turn. Cooperation evolved as a last resort, when alternatives the doctors considered far worse threatened to become reality. What prevailed were voluntary, and therefore unenforceable, guidelines and insistence that, as a profession, doctors must police themselves. This approach, however, could not avert problems that were growing too large to ignore during the 1980s—fledgling clinics learning and practicing on patients, established clinics experimenting unsystematically with new techniques, practitioners of assisted reproduction inflating reported success rates, women and offspring suffering dangerous complications from fertility treatments.

Congressional and public pressure did finally force the specialty's hand. These excesses of "free enterprise" led Congressman Ron Wyden to treat IVF clinics as small businesses, subject to government scrutiny and regulation. His subcommittee focused on two problematic areas: providing infertile couples with accurate information about success rates of specific IVF clinics and establishing quality standards for laboratories that handle embryos. First, he pushed the American Society for Reproductive Medicine into conducting annual surveys and reporting success rates by clinic, identified by name, rather than pooling all numbers into nationwide results. He also introduced legislation requiring embryo laboratories to meet minimal standards, as other types of medical laboratories must do. (Such regulation would not touch in vitro procedures performed in doctors' offices, however, nor would it touch other surgeries and medications that constitute most of fertility medicine's diagnostic and treatment procedures.) As the 1980s ended, the society was working with Wyden's staff, drafting legislation they could live with for clinic success reports and laboratory accreditation. When the dust of compromise settled, the major provisions were voluntary and/or supervised by the society.

Congressman Wyden also forced some attention from the Federal Trade Commission, a government agency whose job is to enforce truth in advertising. At public hearings in March 1989, he lambasted the FTC for its "regulatory slumber," for "turn[ing] its back on the problem of misleading IVF advertising" in a policy of "let the buyer beware." In April the FTC began investigating deceptive or inaccurate statements by IVF clinics, but this regulatory awakening was extremely limited. The agency investigates only if it receives reports about a specific clinic, which neither patients nor doctors tend to make. Its initial case resulted from a radio call-in program a commission investigator happened to hear.

The concrete outcome was that fertility medicine entered the 1990s with only voluntary safeguards that lacked any teeth. While some fertility specialists congratulated themselves for the profession's cooperation with government, others sounded a more pessimistic note. They predicted that doctors would resist the uniform standards and independent evaluations of even a voluntary monitoring process. The brief attention of politicians and the profession scurrying to devise new recommendations would subside, leaving the specialty and its patients in worse shape than ever.

Indeed, even as Dr. Ricardo Asch's Irvine clinic was closing down in 1995, more widespread, if less flagrant, abuses of trust continued. For instance, the long-standing problem of deceptive success claims compelled an official of the Federal Trade Commission to issue a statement to fertility specialists. In the pages of *Fertility and Sterility,* he reminded the journal's professional audience that the FTC's task is to prevent "unfair or deceptive" advertising and other promotional activities by various types of businesses, including providers of health care services. Echoing an editorial written eight years earlier by several physicians about patient exploitation, he reviewed principles fertility clinics should be following. Claims about success rates must be true, supported by reliable scientific evidence, and "must not mislead consumers into believing that the chances of success are greater than they really are." Statements about the safety and risks of assisted reproduction must be substantiated by reliable scientific evidence.[2] By this time, however, the 1994 elections had already brought a conservative, antiregulatory Congress to Washington. If change was coming, the direction was not likely to be toward greater authority and enforcement clout for the FTC, FDA, or other government agencies.

For women and men undergoing fertility treatment, this country's lack of regulations can be harmful to their health and well-being. Aside from harm caused by incompetent or unethical physicians, an ominous result from the previous decade's practices surfaced in the mid-1990s. Though apparently and fortunately rare, a long-incubating side effect of artificial insemination—treatment that became popular with physicians during the 1980s—provides fair warning that inadequate monitoring and regulation can have far-reaching, even deadly, consequences. In March 1995 the *Journal of the American Medical Association* reported seven cases of HIV infection traced to sperm banks that did not screen for this virus or other sexually transmitted diseases, such as hepatitis B.[3] Although the Centers for Disease Control issued guidelines in 1986 for testing human tissue to be "transplanted," including semen, sperm, and eggs, the guidelines were voluntary, with no monitoring provisions. No one can know how many additional HIV cases remain undetected, since sperm banks do not generally keep thorough records of their depositors, customers, or any health screening the facility may perform. No one even knows how many of these facilities exist, who staffs them, how staff are trained, or how donors are selected. In other countries—for example, Australia, New Zealand, Great Britain, Scandinavian countries—medical registries keep track of patients, allowing doctors to study their long-term health and to notify individuals who may be affected as health risks become known. In other countries, moreover, stronger regulations govern fertility treatments in the first place.[4]

The regulatory void in which fertility medicine operates here is an American phenomenon. Other countries are far less leery about whether to regulate the burgeoning array of reproductive technologies; rather, arguments arise over how far regulations should extend. Consider the response of the United Kingdom, home to the world's first IVF baby. Following the birth of Louise Brown in 1978, the British government established a commission, with the active involvement of the medical community, to examine and debate ethical, social, and medical issues related to assisted reproduction. With unanimous agreement of its members, the commission established a Human Fertilisation and Embryo Authority (HFEA) to regulate fertility doctors and clinics. This government agency grants licenses to all IVF programs—covering both treatment and research—conducts annual clinic inspections, and has the power to shut down clinics or revoke a doctor's license to practice. Criminal laws apply in cases of serious violation of mandatory requirements. Rather than resist, the medical community generally welcomed and continues to support HFEA activities. In Australia, another country leading in the development of assisted reproduction, the government prodded physicians and the major infertility consumer group to maintain a clinic accreditation and annual audit program as a condition for including reproductive technologies under national health insurance coverage.

The purpose of licensing and monitoring requirements is to maintain minimal levels of staff training and skill and to ensure that treatment and research meet ethical standards, proceeding only with patient consent and confidentiality. But if the Irvine clinic exposé forced greater awareness that this country sorely lacks patient safeguards, it also raised the question of whether protective regulations would prevent such deplorable activities. The university's chancellor, agreeing with DeCherney and other physicians, claimed not. Even if laws exist, "if an individual wants to run a stoplight, he will."[5] That argument, however, has never meant that a community should not install stoplights at busy or dangerous intersections. Fertility medicine is certainly busy and can often be dangerous. Regulations can cut down on this medical community's traffic problems, saving some patients from being injured, since even the rogue physician usually does not wish to be caught and punished.

Less directly, a solid code of regulations, accreditation, and ongoing policing can help restrain the flow of rewards that have fueled the fertility industry to an unhealthy degree. As the Irvine clinic so clearly demonstrated, those rewards include profit, prestige, and, for some doctors, ego boosts that come with directing a medical fiefdom. In the Irvine case, a university medical center courted a big-name fertility specialist, granting him a faculty position, a well-equipped clinic, and full autonomy, while demanding no accountability. Successful pregnancies brought income and gilded reputations to doctors and institution alike. The absence of regulations and independent oversight can only make it too easy for such an enterprise to thrive. Subjecting the process to more scrutiny—starting with a clinic's inception and continuing throughout its treatment and research program—and encouraging ongoing public and professional discussion of reproductive interventions will at least help limit the number of patients subjected to inappropriate treatment and worse.

By the 1995 meeting of the American Society for Reproductive Medicine, even DeCherney had changed his tune, conceding the need for protective regulations. The physical absence of Asch, former star member, could not diminish his demoralizing presence, like a specter hovering around formal sessions and private conversations. As one officer explained, the affiliated group on assisted reproduction was now establishing guidelines "we didn't think we needed" about embryo donation. With some dissension in the ranks—that group's president was still arguing for self-regulation—the society was forced once again into action. Taking another preemptive move, it broke its fifty-one years of opposition to government regulation of doctors. A committee would begin drafting legislation, modeled upon mechanisms used in the United Kingdom, to be used by states that want to impose controls on fertility clinics. "I know regulation is a scary word," said one society staffperson, "but if we're not involved in the process, they're going to do it to us."[6]

In other countries, oversight of fertility medicine extends further than the licensing and monitoring that might emerge in this country from any new round of professional and legislative activity. Governments or fertility societies have restricted certain treatment and research procedures doctors can perform. Differing types of decisions address varying concerns, leaving no doubt that regulation of reproductive interventions is no simple matter. Britain's HFEA was quick to target one of the clearest causes of complications for women and offspring—the number of embryos a doctor transfers during any single treatment attempt. With a few exceptions, the HFEA established an upper limit of three; out of twenty-one countries that have regulations or guidelines, all but seven have set a similar limit.[7] In France, a 1994 report by a physicians' group, the Ordre des Médecins, expressed concern about the techniques fertility specialists and embryologists were increasingly performing without adequate pretesting in animals—especially ovarian stimulation and experimental injecting of sperm into eggs (ICSI). "In a few years we may well be in the middle of a scandal of similar proportion to that caused by the thoughtless use of [diethylstilbestrol] and the resulting disastrous consequences," the report concluded.[8]

Beyond minimizing health risks, an incentive for other countries toward restricting reproductive technologies is cost-effectiveness within a national health program. Governments that pay for medical care want value for their money. Immediately, however, questions of access arise. How can medical resources be fairly distributed, particularly treatments that are strongly desired but elective, that bring high cost but low success? Who will be able to undergo such treatments, and how many times? As if medical and cost-benefit assessments were not complicated enough, regulating and rationing fertility medicine slides quickly into considerations of social and moral acceptability. While physicians worry over intrusion on professional autonomy, the public must ask whether access decisions are intrusively defining who is permitted to become a parent.

A few examples help illustrate this thicket of concerns. In determining which medical procedures will be covered under national health insurance, the Canadian province of Ontario considered available medical information evaluated by a national commission; the province decided to cover in vitro fertilization only for women with blocked fallopian tubes, the condition for which this treatment is most clearly and frequently beneficial.[9] This deliberation about cost-effectiveness of government health care dollars is quite different from debates now occupying governments and medical communities where reproductive technologies flourish. One target for regulation is the commercialism that in this country tenaciously grasps fertility medicine, with great potential for economic exploitation. To curtail the business dimension of assisted reproduction, for instance, the United Kingdom bans most forms of surrogacy in which a couple pays another woman to be impregnated, carry, and deliver their child (in the United States the fee is generally around $12,000, plus expenses); that country also severely limits fees paid to sperm and egg donors. The Canadian national parliament established similar restrictions in 1996.[10]

A different type of restriction arises in the decision about whether a given embryo will be allowed to develop. By combining in vitro and genetic techniques, doctors and prospective parents can identify some of the characteristics of a prospective child; they can then decide whether to transfer the embryo to the woman's uterus in hopes of having that child. Such prenatal diagnosis often aims at eliminating, or possibly treating, serious genetic illnesses and anomalies.

However, the same techniques can also identify other characteristics—most obviously a baby's sex. As genetic knowledge increases, the list of physical, and perhaps even mental, attributes that can be identified will surely lengthen. With male infants strongly preferred in various regions of the world, with memories of Nazi eugenics still fresh and images of "designer babies" not far ahead, the United Kingdom prohibits selection of an embryo on the basis of its sex (except for medical reasons) or other physical characteristics.

While attempting to preclude designer babies, however, Britain's HFEA could create designer parents by requiring them to possess certain social characteristics. After a lesbian virgin announced her baby's birth in 1994, the HFEA began considering whether single women and lesbians should receive assisted reproductive treatments through the national health service, or whether to cover treatment only for families consisting of a woman and man who are married. Needless to say, gay and lesbian organizations, as well as many unattached heterosexuals, voiced adamant opposition to any such restriction.

Postmenopausal pregnancies, using younger women's eggs, have raised some governments' hackles. This debate pits ageism and sexism (older men with late-life babies generally elicit smiles rather than disapproval) against health risks for older pregnant women, beliefs that women's natural reproductive lives should not be extended by medical technology—or their identity defined primarily as childbearers—and concerns about anticipated social difficulties for children of older parents. While no mandatory age limit for assisted reproduction exists in the United Kingdom, the HFEA expresses strong reservations against treating women over the age of fifty. In France and in Italy— where some of the oldest women to have become pregnant received treatment from a particularly controversial doctor—postmenopausal pregnancies are now prohibited.

Perhaps no country could better illustrate the unavoidable intertwining of modern technological fertility treatments with strongly held social, moral, and religious beliefs than Italy—nor could any display more concretely the range of conclusions that unwind from this mix. At one extreme, Dr. Severino Antinori offers postmenopausal women the miracle of conception, pregnancy, and birth through medical technology. His patients include women who come, as if on pilgrimage, from countries where the practice is banned. In 1994, his oldest successful fertility patient gave birth at the age of sixty-two. A year later, as she expressed the desire for another child, Italy's national medical association was formulating a doctors' code of ethics that would eliminate that opportunity. Responding to postmenopausal pregnancies, cases of surrogacy, selection of sperm

donors to attain specific characteristics in offspring, and cross-racial egg donation, this set of restrictions constitutes Italy's middle ground. Although the regulations were presented as "an urgent appeal" to parliament for legislation, the
professional organization itself has the power to expel or suspend doctors from
membership, effectively ending their practice of medicine in Italy. The ethics
code aims at limiting artificial inseminations to stable, heterosexual couples. It
forbids assisted reproduction for postmenopausal women, for women whose
partner has died (having previously deposited sperm in a sperm bank), and for
any form of surrogate pregnancy. The code bans sperm selection based on social, economic, or professional standing of the donor, and any artificial insemination based on racial prejudice.

Predictably, one of the most vocal opponents of this doctors' code was Antinori, who described the restrictions as "anachronistic, illiberal, and anti-
democratic."[11] From the other end of the spectrum came equally adamant disapproval. For the Catholic Church this code did not go far enough, because it
failed to prohibit all forms of artificial insemination. In this mostly Roman
Catholic country, with the Vatican in its midst, the priests condemn all medical
interventions involving embryos, telling Italian women and men that any type
of artificial insemination is immoral, sinful, and forbidden.

The Vatican is certainly not alone in its concern about embryos, or in more
general fears about where technology is taking human reproduction. In every
country where assisted reproductive capabilities exist, the idea of embryos does
give people great pause, becoming at times the focus of serious controversy as
disagreement erupts over concepts of their humanness and over the ethics of
treatments or research that use and possibly destroy them.[12] Before dangers of
misappropriated embryos, or of research conducted without a couple's consent, materialized in the Irvine clinic, some American fertility specialists were
warning of ethical and legal tangles attached not only to the immediate reproductive intervention but to the increasing accumulation of embryos stored in
freezers throughout the country.

However, on issues of fertility medicine, the profession, government, and
the public seem always trying to catch up, their deliberations pulled by each
new technique that becomes possible. One technological breakthrough provoking a storm of controversy in the mid-1990s was the ability to remove immature eggs from the ovaries of a deceased woman, mature the eggs in a laboratory, fertilize them, and transfer the resulting embryos to the uterus of an
infertile woman; in a very few years, researchers in the United Kingdom an-

nounced, a similar technique would be possible with ovarian tissue from aborted fetuses. As one British analyst put it, with characteristic understatement, "The technique would obviously end the current shortage of donated eggs."[13] Research that would further develop this technique—through better understanding of egg development, fertilization, and embryo growth—could also increase knowledge about reproductive processes and the causes of miscarriage, as well as contribute to more effective methods of contraception and of detecting congenital abnormalities.

These potentially vast new sources of "donated" eggs and other scientific gains pulled reproductive technologies beyond what many people could comfortably accept. Other people draw the line much sooner—at abortion or at destruction of any embryo resulting from assisted conception. In all such determinations, the progression from laboratory fertilization techniques (including cloning) to, at some stage, human life brings into the debate over reproductive technologies people's most basic beliefs about the nature of becoming and being human. In the United Kingdom, research using fetal or cadaver eggs stopped while the HFEA evaluated medical, ethical, and legal concerns—continuing the oversight process initiated after the first IVF birth.[14] In 1995 Denmark's Ethical Council on biomedical research was advising that country's parliament of a need for greater restrictions on doctors and scientists, beyond already existing regional science-ethics committees.[15] That same year, Canada's Health Ministry called for a "voluntary moratorium" on nine new reproductive technologies as a first step toward creating a permanent nationwide regulatory mechanism for reproductive technologies.[16] One year later, the Canadian Health Department brought to Parliament legislation that will prohibit these procedures and four additional uses of reproductive technologies.[17]

No comparable process exists in the United States. Instead, closely linked issues of assisted reproduction, scientific research, oversight, and regulation disappeared into the quicksand of abortion politics. Beliefs about sin and evil predominated, as in Italy; highly charged moralistic and religious assertions defined the struggle, precluding calmer discussion of how best to resolve conflicting views in a secular democracy. The federal government withdrew from involvement with reproductive technologies, eliminating public forums for medical, ethical, and legal debate. This withdrawal would have a direct impact on women and men hoping for a pregnancy, as well as on the scientific and medical communities. The consequences emerge most pointedly in recurrent arguments over human embryo research.

Keeping Government Hands off Research

As the Irvine clinic scandal broke, Dr. Mary Martin felt disheartened on another front where she has devoted time and energy—reversing government policies banning medical and biological research that could improve what she tries to do each day. In this instance, Dr. Martin was not in anguish over transgressions by one of the specialty's own, although accusations she investigated and her current pessimism over IVF-related research are surely connected. Rather, her disheartenment reflects frustrating years in which fertility specialists themselves feel victimized. Although physicians have enjoyed considerable success fending off perceived governmental threats to their independence, one form of involvement the medical profession welcomes, indeed requires, is funding for research. In seeking support throughout the 1980s for studies of the fertilization process, early embryo development, and implantation, IVF researchers met their match. Pleas for government involvement through the usual funding channels could not overpower an even stronger lobby—anti-abortion forces opposed to any such research.[18]

With the Clinton administration had come the exhilaration of anticipated change. Yet now fertility specialists like Martin felt they were riding the drop of a roller coaster. By mid-decade the lesson was: never take political directions or their medical outcomes for granted. Because of this country's ban on government-funded IVF research, fertility patients may be receiving inferior treatments, facing greater risks, agreeing to more "selective reduction" of multiple fetuses, and undergoing more unscientific experimentation than they otherwise would. Hear the history of how this state of affairs came to be—and know that history, in the form of political pressure to halt certain types of medical research, is already repeating itself.

During the 1970s, in response to accumulating reports of research that seriously violated the rights of human participants (including the Tuskegee syphilis studies), the Department of Health, Education, and Welfare (later renamed Health and Human Services) undertook a broad assessment of controversial biomedical research. As one component of this assessment, the department issued regulations requiring that all proposals submitted for government funding of research involving human embryos—including in vitro fertilization research—be reviewed by an Ethics Advisory Board (EAB). Members were appointed to the board, and it began to consider not only a specific research application, but more general questions surrounding human IVF and embryo transfer research. The EAB commissioned studies by scientists, ethicists, and lawyers, and held public hearings to obtain views of professional societies, private citizens, and consumer groups. In a 1979 report, the EAB concluded that such research and government funding for it are ethically acceptable. "A broad prohibition . . . is neither justifiable nor wise." The question of funding priority for individual proposals was referred to the usual scientific peer review process within the National Institutes of Health.

A public comment period followed. The Department of Health and Human Services received over 13,000 responses, the vast majority pouring in from well-organized groups opposed to federal funding of IVF research because embryos might be destroyed in the process. Meanwhile, after issuing its report, the Ethics Advisory Board disbanded. What may have initially been a bureaucratic mistake during transition to the Reagan administration in 1980 turned into a de facto government stance; each secretary of Health and Human Services failed to resurrect the lapsed board. In a stellar example of catch-22 policy formulation, government funding of IVF research was prohibited, since any research proposal would lack the required EAB review.

By the close of Reagan's administration, talk of fertility patient exploitation was reaching Capitol Hill. The congressional subcommittee overseeing Health and Human Services began to investigate the government's role regarding infertility. In 1987, the Office of Technology Assessment reported to Congress that IVF "never went through a formal or regulatory research stage in the United States to demonstrate either safety or efficacy, in large part due to the lack of Federal direction and Federal funding. . . . An unofficial moratorium on all Federal funding and oversight of IVF research . . . [eliminated] the most direct line of authority by which the Federal government can influence the development of both embryo research and infertility treatment so as to avoid unacceptable practices or inappropriate uses." Throughout that moratorium, the administration ignored numerous requests by scientists and physicians to reconstitute the EAB; of course, it was also ignoring the original regulations requiring that such a board exist. A major theme when HHS staff presented options to the department's secretaries was that "to take no action will avoid controversy."[19]

In 1988, the director of the National Institutes of Health—the hub of government biomedical research activities—tried again to spur action toward funding IVF research. He received no response until public congressional hearings began, focused on the federal role in preventing and treating infertility. As scientists, physicians, and consumers testified to the need for reversing the research moratorium, the Assistant Secretary for Health announced that his department would "do the best we can" to establish a new Ethics Advisory Board before the Reagan administration left office. Everyone went home anticipating a change in the government's policy, if not by the end of Reagan's tenure, then with the incoming Bush administration. In the Senate, supporters of a provision to mandate a new EAB as part of legislation that regularly reauthorizes Health and Human Services dropped this strategy following assurances from the department that initial steps were in progress. The steps soon halted. First, action was deferred to the next secretary. Then the next secretary's appointment became mired in opposition from the anti-abortion movement.

As months passed, it became apparent that the EAB was but one captive of abortion politics. A different ethics panel, established within Congress, disbanded without ever meeting, following disagreements between anti-abortion and pro-choice advocates over choosing the panel's congressional members. In a related action, the Bush administration extended a ban on federal financing of research on medical treatments using transplanted fetal tissue, a decision described by Dr. Brit Harvey, president of the American Academy of Pediatrics, as "like the Middle Ages . . . [interfering] with knowledge that is going to save the lives of fetuses, babies, and adults as well." In the view of Dr. John C. Fletcher, former chief ethicist at the National Institutes for Health, the government was certainly involved, by default, with IVF and fetal research; its role in this entire arena of abortion politics and biomedical policy amounted to "outright suppression of scientific research and public debate."[20]

With the 1980s coming to a close, the congressional subcommittee issued its bipartisan report, concluding: "It is an embarrassment . . . that the last five Secretaries of HHS . . . have ignored HHS regulations to appoint an Ethics Advisory Board." Reflecting frustration felt within and outside government at the influence of anti-abortion forces over scientific and medical policy, the committee's chair, Congressman Ted Weiss, stated, "Infertile couples are spending their life savings on treatment that doesn't work because the Federal Government has not been willing to study infertility treatment the way it studies treatment for every other disease. It is outrageous that our national health agency has ignored the repeated pleas of their own scientists, the medical and scientific communities, and millions of infertile Americans who have repeatedly asked them to fund this research and to appoint an EAB to review all controversial medical research." Demonstrating the inextricable connection of the research moratorium to broader medical questions for fertility patients, the subcommittee recommended not only that the government reconstitute the EAB and fund IVF research, but that it increase research more generally on causes, treatment, and prevention of infertility. Additionally, the report called for a national data bank to gather follow-up health information on offspring of assisted conception as well as on women who received fertility treatment.[21] The recommendations fell on deaf ears. Instead, in the wake of congressional investigation, public hearings, expert testimony, official and unofficial requests, fertility medicine entered the 1990s with only greater certainty that an Ethics Advisory Board was dead.

The government's non-policy policy of forgoing all responsibility for support and oversight of research removed yet another restraint on unregulated expansion of fertility medicine. For researchers, private funding, largely from the pharmaceutical industry, became indispensable, as did patient willingness to pay for treatments that were, in fact, reproductive experiments. As for the ethical dimensions of assisted reproduction, individual medical centers, obstetrics and gynecology departments, and physicians were left to their own devices.

Concerned about the adequacy of these devices for ethical review and decisions about research, two national physicians' organizations did attempt to step in where the government had dropped out. In 1991, seeking to "fill a moral vacuum created by the abdication of the Federal government," the American Society for Reproductive Medicine and the American College of Obstetricians and Gynecologists established a private board to set ethical guidelines and provide a peer review procedure for studies involving in vitro fertilization, reproductive genetics, and use of fetal tissue. The fifteen members of this National Advisory Board on Ethics in Reproduction (NABER) include doctors, scientists, lawyers, ethicists, and representatives of consumer groups; among the fertility specialists participating on this board is Mary Martin. As initially envisioned, this board would invite researchers to submit research proposals for ethical review. However, the panel soon decided they were not ready to evaluate proposals; agreeing among themselves on the basic ethical framework would itself require a time-consuming process of information gathering and discussion. Moreover, if they reached the stage of inviting research proposals, submissions would be voluntary, and—in contrast to the government's power to require changes before funding a study—the board would have no power to require changes in any research. As a result, then, although Martin and the other NABER members held meetings and conference calls and organized educational forums, the most publicized controversies in fertility medicine came as a surprise to the ethics board. They were unaware of so-called embryo cloning experiments that caused an uproar when they were reported at the 1993 annual convention of the American Society of Reproductive Medicine. Nor could such a panel prevent the unconscionable behaviors that occurred at the Irvine clinic.

It is no wonder that when the public finally caught a glimpse inside that fertility clinic, the view—albeit in exaggerated form—was of a medical field awash in private money (physicians reportedly carried cash-stuffed envelopes home from the office) and devoid of adequate protections (the clinic director reportedly exerted "authoritarian" control over treatment of patients, eggs, embryos, and clinic and laboratory staff). Unbeknownst to patients, doctors conducted laboratory experiments as well as studies of surgical procedures and medications. Wealthy women, perhaps nearing menopause, were able to pay the internationally acclaimed fertility specialist to "do something" that would make them pregnant, no questions asked. If the usual means (a young woman agreeing to provide eggs in return for $2,500) had not been arranged, he would arrange an alternative—shuffling "extra" eggs or embryos from some other patient (perhaps even superovulating and retrieving eggs from a woman for that reason only), no permission asked.

While the Irvine clinic revelations might finally bring some manner of regulation on fertility medicine, the likelihood of government involvement with embryo research seemed to be fast disappearing by 1995. In the early, heady days of the Clinton administration, scientists and medical researchers celebrated prospects for reversing the Reagan-Bush ban on government support for studies using embryos or fetal tissue. In one of his first executive actions, the newly inaugurated president initiated steps toward the 1993 NIH Revitalization Act, which nullified the requirement that embryo research be reviewed by a nonexistent Ethics Advisory Board. The NIH director appointed a panel that met over several months to review the pros and cons of human embryo research. Once again, Martin found herself traveling to meetings far from office and patients. In a déjà vu spanning fifteen years, she and her panel colleagues concluded that research using human embryos is justified and worthy of government funding. Among the scientific and medical benefits was the potential for improved diagnosis and treatment of infertility.

With the possibility of government-funded research restored, fertility specialists were looking forward to increased knowledge about the conception process, the development and implantation of embryos, the reasons IVF succeeds or fails. They could now imagine conducting research that for so many years took place mainly in other countries, research that would hasten a better understanding of the causes and treatment of infertility, research that might increase success rates and lower complications of assisted reproduction. "Not only would we gain basic scientific knowledge, about normal and abnormal cell growth, for instance," Martin explains almost longingly, "we would not have to resort to what we do today. Instead of hyperstimulating women to get a large number of eggs and embryos, the research could help us develop ways to succeed with a woman's natural menstrual cycle." For instance, research could help embryologists develop laboratory techniques to assess and improve embryo quality, making implantation and normal growth more likely. Specialists like Martin also hoped for a different kind of payoff. Although she recognized that the amount of money actually available to fund specific studies might be modest, she looked forward to the oversight that comes with the government's research review and funding process. Rather than ignore scientific, ethical, and legal implications of this medical reality, the United States would finally join the nearly two dozen other countries that have established some manner of assessing and regulating reproductive technologies.

The NIH panel report in September 1994 was the good news. In a notable stroke of political timing, the bad news for IVF research that fall was the landslide mid-term election of a conservative Congress actively determined to reverse yet again the country's direction. Already, the Clinton administration had suffered the defeat of health care reform and muted its more progressive voices. For fertility medicine in particular, this new comedown in 1994 meant that prospects once so promising now looked grim, as if the déjà vu would in fact extend, returning the country to Reagan-Bush biomedical policies. By the summer of 1995, with a scandalous Dr. Asch hitting the news, legislation wending its way through Congress included a provision banning federal funds for human embryo research.[22] This provision became part of the NIH's appropriation bill in 1996.

That same year, the NIH enforced this prohibition for the first time, withdrawing its funding from a geneticist whose research included IVF-related testing of DNA from eight-cell human embryos—a technique used before proceeding with embryo transfer to screen for mutations that cause severe disease (e.g., Tay-Sachs, cystic fibrosis). Scientists warned, once again, that such actions discourage talented researchers from studying important embryologic questions and further isolate reproductive research within private fertility clinics, beyond the reach of government regulation or peer review. They noted, once again, the paradoxical (described as "obscene" by one researcher) willingness to allow transfer of many embryos to increase IVF pregnancy rates, relying on selective abortion to reduce the number of fetuses, all the while prohibiting the research on fertilization and implantation that could make this practice unnecessary.[23]

Just as regulations cannot stop all rule breakers, government-funded research, with its accompanying oversight, is not an ethical panacea. However, government involvement does bolster existing restraints of peer review and career rewards within the scientific and medical research network; research and treatment does become subject to more discussion and greater accountability. Martin notes that "an individual can set up a laboratory and clone embryos in his garage if he is so inclined, even though there are no academic or career incentives reinforcing that behavior." But the more eyes on the specialty, the more ethical reviews and restraints, the less likely unjustified research and improper patient treatment become.

Fertility medicine is a matter of probabilities in more ways than patients commonly recognize. Beyond likelihoods of success or failure or of medical complications are chances for exploitive and unethical treatment. Government funding of research, even in combination with more direct regulation and monitoring of physicians and laboratories, will not provide fail-safe protection for women and men undergoing fertility treatment. However, this involvement can make patient mistreatment less likely.

Forcing the Real toward the Ideal

As of the mid-1990s, even as upheaval within fertility medicine and the need for major changes became undeniable, the odds for improved patient protection and treatment were still not favorable. There was no government funding of embryo research, no well-enforced regulation of doctors or laboratories, no registries maintaining comprehensive records of immediate and long-term health effects related to fertility treatments, no public debate about the manner and direction of reproductive interventions. Beyond this decade into the twenty-first century, moreover, some additional characteristics of health politics and policy in this country may further reduce women's and men's reproductive chances.

Failing to Look Upstream

When the Office of Technology Assessment reported to Congress on infertility in 1987, its investigation could find no federal government support of "identifiable activities expressly directed toward prevention of infertility." During the Clinton administration's attempt to formulate health care reform, prevention became an accepted medical watchword, especially as a potential cost-cutting approach. Rather than continue devising complex ways to save people from drowning, argued some economists and health care administrators, we should "look upstream to see who is pushing people in."

Present and future generations of women and men could certainly benefit from shifting the medical gaze upstream—toward determining what compromises their fertility, pushing them into the pool of patients needing medical help to conceive a pregnancy. As Chapter 6 suggested, preventing infertility entails more than lifestyle choices that are within the individual's power to make. A preventive approach requires knowing and attacking environmental causes, iatrogenic (medical) causes, the presently unknown causes of infertility; it also requires government prodding, most concretely in supporting preventive research and health care. The pharmaceutical industry, a major source of funding for research in fertility medicine, is far more likely to support studies of treatments that use their products—heroic medical efforts to rescue "desperate" fertility patients—than studies of ways women and men can stay out of the stream. Nor do fertility specialists make their careers by preventing infertility. An additional component of prevention will also depend on government support—registries that document the long-term health consequences of current treatments for women and offspring. By maintaining thorough records of patients, prescriptions, and procedures, researchers can attempt to identify health problems early and prevent similar iatrogenic outcomes in the future.

While prevention may be in danger of joining human embryo research as a casualty of political backtracking, its salvation could be the mounting concern with health care costs, a concern not easily dissipated by political reversals. However, the prevailing means toward controlling expensive medical procedures brings mixed prospects, at best, for fertility patients.

Managing Costs, Care, and Consumers

Return for a moment to Dr. Martin's office, the outer office where a persistent ringing of telephones punctuates the typing of two staffpeople. You need hear only the office side of the conversation to gain a lesson about health economics in everyday life.

"No, we don't have any discounts here," is one response. The caller has seen a newspaper advertisement offering a reduced IVF fee to infertile women who participate in a research study. Now she is comparison shopping before deciding where to seek fertility treatment.

Another caller is already Martin's patient. "We don't know what the supply will be in the fall . . . We could schedule you in August," is the answer to this patient's inquiry about a shortage of Pergonal, the most commonly used fertility drug for superovulation before the various forms of assisted reproduction. "But Dr. Martin will be away part of that month." The caller is worried. She and her husband have planned a summer vacation, a break from fertility treatment, before starting again, hopefully refreshed, in the fall. Now they have heard from their pharmacist of the Pergonal shortage. Perhaps they should stay home, take a vacation some other time, in case the drug is completely unavailable later. "So your period would be due when?" asks the staffperson, as the caller now tries to figure whether her menstrual cycle will synchronize with the doctor's travel schedule. She would be disappointed to have another physician—someone she doesn't know as well—transfer her embryos.

Martin has, in fact, met recently with a representative of Serono Laboratories about this Pergonal shortage, as have many fertility specialists. She was "suspicious," thinking the drug's manufacturer might be holding back this drug as a way of getting doctors to switch to a newer Serono product, thus beating out a European competitor. Serono has a bad image with patients because Pergonal is so expensive in this country, costing twice as much here as it does in Mexico, for example. The expense of fertility drugs jacks up the price of treatment considerably for fertility patients. Doctors charge a basic fee, with the cost of medications added (approximately $2,000 per cycle in 1997); medications are generally not covered in the few insurance plans that include some type of fertility treatment. As Martin puts it, Pergonal is Serono's "gold mine," used by 30–50 percent of patients receiving a fertility treatment. After meeting with the representative, she thinks the shortage probably is what the company claimed— product shortfall, until their synthetic version of the same drug is ready to be marketed. That version still awaits FDA approval. This wait, of course, could be another motive for allowing, or creating, the shortage that has patients anxiously calling pharmacies all over the country.

As for insurance coverage more generally, one of the office staff fielding the doctor's phone calls has just returned from a long, tedious meeting where personnel from departments throughout this medical center received an update about the hundreds of insurance plans, varying forms, and requirements their patients may have. "Makes me want to rethink single-payer," she comments, referring to dormant, if not dead, efforts to establish a national or state health insurance plan that would eliminate private insurance companies from the medical action. Whatever their particular insurance or financial means, people with fertility problems will be caught in a managed-care squeeze that increasingly defines this country's efforts to cut medical costs. Women and men considering fertility treatment need to understand how these pressures may be affecting their own care, for better or worse.

The collapse of health care reform during the early 1990s left unresolved basic questions about who will receive what medical services and how the cost will be covered. In all aspects of medicine, determining the efficacy of medical procedures and distributing them fairly remain essential and formidable tasks. In fertility medicine, present operating principles are relatively clear: those who can afford to pay out of pocket for diagnosis and treatment or can afford an insurance plan that at least partially covers infertility receive medical services. The quality, appropriateness, and consequences of care for individual women and men are far less apparent.

Fertility medicine has always been skewed toward those able to pay when their health insurance will not. Obtaining insurance coverage has been an ongoing struggle for individual patients and the consumer organization Resolve; insurers balk at interventions they define as elective and experimental—not to mention expensive—for a condition they often designate as "preexisting."[24] Failure to establish a national health insurance program in the 1990s took the wind out of efforts to mandate insurance coverage for infertility, efforts that had been proceeding state by state. Patients and physicians still find themselves waging individual battles with a vast array of health plans. However, health care trends now prevailing in this country have shifted financial incentives for many physicians, changing the medical strategies with which fertility patients must contend. While the need for patient vigilance remains constant, the potential dangers of undertreatment as well as overtreatment are somewhat altered, depending on one's insurance status.

The major trend in the aftermath of failed health care reform is rapid expansion of managed-care plans that pay doctors' groups and hospitals a set, capitated annual fee for each enrolled patient, no matter how many medical services that patient actually receives. This creates an incentive to spend as little as possible "per capita." Physician income does not rise with every visit and procedure, as in the fee-for-service payments (whether by patients or third-party insurers) that characterized American medicine in the past; indeed, some managed-care plans penalize doctors who perform too many procedures, as determined by the plan's managers, and reward those who come in under budget. The most prominent strategies for controlling cost—enroll patients who are not likely to use many services, perform fewer medical procedures, and refer patients less often to specialists—strike directly at the practice of fertility medicine.

What could be the consequences for women and men with fertility problems? For a proportion of patients in managed-care plans, fewer procedures and less specialized care will in fact mean avoiding medical interventions they don't need. With time and, perhaps, less invasive treatments, they will have a baby. Or they will stop pursuing treatments that, in their case, continue to fail. In this scenario, doctors and patients share an interest in performing only those diagnostic procedures that are useful, in trying treatments that have been proven effective, in not prolonging treatment that fails, in avoiding harmful—and costly—complications. Preventing infertility in the first place can also reduce medical expenditures. These are examples of managed care working at its best, actually reducing unnecessary, expensive, and potentially harmful medical interventions. However, there seems no reason to assume the best.

As the managed-care trend gains momentum, ample indications suggest that the paramount concern of management is too often simply the lowering of costs, with little regard for providing what individual women and men actually need, to all who need it. This shift in financial incentives for doctors leaves patients shortchanged. Within managed-care plans, patients may face a problem now endemic across the American medical scene—cut-rate medical care. Certain diagnostic and treatment procedures may not be covered by their plan. Procedures that are included may be applied in assembly-line fashion without first determining which individuals need what. To attain quick success, doctors may use more aggressive treatments that carry more risks.

Patients with complex, prolonged infertility—those most in need of medical intervention—are likely to experience the greatest difficulty obtaining it. A physician who is a specialist on their particular problem may not be on their plan's list of available choices. Medical school faculty—who may be most knowledgeable and experienced in treating certain conditions—already feel the pressure; as one university hospital director reportedly stated to his faculty, "[We can] no longer tolerate patients with complex and expensive-to-treat conditions being encouraged to transfer to our group." [25] Women and men who can benefit from a specialist's care will face a frustrating financial bind. Referral from their internist or general ob-gyn to a fertility specialist, even one on the plan's list, may be hard to come by. Do they settle for whatever treatment is covered, performed by a physician who may have less experience, skills, and knowledge? Do they pay extra, perhaps at great sacrifice, to go outside their insurance plan? While fertility specialists hammer home the message that "we can get you a baby," and while fertility patients want to know that "we did all we could . . . we took the extra step," they may have to pay dearly for that step and, perhaps, that baby.

The bind produced by today's managed care is even more complicated, however, entangling as well those women and men willing and able to pay for the medical extras. Fertility specialists who see their patient pool shrinking, as managed care limits referrals, may inflate claims about the need for sophisticated and invasive procedures only they can perform. The managed-care patients can then try arguing their way to a referral based on the need for specialist care their insurance plan's physicians cannot offer. At the same time, with fewer insured patients, specialists will solicit greater numbers of what has always been their assured clientele—women and men able to pay out of their own pocket. As doctors compete for fertility patients, the patients may need to be even more wary of deceptive advertising and aggressive treatment. To maintain high volume, doctors will be particularly eager to attract the easiest cases—including many subfertile couples who could conceive a pregnancy without treatment. They may also repeat unsuccessful treatments too many times. For these patients, fertility medicine will maintain, and even intensify, the fee-for-service incentives of the past.

Physicians are certainly aware of this dynamic. In the view of Dr. Norbert Gleicher, head of a large group practice of infertility specialists in the Chicago area, "Certain providers have strong financial incentives to take patients to IVF, which may lead patients there who don't need it." And the medical director of Illinois Blue Cross–Blue Shield comments: "In the fee-for-service sector, as long as a woman is willing to go on, the doctors might say, 'Let's keep trying.' Obviously one makes more fees that way."[26] Overall, this trend will reinforce excessive use of more invasive and risky fertility interventions. As in previous generations, wealthier patients with greater access to information, specialists, and treatments will disproportionately reap the benefits of medical progress—and the futility and harm it can bring.[27]

Bringing Fertility Treatment to Managed Care

The impact of managed care, and of cost-cutting more generally, cannot be emphasized enough. Two panel presentations at the American Gynecological and Obstetrical Society's annual meeting, held in 1995, provide a glimpse of what patients may increasingly face at the doctor's office.

One presentation tells doctors how to develop an infertility managed-care plan. As noted, managed care theoretically holds potential for improving some aspects of patient care; it is hard to argue, for instance, with the stated rationale for this alternative to the usual fee-for-service system—"that many couples [presently] undergo diagnostic and therapeutic interventions that contribute little to successful outcomes."[28] At the same time, this "how-to" prototype suggests a less than promising picture of what the reality—the managed-care "product," as such plans are called—will be. Consider the following aspects of the plan:

With its predominant emphasis on costs, break-even points, profit margins, and financial advantages for an insurance company, the plan offers patients a standard package that must be quick (completed within fifteen months), low cost (compared to present fee-for-service), and high volume.

Calculations of cost per pregnancy determine which specific procedures doctors can perform; any procedure with either low probability of pregnancy or high cost is eliminated.

The plan must be simple and uniform, since "multiple pathways for treatment extend the time to pregnancy and increase the costs." While acknowledging the difficulty of providing a standard protocol for fertility problems, these panelists propose replacing many of the other diagnostic and treatment procedures with in vitro fertilization.

Once the participating doctors agree on a standard package, "it cannot be violated. Violations will result in increased costs (and decreased profits) to the physicians or institution providing the infertility services."

Managed care "encourages early treatment for infertility," and should be considered a "lifetime plan" (i.e., a onetime, all-or-nothing chance, with no further insurance coverage if patients do not conceive during the 15-month protocol).

And this final piece of advice to doctors "when marketing a managed care plan" to insurance executives: "The financial advantages to the insurance company must be presented within the first 5 minutes. Otherwise, executive attention will be lost."[29]

The second presentation reinforces all of the above, but focuses on a prevalent fertility problem—fallopian tube disease—asking, "Is there ever a role for tubal surgery?" Their answer: "Hardly ever." IVF will take over "not only because it is simply the most alluring technique available, but because it meets the demands placed on all fertility therapies in the market today." Those demands are to achieve a pregnancy "in short order at the lowest possible cost for the greatest number of individuals."[30] Unlike so many previous reports on tubal surgery, this discussion emphasizes the low rates of successful pregnancy and the high rates of ectopic implantations following such treatments. Given the increased numbers of IVF programs in all regions of the country, compared to years past, almost any woman can now undergo assisted reproduction, with minimal diagnostic investigation.

Despite the emphasis on cost cutting and "one plan fits all" care, there are potential benefits to managed care, as noted above. More fertility specialists are acknowledging what has been apparent for a decade and more: that too many doctors are doing too much to too many patients (although in a tricky bit of reasoning the enlarged number of IVF programs becomes a reason for replacing surgery with IVF). During coming years, economic demands may achieve what patient needs could not: concerns about expense may speed the demise of ineffective tests and treatments and cut down on excessive attempts at treatment that is not succeeding.

The overriding requirement cited by both panels is to reduce "superfetation." With this newly coined technical term for large multiple pregnancies and the undeniable evidence of cost analyses, the managed-care reality for doctors is that insurance companies will not stand for this persistent complication of controlled ovarian hyperstimulation. In fact, one panelist affirms, a managed care plan's "most important selling point [for insurance executives] is the potential to control superfetation." Warns another, insurance companies will take capitated fees away from IVF programs that "have high pregnancy rates based on placing many embryos back in the uterus." More difficult will be reining in aggressive use of fertility drugs unrelated to in vitro treatments.[31]

Faced with the ultimatum of cost, fertility specialists may attempt to impose some order on the way treatments develop and spread. Researchers in a limited number of centers, all with institutional review boards, would evaluate the efficacy and safety of new procedures (an idea voiced during assisted reproductive technology's earlier years) and determine training requirements. The profession might restrict certain of the more complicated procedures to these centers rather than allow widespread dissemination. (Panelists mention ICSI and superovulation, although retrenching on these already widely used treatments seems highly unlikely.)

There are also the risks that come with managed-care infertility plans. All roads seem to be leading to a uniform treatment package, and especially to IVF. This standardization brings its own compromises to informed consent and its own coercive pressure to patients who cannot pay for a freer choice among the reasonable alternatives. With managed care, time is also becoming a scarce commodity. Neither time nor money will be spent for patients and doctors to discuss a full range of options or to devise together a treatment plan tailored to an individual's condition and age (including waiting an adequate amount of time for spontaneous pregnancy or taking a break before returning to treatment or altering a tentative diagnostic/treatment schedule as seems appropriate to patient and doctor in open, ongoing consultation).

In fact, the emphasis on early intervention and limited time for treatment may mean treating more aggressively patients for whom no treatment or minimal treatment will result in pregnancy. Taking a longer time to become pregnant is not in itself undesirable, if pregnancy occurs with minimal or no treatment after, say, eighteen months rather than ten or fifteen months.

The short and narrow road also leaves no room for flexibility in responding to the unexpected or idiosyncratic in a patient's course of diagnosis and treatment. Even potential changes of protocol are defined by the protocol, which is in turn defined by economics. For instance, if more than four eggs mature (as seen by an ultrasound scan of the ovaries) after superovulating a woman who is set to undergo intrauterine insemination, the managed-care physicians "give her the option of canceling that cycle or converting it to IVF [with the transfer of fewer embryos after egg retrieval] at one half the cost because we want to try to indemnify what they have already invested in the stimulation cycle to prevent superfetation."[32] Rigidly managing fertility care undermines vital dimensions of a good medical relationship—including a doctor's clinical judgment (when unpredictable events require alterations in a treatment) and a patient's trust that her best interests are foremost in the doctor's considerations.

Doctors' financial obligations to corporate executives and stockholders come at the expense of medical obligations to patients. In fact, individual patients are missing from the managed-care picture, except for their substantial cost-sharing role ("to facilitate rational decision making in executing the treatment protocol"). Most notably absent are patients with complex, unusual cases, whose enrollment will surely not be encouraged. ("Profits are made on simple ovulation-induction cases; losses are made on insoluble complex cases.")[33]

Whose Cost-Benefit?

Concern about the expense of medical procedures is pushing physicians to try combining interventions in ways that may not benefit, and could harm, fertility patients. One example is a suggestion that "the complete reproductive surgeon and endocrinologist can achieve greater success and reduce costs" by performing certain types of tubal surgery *and* an assisted reproductive technology (e.g., retrieval of eggs for IVF or GIFT) during a single laparoscopy or laparotomy.[1] Whatever the potential merits (by no means yet clearly demonstrated) for "a relatively few and highly selected patients," it is highly unlikely such attempts will be limited to those few patients or to the few specialists who might have all of the skills required.

Another example demonstrates the recurrence of cost-driven and unsystematic experimentation on women—a mixing and matching of interventions that defies adequate evaluation, combining an IVF cycle (including superovulation) with diagnostic laparoscopy. The rationale offered? If no IVF pregnancy occurs, this fertility evaluation/treatment will at least yield information about the sperm's ability to fertilize the eggs (and, taken the next step, about need for more advanced gamete micromanipulations if fertilization does not occur). A published report on this dual procedure also provides an example of the kind of interchange that could become more common if observant, well-informed, and vocal patients participate in a more open medical field.[2] In a subsequent letter to the editor, published by the journal, a former fertility patient who works as a librarian for the consumer group Resolve presents her critique. Among the comments from this unusual, non-physician correspondent: "No evidence is given by the authors to support [the] conclusion . . . that IVF at diagnostic laparoscopy has utility as a therapy." The letter writer goes on to cite studies showing that a large proportion of couples do conceive a pregnancy after initially failing the test of sperm in a laboratory dish; the combined procedure, therefore, does not provide useful diagnostic information about the sperms' ability to fertilize an egg or about the need for even more invasive micromanipulation of the couple's sperm and eggs. Furthermore, patients generally undergo a diagnostic laparoscopy fairly early in the pregnancy quest; among those who do conceive with the combined IVF-laparoscopic treatment are the relatively more fertile women who might well have become pregnant without the IVF treatment. After summarizing additional weaknesses of the published report, this correspondent concludes, "I had hoped [the authors] would provide empirical support for the utility of IVF at diagnostic laparoscopy. Empirical evidence would seem to be a prerequisite to justify its risks and [its physical and emotional] costs."[3]

---

1. Novy 1994.
2. Gindoff, Hall, and Stillman 1994.
3. Byer 1994. See also Hershlag et al. 1992; Kundin, Sjögren, and Hamberger 1996.

Doctors appear to be giving up on trying to understand why patients do not conceive and to tailor fertility treatment to patient characteristics—for instance, to various types of ovulation disorders or tubal disease.[34] Rather than intensify scientific investigation of causes, improve admittedly inadequate diagnostic techniques, and develop interventions that more specifically target a problem, the strategy is to eliminate diagnosis (and save the costs) and point everyone toward IVF.

And, finally, the managed-care infertility plan looks very much like a policy of "one chance, one child"—except, of course, for those who conceive twins and triplets!

Whatever happened to letting patients decide? In this managed-care era, patients can choose neither their doctor nor their treatment plan. Doctors are scrambling to survive in the medical marketplace, and not only as individual specialists. In part, the current maneuverings reflect a turf battle, as the subspecialty of reproductive endocrinology positions itself to take infertility away from the general obstetrician-gynecologist.[35] It is not at all clear whether the "fittest" doctors surviving at this century's end will be those with the greatest medical abilities or those with the lowest bid. The outcome will not only determine which doctors survive, but will also define for large numbers of patients the very nature of trying to have their baby.

The Work to Be Done

In an ideal medical world, safe and effective fertility treatments would be available to all women and men following accurate diagnosis of a particular problem. Most patients would be helped by relatively noninvasive interventions, at minimal risk; patients with more complex fertility problems would be referred to a specialist with greater knowledge about the condition and its possible treatments. Doctors would take time to determine the needs of individual patients and to provide care appropriate for that individual. Ongoing research, with carefully reviewed ethics and methodology, would provide the biological underpinnings of a continually improving diagnostic and treatment repertoire. Beyond fertility patients, the public at large would develop an understanding of—and participate in a professional-lay dialogue about—medical developments that can affect reproduction for all women and men.

As Dr. Martin's anguish attests, that medical world is far away. Current economic and political trends in the United States seem to be pushing it even farther off. What steps might be taken now to move fertility medicine—its patients and doctors—in the right direction? Most generally, the profession and public need to address more deliberately the medical and social issues raised by new reproductive interventions and the broader political issues of health care.

There will be no easy solutions that leave everyone happy; nor can mechanisms that work in other countries necessarily be duplicated here. However, experience leaves no doubt that physician self-policing, voluntary professional guidelines, and *revised* voluntary professional guidelines do not adequately protect patients. And abortion politics has prevented the open, uncensored scientific and societal debate that should contribute to the development of reproductive health policies.

Some specific needs are fairly clear:

To ensure minimal training and ongoing competence of physicians performing any type of fertility treatment and to maintain quality standards for embryo laboratories;

To increase biological knowledge about causes, prevention, and treatment of fertility problems while strengthening safeguards against inappropriate and unethical experimentation;

To minimize opportunities for physicians, other personnel, or business interests to exploit patients for financial or other gain;

To enlarge opportunities for laypeople, physicians, and scientists to assess the nature and direction of new reproductive technologies.

Less obvious are the means that can lead to these ends. Certainly they will require the combined efforts of patients, doctors, and government, using a variety of approaches that are less novel than neglected.

Independent Monitoring

Fertility medicine can no longer enjoy the liberties of an exclusive professional domain. Rather, laypeople and their government representatives must insist on quality assurance mechanisms that regularly verify the competent and ethically justified performance of physicians, fertility clinics, and embryo laboratories. Such mechanisms include, for example, training and credential requirements for surgical techniques and assisted reproductive technologies; accurate records of patients, their fertility treatments, and—in cases of assisted reproduction—the source and disposition of eggs, sperm, and embryos; annual reports that thoroughly document rates of treatment success and complications, using valid and consistently applied measures; on-site inspections of fertility clinics and embryo laboratories by qualified evaluators; mechanisms for improving or closing clinics and laboratories that do not meet quality standards. Legitimate requirements of patient confidentiality should not become a smokescreen to impede the monitoring of medical practices and records.

Enforced Regulations

The great potential of fertility medicine for physical and psychological harm—and for exploitive financial manipulation—requires the power of law to provide a safety net for patients when professional guidelines and ethics fail. Physician autonomy is not so zealously protected in other countries. Medical practices that result in excessive risks are subject to government or professional regulation—for example, limiting the number of embryos transferred after in vitro fertilization. Other countries are far less tolerant of the commercialization rampant in the American fertility business—the for-profit clinics, egg brokers, rising fees for various "donor" and gestational relationships, excessive costs of fertility drugs.

Support for Research

Assisted reproduction will continue in doctors' offices throughout the country, whether there are systematic, scientifically controlled studies or not. The longer an ostrich-like federal policy of noninvolvement prevails, the more women and men will undergo unnecessary, ineffective, and harmful fertility treatments. Allowing fertility medicine into the ranks of research support and review may at least increase the number of valid and useful studies that ultimately help patients. Additional safeguards for current and future patients will come with mechanisms for reporting harmful side effects that arise immediately and for documenting the long-term health of fertility patients and their offspring.

Concern with cost-effectiveness will also continue. Fertility medicine can use this pressure to redirect and fortify biological and medical research aimed at protecting people's natural fertility and improving outcomes for those who do require medical treatment. Academic medical centers can become the locus of systematic studies to evaluate existing and new reproductive procedures, as well as a consistent source of clinical care for patients with complex or unusual fertility problems. Researchers can use the managed-care trend itself to document outcomes, over time, when patients undergo fewer medical procedures compared to their fee-for-service counterparts. Fertility specialists can maintain accurate statistics not only on procedures and outcomes but also on the rate of spontaneous pregnancies that occur in their patient populations.

Whether a study is government-funded or not, whether the researcher is affiliated with a hospital or medical school or in private practice, all human studies of fertility interventions should be evaluated by a review board that is independent in its membership (i.e., not selected by the researching physicians) and its deliberations. Legislation extending federal requirements for informed consent and IRB review to all research using human subjects was introduced in Congress in 1997 but is meeting opposition from pharmaceutical manufacturers, who provide much of this country's private funding.[36] This legislation, the Human Subject Protections Act, would also impose criminal penalties on violators. Beyond improved scientific methods and knowledge, these steps will open ethical dimensions of reproductive medicine to increased scrutiny.

Opening the Field

Greater openness throughout this specialty may be the most far-reaching protection for patients, and the most divergent from usual medical practices. Whatever the formal, official mechanisms established by government or profession, the needed safety net of monitoring, regulations, and research can never be so fine that no patients slip through. Fertility specialists—even famous, internationally visible ones—will at times run medical stop signs; a researcher may clone adult cells or embryos in his garage. However, the more eyes watching the medical enterprise, the more ears hearing what is going on—and the more doctors become aware that these eyes and ears remain vigilant—the better the prognosis overall for patients.

Fertility medicine is the territory of patients and doctors alike. Opening up this medical field requires breaking down internal barriers that separate the professional from the layperson—especially, allowing patients a fuller view of doctors' knowledge and actions. At the same time, barriers enclosing patients and doctors together in a world of their own—consumed by the pregnancy quest—need to dissolve. Opening up fertility medicine requires inviting the view of physicians and scientists with a broader medical and biological perspective, as well as widening the general public's view.

What would greater openness mean?

Exposing the controversies, uncertainties, and conflicting opinions about diagnoses and treatments, as well as the bad outcomes that do occur.

Agreeing that uncertainty does not inevitably mean indecision and that options (including no treatment) are sometimes a medical "toss-up";

reaching a medical decision, however, does require that a patient and doctor together give careful consideration to the range of possible outcomes for that individual.[37]

Increasing opportunities for public dialogue about ethical concerns surrounding treatments, research, and the ways doctors use treatments and research.

Exploring how perspectives of medically trained people may diverge from those of laypeople, leading to medical interventions patients might rather not pursue (for example, "prophylactic oophorectomy," the removal of ovaries of women who previously took fertility drugs, as a "preventive" response to the increased risk of ovarian cancer; using fetal reduction as a way to manage large multiple pregnancies that are one "side effect" of ovarian hyperstimulation; promoting postmenopausal pregnancies because "the age of the uterus" apparently does not preclude it).[38]

Abolishing insular medical fiefdoms in which the doctor's autonomy, free of independent oversight, is the strongest rule of behavior.

Emphasizing the "do no harm" rule of medicine, including cautioning patients about potential risks—even when those cautions focus upon an individual doctor.

What Might Greater Openness Look Like?

Information

As will fertility interventions themselves, public access to medical information will increase all the more as computers bring scientific and medical journals, print media, and "conversation" networks into the home. Presently, some patients undergo treatments with only minimal information, while many face a glut of largely promotional material—brochures produced by a particular fertility center, pamphlets funded by a fertility drug manufacturer. In panel presentations, doctors often seem to be selling their approach (and a future appointment at their office), rather than discussing medical complexities and uncertainties; the audience certainly does not hear doctors' disapproval of a colleague, no matter how strongly felt.

Support groups frequently aim primarily to help patients cope and comply. One physician, summarizing benefits of such groups, notes that patient participation reinforces medical services (increased satisfaction, improved attitude, better compliance with physician instructions, fewer referrals requested to other physicians); saves the doctor time (fewer questions and phone calls to the doctor); helps patients handle problems that arise with finances, stress on personal relationships, and fears about treatment. Most reassuring for the physician, support groups that are guided by a facilitator avoid discussing care by, or criticizing, individual physicians.[1]

To encourage greater give and take, patients and doctors in local communities would need to follow a somewhat different path. They would exchange and analyze information in a variety of forums—face to face and written—that emphasize dialogue about the pros and cons of treatments, conflicting medical opinions, varying approaches taken by physicians in that community as well as in nearby research centers. Unlike presentations by a single fertility clinic—or most panels of specialists from different clinics—meetings in which patients (including prospective patients who are choosing a doctor or fertility clinic) and doctors participate would encourage follow-up of statements that other participants think are inaccurate, misleading, unclear, or open to disagreement. Meeting participants could discuss real or hypothetical cases in an effort to think more clearly about complicated issues: weighing known and potential risks and benefits of a medical intervention; considering when it makes sense to escalate treatment, "try something new," or stop fertility treatment; examining the "fine print" of various financial plans or extra IVF cycles many clinics offer; assessing the ethics and design of a study patients may enter.[2]

In discussing specific diagnostic and treatment techniques, laypeople and doctors could move toward shared awareness of certain medical realities. For example, doctors could provide a perspective on medical "fads"; a patient told she needs a treatment because a sonogram or hysteroscopy shows uterine abnormality or inadequate endometrial lining might learn that, while many doctors like to use this technology, such diagnoses are not well established. Doctors and patients could discuss options that are, medically speaking, a "toss-up," allowing patients to consider their personal convenience and desires; a young woman for whom tubal surgery brings a chance of pregnancy comparable to IVF might prefer conceiving naturally and trying to have several children spaced over several years.

Initiating this type of exchange may require nudging and some legwork by patients. Such activities are unlikely to happen unless patients start to organize them at the local level; individuals who might never consider themselves "activists" may, in some instances, be the very ones to set the wheels in motion. Patients can ask physicians at a nearby university or other large medical center to help spearhead these efforts, provide physical space for meetings, encourage involvement of other local physicians—with a goal of establishing physician participation as the norm. Once patients meet each other, they can identify sympathetic doctors who are concerned about problems within their specialty, who do want increased regulation and oversight of fertility medicine, who want to see well-designed and ethically sound research that could contribute to improved outcomes, and who themselves need ways to harness the energies of laypeople to more adequately inform and safeguard fertility patients.[3]

The type of dialogue envisioned here could help fertility patients and the specialty step away from relying primarily on reported "success rates" to evaluate or choose a fertility clinic. The emphasis would instead be on far more nuanced characteristics of the patient populations selected and medical procedures performed. In some instances, a doctor might be criticized, especially as consensus grows within a community that this doctor does not treat patients well.

Laypeople with access to increasing amounts of medical information can surely understand that doctors have differing interpretations of such information, form conflicting opinions about uncertain medical knowledge, bring a particular philosophy of intervention and varying personal styles to the practice of medicine; patients can appreciate that unfair rumors must be distinguished from well-founded criticism. Only as all aspects of fertility medicine receive an open airing—including the actions of individual doctors—will these distinctions become more clear, with patients better able to choose a physician who meets their individual needs and better protected from inappropriate or unethical treatment.

These new forums could additionally become one step toward the broader goal of ongoing public debate—involving laypeople, doctors and scientists—about difficult reproductive issues and uncertain reproductive directions. In time, fertility medicine might produce fewer "surprises"—as doctors and scientists have described, for instance, the rapid expansion of egg donation and payment of young donors, the offer of ovarian cryopreservation for women facing cancer treatment, the accumulation of "abandoned" frozen embryos, the real possibility that humans can soon be cloned.

Places and Procedures

The in vitro laboratory represents, in concrete form, medical territory and practices that exist behind closed doors. Physically removed from public view, manipulations of eggs, sperm, and embryos also lie beyond the scientific grasp of most laypeople; many physicians have only a general understanding of the embryologist's techniques. An essential step toward opening up the process of assisted reproduction is to impose mandatory requirements for training personnel, for licensing fertility programs, and for making independent inspections on a regular basis. Greater openness to laypeople will, of necessity, have limits; the goal of patients' access should be greater physician accountability. Some fertility centers do invite patients to visit the embryo lab, even to view their own embryos. Unfortunately, encouraging "more eyes" on the process in this manner may play excessively on patients' reproductive hopes, manipulating in the extreme some notion of "attachment"—pushing even further a techno-psychological gimmick already seen in the claim that ultrasound images taken during early pregnancy help promote parental "bonding" with the future newborn. Embryo laboratories cannot be forbidden territory for patients. However, safeguards that can result from having more eyes on the process, including those of patients, need to focus on monitoring and documenting: to identify where doctors and staff received training, to verify precise numbers and allocation of embryos, and to ensure doctor compliance with informed patient decisions. (How many viable embryos do I have? How many were transferred, how many frozen or destroyed, used for research, donated to another woman—as agreed through my informed consent document?)

Many assisted reproductive procedures and most other fertility treatments occur within the doctor's suite. This professional domain is even more resistant to outside observation or evaluation by other physicians or government agencies. Unlike procedures performed in a hospital, peer review and quality assurance is an extremely difficult proposition. (Even within hospitals, the impact of peer review is limited; there is no public disclosure of conclusions about a reviewed colleague, and serious sanctions are rare.) Similarly, research conducted outside of hospitals or academic medical centers may never receive the methodological and ethical scrutiny of an independent review panel. The closest, most consistent view will come from the lay public, the women and men who enter the private suites as patients.

Your Individual Case

Questions and observations by individual women and men will form a wedge for opening fertility medicine to greater oversight and public discussion. As more patients insist that doctors meet certain requirements—and as doctors become aware that patients will take this approach—significant change may finally emerge. Before agreeing to diagnostic or treatment procedures, patients should, of course, discuss with doctors the risks, benefits, and alternative options; they can also ask doctors to describe the internal checks and peer reviews built into their practice. If their doctor proposes a research study, patients can refuse to participate unless the study has passed evaluation by an independently selected review board. Before signing on and paying for treatment, patients can schedule periodic reassessments of their case—appointments at which the doctor reviews with them the procedures completed, the likelihood of success in light of those outcomes, the alternatives still available (including stopping treatment), and the opinion of another physician who is not affiliated with that patient's current doctor.

1. Nettles 1995.

2. As an extension, interested patients could participate on ethics committees established at medical schools or hospitals to discuss cases involving fertility medicine; Seibel 1996 describes such a committee.

3. Models of patient activism—particularly regarding pressure for more research—now exist in the efforts of DES Action, AIDS patients, and organizations focused on breast cancer.

A Revised Etiquette for Physicians and Their Patients

The last step listed above may be the hardest of all, for it runs counter to the informal but sturdy professional etiquette that has long shielded incompetent or unethical physicians. Doctors may ignore voluntary guidelines and defy regulations; the ethics of reproductive technologies are murky, left to individual determinations. Yet one code of behavior gains general obedience: a doctor does not publicly speak ill of another doctor. Reluctance to testify in malpractice cases, a well-known phenomenon, is but the tip of this iceberg. Criticism of a colleague, if voiced at all, stays within bounds of private conversations among fellow physicians. For some doctors, this etiquette seems a shackle from which they cannot escape. But even they rarely try; most doctors toe the line. In the most serious instances, this "shackle" contributes to a conspiracy of silence, an effective protection for doctors at patient expense. Women and men who may be harmed are too often the last to know.

A revised etiquette would mean physicians are less tight-lipped, not only about the outright charlatans, but also about colleagues whose questionable practices are more subtle and amorphous—the consistently exaggerated claims; the continually aggressive overtreatment; the testimonials of true believers who, like the Wizard of Oz, generate far more smoke than substance.

Patients too must change. Just as doctors must be willing to discuss openly with patients the full range of complexities attached to diagnoses, treatments, and, at times, a colleague's actions, patients must be willing to live with medical uncertainty, accept physician fallibility, shed attitudes that can only reinforce the ways doctors have long behaved: reverence for the expert, timidity, apprehension about treading on physician territory. Most importantly, men and women desiring a pregnancy need to step away from the image of "desperation," whether truly felt by the patients or imagined by their doctors. Patients need to understand how the fertility enterprise helps generate and sustain this attitude, too often causing them, along with their doctors, to lose sight of "do no harm"—leaving patients highly vulnerable to the worst in medical care.

•

In the end, it all comes back to individual women and men seeking medical care for a fertility problem. They are ultimately the ones most concerned about what happens in their own case, more than even the most caring of physicians. The concluding chapter, then, examines what patients can do to master great quantities of incomplete, often contradictory information, and problems that seem beyond their control.

9 Finding What You Need

Now and then I still receive phone calls from women who have experienced un-relenting reproductive problems and, in many cases, other health problems, some mysterious. They explain that the consumer organization for which I worked in the past, DES Action, gave them my name. The women on the phone all ask the same question: Am I having these problems because my mother took diethylstilbestrol when she was pregnant with me? Aside from the health effects already documented in follow-up studies of women who took this hormonal drug and of their offspring, my answer is, "No one knows." It is unlikely anyone will ever know the full range of harm caused by this ineffective reproductive treatment. I've grown resigned to that pervasive, boundless unknown for my-self and for the strangers with whom I share such an unwanted and irrevocable bond—the generation of DES daughters and sons. I accept the possibility of fu-ture health problems and the impossibility of ever knowing for sure. And I ac-cept the depth of my feelings about the impact DES exposure has had on my life. What I cannot resign myself to is that the same patterns of reproductive treatments that have caused so much harm in the past should continue.

When I receive these phone calls, I think again of those women and men who, in 1989, attended the fifteenth anniversary celebration of the infertility organization Resolve described at this book's outset. I often wonder what fol-lowed for these relatively well informed fertility patients. To whatever qualms I had then about unmentioned controversies and uncertainties, "massaged" suc-cess rates, patient exploitation, the lack of government regulation and research, I must now add yet another, more pointed question. One of the fertility spe-cialists selected to educate these consumers as the 1980s ended was Dr. Ricardo

Asch—an expert who would also speak over the following months at the American Society for Reproductive Medicine's annual convention and at numerous professional meetings around the world. During the ensuing years, did some of these couples find their way to the Center for Reproductive Health, at the University of California, Irvine, to undergo an assisted reproductive technology performed by this internationally famous specialist?

This possibility captures, with painful irony, questions of tremendous consequence for all women and men seeking medical advice about their fertility. The flagrant violations identified at the Irvine clinic brought to a head problems long festering beneath the hope-glazed and increasingly technological surface of this specialty. These revelations also forced recognition that, by the mid-1990s, American fertility medicine was a different enterprise than just a few years before.

In this final chapter, I sum up considerations that, in my view, can most help fertility patients obtain the best care for their individual needs. To repeat my primary caveat: I am not a medically trained professional and would never give medical advice about any individual's diagnosis or treatment. Rather, I give here my thoughts and cautions, as when answering the phone call from a stranger or questions from a friend. The ways in which fertility medicine is now different seems a necessary starting point for my conclusions. Readers can then take their next steps knowing they face a medical specialty always in motion, always laden with uncertainty, but pushed, as this decade and century end, to a crossroads. After summarizing changes of greatest import to people who are considering fertility treatment, I review main themes and patterns that can frame an individual's decision process—an overview, in a sense, of what has *not* changed over the years. I then suggest key questions for individuals to ask themselves, their doctors, and others involved in their care. Think of the following summary as layered, like an onion, the more general themes and questions surrounding a core of individual concerns about a particular diagnosis and treatment.

Fertility Medicine's Changed Circumstances

Neither the profession nor patients can maintain an unequivocally rosy picture of the specialty's progress. In vitro fertilization and its spin-offs have grown into big business. Assisted reproductive technologies can improve the chances of pregnancy for some people or shorten the time before they conceive; however, the commercial reach and the potential for exploitation of these technologies are formidable, embracing not only fertility patients themselves, but a newly recruited class of young women paid to provide eggs for other women and their partners. Physicians are acknowledging to themselves that the specialty has serious problems, that many common practices are inappropriate, and that the progress of assisted reproduction is slow.[1] Moreover, persistently low success rates and the inadequacy of existing research are finally becoming public knowledge. By mid-decade, even a *Newsweek* cover story would trumpet the reality murmured years earlier by a critic within the field regarding many reproductive interventions, that "the emperor has no clothes."[2] Months later, fertility clinics would appear as one more product evaluated by Consumers' Union, alongside road-tested automobiles, compact discs, refrigerators, and boxed chocolates—a far cry from the professional medical demeanor long insisted on by many of the specialty's practitioners.[3]

At the same time, this specialty has progressed to the point where the pregnancy quest has no clear end. Even after menopause, with hormonal manipulations and donor eggs, women can hope to become pregnant.

Neither the profession nor patients can ignore the potential for harm to patients— physical and psychological—even in the hands of top specialists in the field. The Irvine clinic scandal threw a spotlight, at least momentarily, on the dangerous lack of regulation and oversight in fertility medicine. However, the politics of health care and medical research have taken a particularly volatile course during this decade; concrete outcomes in the form of government regulations, research funding, and ultimately what happens to patients are hard to predict.

The shifting economics of health care in this country exerts significant pressure on fertility medicine, with significant impact on patients. Most prominently, large managed-care corporations are increasingly calling the shots—defining limits on medical procedures and specialty care to lower costs. Fertility patients will be pressed more and more to pay for treatments themselves; they will contend not only with difficult medical issues, but also with solicitations and financing deals from fertility entrepreneurs. Those with more complex fertility problems are likely to have the most difficulty finding appropriate, affordable medical care. Whoever is paying—patients or insurers—economic pressures have also made obvious the long-ignored need for systematic research to determine what medical procedures are effective for whom.

From this decade on, patients and doctors live with an unprecedented explosion of information available through a profusion of easily tapped outlets. Doctors face a constant task of keeping up with and evaluating new information. Patients face a dual task: to find and interpret information relevant to their decisions about fertility treatment; and to find a doctor who keeps up with and evaluates information of greater quantity and sophistication, explains this information fairly, and openly discusses the pros and cons with patients.

These changed circumstances are not lost on fertility specialists. Consider solicitations for new patients. Newspaper advertisements have become common—a full-page photograph of a young couple headlined "No Couple Should Have to Go through Years of Labor to Have a Baby"; two half-full glasses of wine in front of a fireplace captioned "It's one way to make a baby. But there's a lot to be said for gamete intrafallopian transfer." Not long after the Irvine scandal breaks, however, the newspaper advertisement for one California fertility program is noticeably changed in tone. Before Irvine, a bold headline reads, "Infertile Women Needed for Research Study"; the study will "help doctors evaluate a new technique of IVF." After Irvine, a new, visually subdued advertisement seeks infertile women for "a clinical investigation . . . using standard techniques in a caring, personal environment . . . [with] no experimental medications or procedures." A few months later, the clinic's advertisement advises prospective patients: "Check our credentials, learn all you can about this and other fertility programs." And the next time: attend a free seminar to hear fertility specialists and "an expert in managing health care costs." In the same city, another fertility clinic unveils a new financial package. "In response to media reports about 'low IVF success rates' and the insensitivity of the insurance industry to the plight of the infertile," this clinic is now offering a money-back guarantee. A lead story of the newspaper's business section (headline: "A Fertility Clinic Offers Guarantee") outlines the new payment deal. Certain eligible couples, under certain specified conditions, will receive a 90 percent refund of their up-front basic fee (diagnostic tests and medications not included) if they do not achieve a pregnancy, lasting more than twelve weeks (note that they do not "guarantee" an actual baby), after transfers of all embryos (fresh and thawed) derived from a single egg-retrieval. This brash display of medicine as a business proposition adds an economic gamble (the up-front payment is $5,000 more than the clinic's standard single-cycle fee of $7,500 for women under thirty-five years of age) to fertility patients' already difficult medical gamble. Beyond taking the basic risks of any IVF treatment, moreover, these physicians will surely employ an aggressive superovulation and embryo transfer regimen in order to minimize fee refunds and maximize financial returns.

Another Change: The Internet

The unimaginably vast expanse of communication available through the Internet brings remarkable change even as it plays out some of the ongoing themes and patterns of fertility medicine. The most obvious change is people's ability to tap into libraries and medical databases worldwide, to have the information they seek displayed on their home or office computer screen. Beyond this boundless new access to information about diagnoses and treatments is the Internet's amorphous and anarchic tangle of solicitation, opinion, voiceless and faceless conversation.

Established print medical journals, nascent online journals, health web sites, commercial and nonprofit organizations, online conferences, news groups, bulletin boards—in greater numbers by the day—are accumulating thousands of "visits" by people wanting information, in this case, about infertility, sperm or egg donation, surrogacy, and related topics. Any individuals or organizations with computers and modems can create their own web sites, which will appear alongside all the others in this chaotic mix. Log onto one web site and a profusion of links leads into a maze of additional sites linked to still others. So much information is thrown onto the Internet from all manner of sources that it is often difficult to judge the caliber of this information or discern the authority with which some of the voices speak.

As with sources of information discussed in Chapter 7, patients and doctors will need to be savvy about how even well-established medical authorities use the Internet to shape information. The ASRM announces a new direct link from its web site to "highlighted articles" published in *Fertility and Sterility.* Yet these articles, highlighted also in press releases, are not selected randomly. Over time, the choices become predictable: articles reporting that fertility drugs do not cause ovarian cancer; studies reporting no long-term problems for IVF offspring; reanalyses of data showing sperm counts are not dropping in all parts of the world. Such reports may contribute to knowledge about fertility medicine. However, just as medical journals reflect a bias, overall, toward publishing studies with positive treatment results (with pharmaceutical funding well represented), this additional winnowing will further skew the information doctors and their patients receive.

Fertility clinics have jumped into the fray. Without ever leaving home, current and prospective fertility patients can learn about a particular clinic—that is, learn all the clinic wants them to know about their services, view photographs of its buildings and doctors, read complimentary news clippings about the clinic's achievements. Clinic personnel need only create the web site—a computer-age advertisement designed with the latest in public relations techniques. For example, one San Francisco clinic not only provides descriptions and explanations of its various diagnostic techniques, treatments, and financial plans, answers to important questions, and information on becoming a long-distance patient; it also provides a collection of "success stories." By clicking on "SUCCESS" the web site visitor finds poignant vignettes—brief online soap operas of sorts, with such titles as "Barbara's Story: How Overcoming Antibodies Finally Got Me Pregnant," or "Lia's Story: Heparin and Aspirin Defeated the Antibodies That Made Me Infertile," or "Cristal's Story: My Best Friend Had My Baby for Me"—portraying patients' past tribulations, culminating in recent joy, thanks to one or another medical intervention at this clinic.

Another example is the Genetics and IVF (GIVF) Institute of Fairfax, Virginia, which in early 1996 added "an important new service" to its Internet menu of available reproductive treatments and tests—ovary cryopreservation (freezing and storing) "for reproductive age women anticipating chemotherapy or radiation treatment" (see Chapter 5). People visiting this web site learn that the GIVF Institute is "the first medical facility in the United States to offer this new option to patients." (They learn also that this achievement was reported in the *New York Times*.) The explanatory page—a page more carefully worded than cautious—continues, "The cryopreserved ovarian tissue *can be later replaced* in the ovarian bed *with the purpose of* restoring reproductive and endocrine function after disease treatment and remission" (emphasis added). Although technically true—the tissue can later be replaced—no one knows whether the ultimate purpose can ever be achieved in humans. Internet users learn nothing of the new service's complexities, especially for cancer patients, or of the controversy and disagreement engendered within the specialty by the Institute's "pioneering" offer to remove and freeze ovaries of these women. The web site's explanation fails to mention that the British researcher who developed this technique has stopped removing human ovaries from women and girls pending further study. Although it acknowledges that "experience with this method in women is just being initiated," the GIVF page concludes that "the rationale has strong support from . . . remarkable [animal] results."

This clinic will surely provide details about risks and benefits of this experiment to obtain a woman's informed consent, just as the previously mentioned clinic will enumerate less gratifying possibilities than the online "success stories" before a patient signs the legal forms and pays. Yet, these technologically intriguing, elaborately designed invitations sent into people's homes may be all the more alluring as commercial enticements than their more modest counterparts, the newspaper advertisement. Bold statements here allow no immediate question or contradiction. Newspaper advertisements, at least, generally link more closely to actual providers and facilities known within a community of other doctors and patients; newspaper advertisements often lead to public meetings where prospective patients can question a doctor, perhaps hear or express skepticism or a whisper of less-than-successful stories. While Internet browsers may venture deeper into the web, they may never encounter face to face the doctors or other patients until arriving for a "free consultation" or initial appointment—often the first step toward signing on for much more.

However, the Internet can also bring more to fertility patients who do venture beyond a clinic's web site. Also without leaving home, laypeople can now click into medical controversies and disagreements previously secluded in the unfamiliar, forbidding territory of medical school libraries or professional meetings. The journal Human Reproduction, for instance, publishes online its regular print "Debate" articles, with web site comments on such topics as egg donation, ovarian stimulation, ICSI and other issues of male infertility. And fertility patients can share with each other their experiences, concerns, questions, and answers. Any time of day or night, unrestricted by geographical boundaries, a support group is available to any subscriber who logs on. On the one hand, a danger lurks in this continuous stream of computer conversation, as it does throughout the Internet. People are getting and giving advice cloaked in the anonymity of E-mail monikers. Internet advisers assert their opinions of others' needs with surprising authority; yet here all the information is anecdotal, message after message, even more than with conventional information gathering. Even more than from doctors, a drug's manufacturer, or the media, sources of this information are unknown, untraceable, and unaccountable.

On the other hand, a wholly new forum is emerging that could help pry the lid, at least partially, off the workings of fertility medicine. Here patients do express and "hear" skepticism. Far from local communities (where patients and doctors need still to face each other with greater openness), the anonymous communication between laypeople flies with exhilarating abandon. For example, the fertility clinic whose web site offers "success stories" also offers a variety of financing plans. The clinic's commercial reputation begins to spill onto the Internet. One participant in an infertility news group complains that these doctors refuse to accept insurance reimbursement (even as their advertisements bemoan the insurance industry's "insensitivity . . . to the plight of the infertile"). They require advance payment in full, this message informs others across the World Wide Web—a lump sum the message sender clearly does not have. Additional dimensions of this clinic's performance may soon appear, as another message from another part of the country asks: Has anyone out there had experience, good or bad, with this clinic? The inquirer is preparing to fly to California for treatment. "The attraction," concludes this woman or man, demonstrating the clinic's advertising success, "is a 90 percent refund policy." Sprinkled throughout the free flow of Internet postings come patients' comments—favorable and not—naming other doctors and clinics as well.

Ongoing Patterns and Themes to Keep in Mind

Physicians often ignore the well-known occurrence of "treatment-independent pregnancies" among "infertile" couples when using, evaluating, and claiming success for a fertility treatment. Few couples seeking a doctor's help to become pregnant are completely unable to conceive on their own. Rather, their chance of conceiving each month is below a range that is considered normal fertility; for example, they may have a 15 percent chance each month compared to an average of 20–25 percent. For these subfertile patients, treatment that is appropriate for the underlying cause of their reduced fertility increases their chances; if they do conceive, it may occur sooner than without treatment. But the baseline (or "background") rate of spontaneous pregnancies complicates doctors' claims that a treatment was responsible for a pregnancy that might have occurred anyway, and complicates patients' decisions about whether to undergo treatment. More obvious examples of treatment-independent pregnancies are those that occur while couples are on a waiting list for treatment—or many years after fertility treatment has ended. Ignoring such pregnancies is not a new phenomenon. A 1983 report in the *New England Journal of Medicine* cautions physicians about this problem, harking back a hundred years to "Lectures on the Sterility of Women," published in the *British Medical Journal* of 1883: "A reputation for curing sterility is spoken of as if it were founded on substantial claims. . . . [A] coincidence has been regarded as a consequence."[4]

Physicians use fertility treatments that can help certain subgroups of women and men with fertility problems more widely, on individuals who gain no benefit. This expanded use also means that untrained or inexperienced practitioners are performing the treatments, raising the risk to patients.

Much in the development and daily practice of fertility medicine constitutes experimentation on women. Doctors try out new reproductive interventions in a trial-and-error manner, with no scientific controls or oversight; they use existing procedures, intended initially for a limited target group, on women with very different fertility problems. In this manner, unproven treatments gain acceptance, even popularity, as standard medical practice.

Doctors and patients often continue to try a treatment after many failed attempts suggest this intervention is not appropriate for that individual. Many specialists now think that if a particular treatment can help an individual, success will generally come during initial attempts—a kind of window of opportunity, usually during the first three treatment cycles, usually *not* after six failures.

Development of a reproductive intervention tends to begin with an aggressive course of treatment—for example, high medication dosages, invasive procedures—followed by more conservative modifications that carry fewer risks. Patients receiving treatment during the more aggressive stage may be receiving an "overdose"—overly invasive and risky. Physicians often become unduly enthusiastic about applying new medical procedures; with time, and less than promising results, a medical fad wanes. In recent years, the rapidly changing areas of immunologic and male infertility have attracted fertility specialists' enthusiasms. Some of the new diagnostic and treatment procedures will prove useful, others will eventually fall by the wayside. Patients need to demand evidence that a treatment has been shown to be effective, that it is appropriate to their condition, and that benefits outweigh risks. If a procedure is unproven, doctors need to explain clearly to patients the reasons for a proposed experimental use in their case.

Whatever the shifts in health care financing and incentives, the recurrent answer to the question "What drives developments in fertility medicine?" is "The marketplace." This answer takes many forms—IVF entrepreneurs; frenzied expansion of laparoscopic and laser surgery; widespread advertising of a highly experimental, unproven procedure of removing and freezing women's ovaries to preserve fertility for some future time; the cranked-up pace of health care, as medical personnel and insurers strive for greater volume. To a fertility patient, this market-driven pressure appears not only as full-page newspaper ads, radio and television spots, toll-free phone numbers, E-mail and web sites, but as financial lures. Prospective patients who attend one clinic's "free seminar" will learn about a "third cycle free" for "eligible" patients; at the conclusion of this informational seminar a "free [ART] cycle drawing" will be held—a novel reproductive door prize or, perhaps more aptly, a game of Jeopardy. With different clinics offering various financial deals, fertility patients must calculate the real costs and bigger discounts, as they do with airline tickets, credit cards, car rentals, or telephone rates. Along with consent documents for their protection, patients will sign medical contracts detailing eligibility and limits on offers that protect the clinic's side of the bargain.

The marketplace also requires closely squeezed appointments with rushed doctors, uniform treatment protocols geared toward high volume and scheduling efficiency rather than individual medical needs, mistakes made by a too busy staff. Not to mention mistakes never apparent to patients—in medications they take, or during a surgical procedure, or within the embryo laboratory. And, as in other marketplaces, there are the nonmistakes—the intentional deceptions, and even thefts, of which buyers must beware.

Health-care workers as well as patients are expressing their concern about these market forces. Patients at the prominent New York Hospital–Cornell Medical Center in vitro fertilization clinic were probably not aware of the laboratory director's displeasure during the early 1990s with the ballooning numbers of egg retrievals and embryological procedures performed each day (weekends included)—until 1994, when he and much of the laboratory staff left to join more modestly sized fertility programs.[5] The director asserted that an expanding workload, intended to increase clinic income, placed unreasonable demands on the embryo laboratory's staff and facilities, threatening the quality of their work and jeopardizing chances of establishing pregnancies for women undergoing assisted reproduction.

In California, pharmacists were expressing similar concerns about workloads expanded to safeguard profitability of managed-care health insurance plans. At one of the largest HMOs, Kaiser-Permanente, state inspectors found in 1995 that "the goal of the pharmacy seems to be speed." As one pharmacist described his last several years, "Call it downsizing, consolidation, cost savings, whatever. . . . There is more pressure to turn out more prescriptions, with less personnel. When you're working under this kind of stress, it cuts down on the time you have to double-check things." The outcome is staff fatigue and mistakes that can harm patients. Whether for pharmacists, doctors, nurses, or other personnel, more work done more quickly is a deliberate managed-care goal. When attempting to cut costs, explains one health care analyst, "you don't *want* your staff to spend a lot of time per patient."[6]

The latest forms of patient exploitation may generally be more subtle than during the 1980s, but the problem persists nevertheless. Physicians still calculate success rates in ways that make their program appear more successful than would other, more comprehensive descriptions; patients still accept low success rates as the norm. Doctors and patients still perceive "no harm in trying," though potential harm may not be immediate or obvious. Serious medical issues are increasingly overshadowed by economic incentives.

But the latest exploitation—intensified by assisted reproductive technologies—derives from the expansion of information and of hope. Doctors tread fine lines between explaining complex medical procedures and soliciting customers for them; between advising, convincing, and coercing; between maintaining an optimistic outlook and manipulating unrealistic hopes. Fertility patients remain exceedingly vulnerable—pulled by the hope that, whatever the odds, they could be the successful case. By the mid-1990s, a different Resolve conference, on the other side of the country, again captured the trends. Attendees at this conference seemed almost smothered with information—tables laden with packets of written material from various fertility clinics in the region; displays mounted by Serono Laboratories, by egg and surrogacy brokers; a program filled with so many fertility specialists from the various clinics, speaking on so many panels, it made your head spin. Capturing succinctly, if unintentionally, the informational risk for patients was this comment in the opening remarks of the region's Resolve president: that during her many years of involvement as a patient and as a Resolve member, support group leader, and officer, so much about infertility and its treatments had become "blindingly clear."

A decade after fertility specialists began expressing concern about deceptive success claims and overuse of assisted reproductive technologies, after considerable argument within the profession over how to report and compare IVF clinic outcomes, with a scandal over misappropriated eggs and embryos still emerging, a statement published in the *New York Times* by a New Jersey fertility center displays just how confused and confusing these fertility treatments remain. This lengthy statement takes exception to the first article of a four-part series in the *Times* on "The Fertility Market" and protests most strongly a "scorecard" included with the initial article (aptly entitled "Conflict and Competition"), listing success rates for the dozen busiest IVF clinics in the New York City region. Intended to remedy a "false impression of our actual success rates," the explanation offered to *Times* readers is far more blinding than clear.

The statement seeks, first of all, to clarify its IVF success rate. Although second highest in number of egg retrievals performed, this busy clinic scores lowest in "rate of live deliveries per initiated cycle" (i.e., the proportion of deliveries with at least one live-born baby out of all IVF attempts started that year; see Chapter 3). According to these IVF practitioners, the reason for this apparently dismal track record is

> our common practice of deferring the embryo transfer on the retrieval cycle, freezing the embryos, and then transferring the frozen embryos on a subsequent cycle. Thus the statistic of "pregnancy rate per initiated cycle" does not add in any pregnancies achieved when the deferred frozen embryos are transferred for the first time. [The] scorecard correctly showed that we had the highest number of frozen embryo transfers in 1993 (293) with the next highest number by another center being 141. In contrast to many other IVF centers . . . our success rate with frozen embryo transfers is equal to that of our transfer rate with fresh embryos. It is our intent and purpose to stimulate as many eggs as possible, to provide a patient with multiple transfer opportunities from only one retrieval. This saves the patient from the annoyance of ovarian hyperstimulation, the risk and expense of fertility drugs, and the extra expense of retrieval versus the inexpensive transfer of frozen embryos. However, the patients who would expect the highest pregnancy rates on a retrieval cycle are the ones who stimulate the best, and these are exactly the same patients who are most likely to have the fresh transfer cycles deferred to freezing because of the risk of ovarian hyperstimulation. Thus, this leads to a false impression of a poor success rate by our IVF center when only mentioning pregnancy rates per initiated cycle, without explaining that deferring the fresh transfer to a frozen transfer counts as a zero success for that couple using that method. Furthermore, in women over 40 we have found they frequently do not attain adequate uterine lining thickness and commonly defer fresh embryo transfers for subsequent frozen embryo cycles.

Following this breathtaking clarification of fresh versus frozen embryo transfers, the statement proceeds to numbers and percentages. Bold print cites an approximately 20 percent live delivery rate per embryo transfer procedure (not per initiated cycle, as in the *Times* article), whether fresh or frozen embryos, during the year *following* the SART Registry data reported in the original article. The statement describes these rates as "equal to or better than the delivery rate of a normal fertile woman," an often used though inappropriate comparison with assisted reproductive technologies.

The focus then shifts to the high cost of IVF, another topic covered in the "Conflict and Competition" article. Complaining that the reporter emphasized expense without contacting their center, the statement continues, "Had he interviewed us, he would have discovered that our charges are very reasonable, even though these rates have almost doubled this year related to decreased disbursements from managed health care, for non-IVF services we perform in our reproductive endocrinology practice." A listing of fees follows.

Discussion of cost not only cites the economic drain of managed care but also slips quickly into the murky arena of IVF ethics. Acknowledging that even their "reduced prices" are beyond the reach of some patients, this fertility center offers

> a donor oocyte program where a patient willing to share half of her eggs with another woman (anonymously) would receive her medication at no charge and the $1,875 IVF charge would be waived. The recipient in the program also pays less, because they already benefit from our inexpensive IVF charges, and now do not have to pay $2,000 to $3,000 for an oocyte donor. From our own ethical view, this is the ideal way for a donor oocyte program to run since young women are not subjected to the risk of ovarian hyperstimulation and the risk of retrieval just for financial remuneration. In our center, the women undergoing these risks have to do so anyway as infertile women needing IVF, . . . [but] without the recipients' financial assistance, a baby through IVF would be denied to them.

While congratulating itself over its ethical concern for young egg donors, the clinic ducks the ethical question of financial pressure on women who perceive the choice of sharing half their eggs as the only way they can have a baby. Far from "ideal," this solution merely exchanges one set of troubling ethical issues for another. In addition, these women will likely face an even more aggressive superovulation regimen, with even greater risks, in order to have "as many eggs as possible," including enough eggs for the other recipients.[7]

The statement concludes with a brief foray into the thicket of patient selection, particularly by age, noting that

> our program is willing to accept more difficult medical cases, even those with elevated follicle stimulating hormone (FSH). These patients do not stimulate as well as those with low FSH levels and may take many cycles

to achieve a pregnancy. . . . Obviously a center that can offer many [egg retrieval] cycles to poor risk patients may show a lower pregnancy rate per transfer than a center who purposely excludes even one cycle of IVF because of potential poor response.

Not mentioned is the question of just how low a patient's chances should go before doctors advise against or refuse to provide IVF (let alone repeated attempts, for example, to women whose FSH levels suggest that they are approaching menopause and that such attempts are futile). Rather, these IVF practitioners contend, "By charging less for retrieval cycles, having success with inexpensive frozen embryo cycles and an almost free shared oocyte program, we allow an individual or couple multiple opportunities to achieve a pregnancy, thus a good pregnancy rate per patient registered. This is not a category required by SART." Finally, although this IVF center claims "we have never marketed our IVF center, since our excellent reputation and good name brings an abundance of patients," the statement does close by noting their program's "convenience of offices" (phone numbers included) in New Jersey, Pennsylvania, and Delaware—offices where, "in addition to IVF, we treat other types of infertility and reproductive endocrinological problems."

By the end of this statement, it is hard to decipher who is misleading whom about what doubtful information. The prominent fertility specialist quoted in Chapter 3 may have had a point when he argued that the SART Registry's clinic-specific reports would merely replace misleading information with a supply of "different but equally misleading information."

●

I summarize these patterns to emphasize the need for caution when embarking upon fertility treatment—an emphasis intended to temper the overly optimistic picture often conveyed by physicians and the media. Clearly, the positive side of fertility medicine during the past three decades is that more treatments have been developed for women and men who have fertility problems. The difficulty comes in matching these treatments to individuals who may benefit.

Keeping in mind these characteristics of fertility medicine that require patients to be wary, how can individuals identify and benefit from the positive options that may in fact exist for them? To help focus the search for information, I have attempted first to distill concerns discussed in previous chapters into five basic questions about fertility. These questions assume the reader has some type of problem that is lowering chances for a successful pregnancy; they aim at helping that individual think about whether to pursue medical treatment at this time and, if so, how aggressively.

Five Basic Questions about Fertility

Does your condition mean you cannot conceive without medical treatment, and, if so, is there a treatment that can overcome this problem? Women and men within this category of complete infertility (approximately 5 percent of couples who are attempting to conceive) have a good chance of conceiving a pregnancy following appropriate treatment (for example, effective treatments exist for certain women who do not ovulate or have completely blocked fallopian tubes, for some men with no sperm in ejaculate).[8] Determining the benefit of treatment is more complicated for women and men with milder problems, whose chance of becoming pregnant spontaneously falls somewhere along the lower end of a fertility continuum (the cut-off between normal and subfertile is arbitrary). If you are within this much larger category, the following two questions about time become crucial when considering medical intervention.

What is the duration of your inability to conceive? That is, how long have you been trying for a pregnancy, timing sexual intercourse to the fertile days of the woman's menstrual cycle? The best estimate of a couple's likelihood for conceiving without treatment depends on the length of time they have been trying. Particularly with mild problems detected during a fertility evaluation, the diagnosis of a specific condition—or combination of problems that could lower fertility—does not necessarily predict your chances for a spontaneous pregnancy. Couples with long-standing (more than three years) unexplained infertility are more likely to need medical treatment than couples who have been trying to conceive for less than two years.

How much time do you have left to conceive spontaneously, given the woman's age? As one specialist put it, this consideration involves the amount of time available "for chance to have its way."[9] Obviously, women in their late thirties or older do not have as much leeway to wait for a spontaneous pregnancy as women in their twenties and early thirties. In general the best prognosis for pregnancy without treatment (and for success if treated) goes with younger age, short duration of infertility, and a previous spontaneous pregnancy or treatment success.

What are the risks of treatment, and how much risk are you willing to take for the benefit you gain? The medical precept to "do no harm" demands particular adherence when considering reproductive interventions, since patients are generally healthy when treatment begins. Even in the best of circumstances—with effective treatment appropriately prescribed—the benefit is an increased *chance,* not certainty, of a successful pregnancy. In all circumstances, medical procedures carry risks—some known, some hinted, and perhaps others unknown. Deciding how much risk you are willing to take depends on answers to additional questions:

How severe is your fertility problem? Is medical treatment the only way to have a chance for pregnancy? If pregnancy is possible without treatment, how much would treatment raise your chances?

How serious are potential complications or long-term harm from treatment, and what is their likelihood?

Has a proposed treatment been proven effective, or is it an experimental attempt to "do something"?

Does a safer, less invasive alternative exist that brings enough benefit?

What are your "time" answers (see above): the length of time you have tried to conceive without treatment and the amount of time you have left to try?

Patients diagnosed with relatively mild abnormalities, or unexplained infertility of relatively short duration, need to consider most carefully the "iatrogenic risk"—the possibility that medical intervention itself will harm health and/or fertility, creating a greater problem than originally existed. Describing a "prominent principle" in reproductive medicine, one specialist contends that physicians "are most likely to achieve beneficial outcomes when departures from normal are more than slight. Most of our treatments can have side effects [that] are more likely to tip the balance unfavorably when the condition being treated is relatively trivial."[10]

How much risk you are willing to take is, of course, also a matter of how you see the alternatives within your own life. How important is it to have your own genetic offspring? Would you consider adopting a baby? Can you foresee a contented life without children? These are questions to ask yourself and discuss with your partner.

Finally, the fifth of my questions is for you to ask yourself periodically after fertility treatment has begun—

To what extent are you propelled by the momentum of fertility treatment, the month-by-month pull of the process itself? You may need time to pause, reassess, seek the opinion of a different, uninvolved physician. You may find yourself repeating a treatment that has failed too many times or agreeing to a treatment that seems a bit too much, overlooking the risks each attempt brings. "The goal for any infertile couple," concludes one group of fertility specialists, "should be either a live birth or the ability to feel that they have exhausted all *reasonable attempts* to achieve a pregnancy" (emphasis added).[11] The who and how of defining "reasonable" is, of course, the hard part; this decade's cost-cutting trends have at least forced the question of how many treatment attempts for which types of fertility problems are enough.[12]

The momentum of fertility treatment is hard to resist, however. For some patients, trying one more time or escalating to a more invasive intervention is a reasonable decision. Others ignore indications that they are heading not only toward further disappointment, but toward drained physical, emotional, and financial resources. One fertility patient, herself a physician, expresses a common predicament. Drawn by a newspaper advertisement to attend an informational meeting at a large hotel, she took advantage of a "free consultation," which in turn led her to begin a diagnostic workup at that clinic. With IVF treatments begun, she is of two minds: "I hate being caught in this situation. I should know better than to go for such a big sell, to sign up for whatever they say. . . . But it's knowing I did everything possible. That I took the extra step." Only later, after the IVF cycle failed (with transfer of five good-quality fresh embryos), did this couple's doubts prevail. Her doctor was recommending heparin and aspirin (this immunotherapy in spite of negative results on immunologic tests) and the transfer of all seven frozen embryos; if that didn't work, based on a hysteroscopy required during the initial infertility evaluation (during which the doctor performed a uterine scraping procedure not discussed beforehand), their best option was to hire another woman, a surrogate, to carry their desired pregnancy. Upon consulting several other specialists, they found none agreed with these recommendations or with the diagnostic methods employed. When her doctor "refused to consider any changes at all, we were left with no other option except to hand carry our seven embryos in a liquid nitrogen bank" to a fertility clinic at the nearby medical school (a clinic that does not advertise or hold "free information meetings" for prospective patients) where, on their next try, the transfer of two thawed embryos resulted in the birth of their daughter.

Depending on an individual's fertility problem, there may in fact be times when less aggressive therapy is as likely to bring success as the more aggressive "extra step." In some cases deciding against treatment offers approximately the same odds of pregnancy as pursuing a medical intervention. Nor does pausing or stopping treatment after failed attempts eliminate the possibility of "treatment-independent pregnancies" among subfertile patients; in fact, repeating a treatment that has failed many times may offer less chance for success than trying to become pregnant without medical treatment One woman, a biologist, did stop IVF treatment when she could get no reason from her physician—a top medical center specialist—for changes in her treatment protocol from one attempt to the next. "They couldn't give us straight numbers. We were experimental subjects, without them saying so," she now comments. She and her husband decided to stop when they realized that even the best numbers, the highest chances of success, were still not very good. And her husband adds, "We knew we were interested in adopting, which may have influenced us."

Looking back, many former fertility patients see their years of treatment differently than they did while caught up in this medical world. A woman who found a doctor willing to prescribe massive doses of fertility drugs after her first doctor refused, now says, "It was crazy." Another speaks about risks she previously took, "We may not need to do everything [the doctors offer]. . . . I thought pregnancy was all I wanted, but I also want to live." Says another, "Had I known the low success rate for my age, I would never have done it."

A "had I known" test might be one way to reevaluate and double check momentum's pull. Of a specific diagnosis or treatment, do you know what there is to know? In light of medical uncertainty and incomplete knowledge, where do you draw the line? What chances are you willing to take? What is the least benefit you should gain? What is the greatest risk you want to face? How do these months or years of fertility treatment fit into the whole picture of your life, including before you began trying for a pregnancy and after you stop?

The tantalizing thought that "this time they may be right, this new breakthrough may be the answer for me" can endlessly postpone the decision to take a break or to end fertility treatment. The "desperation" some fertility specialists see in patients is, at least in part, a creation of their profession's own making. Fertility centers promote new reproductive technologies as a way "to have your own genetic child." Some specialists offer an option using donor sperm, donor eggs, and a surrogate to carry the pregnancy. Hearing this scenario during an informational meeting for fertility patients, a man leans to his partner and asks, "How is that different from adopting?" Of the new possibility for postmenopausal pregnancy, a woman says to a room full of other women, all former or current fertility patients, "The medical community won't help us stop. It's our responsibility."

While I do not deny the disappointment and sadness that come with fertility problems or trivialize the difficulty of this experience, patients and doctors should be aware that highly charged negative reactions—the depression and anger, the "desperation"—are not universal. Psychologists working with fertility patients find a heterogeneous group; many individuals show great resilience in handling the ups and downs, in rethinking family options if no successful pregnancy occurs.[13]

At the same time, the question of professional responsibility remains. Physicians can temper offerings that fuel desperation, requiring heroic, often futile, and potentially harmful medical manipulations. Endless possibilities may well undermine, rather than support, patient resilience in assessing their options realistically. The medical community's responsibility extends, moreover, beyond a doctor's own patients. It is one thing for a doctor to convey needed information about risks and benefits of any particular procedure—to help an individual understand her chances, for example, of conceiving a large multiple pregnancy likely requiring fetal reduction in order for any baby to survive, let alone survive in good health. It is something else for doctors to exercise restraint as a medical community, to refrain from pushing developments that rely on risk-laden interventions aimed at pregnancy, no matter the patients' personal or financial costs. Within professional ranks, doctors can discourage the cavalier view of complications arising in pursuit of "success." Doctors can restrain the hard sell of egg donation that so enlarges demand for a supply of young donors; the specialty can redirect efforts toward developing less onerous medical responses to a loss of fertility that comes as women age. Recognizing the potential for physical and emotional harm, doctors can choose not to always forge ahead into the vast reproductive unknown. A shared medical philosophy can emphasize gaining more of the missing biological knowledge before employing whatever intervention becomes technically possible. The way fertility medicine develops cannot be left to doctors alone. However, neither should doctors be let off the hook when it comes to accountability for what the profession is doing now and responsibility for where it ventures next.

•

In truth, even the basic questions about fertility expand to encompass a fairly large handful. And there are other questions to grasp, questions focused on particular diagnoses, treatments, and doctors. As you consider medical interventions, questions in the following sections may help you evaluate a proposed treatment and choose a physician who best meets your needs.

Understanding Diagnosis and Treatment Options

People differ in the amount of medical information they want and in the way they reach decisions about treatment. At a minimum, fertility patients need to avoid handing themselves over, expecting a doctor to make the right decisions for them. They need to keep in mind two main purposes for consulting a fertility specialist in the first place: first, to learn their likelihood for a successful pregnancy without fertility treatment, in approximately what amount of time; and, second, to know what treatments might be appropriate in their particular case—what they would gain and what risks they would take. Doctors and patients need to discuss the reasons for a recommended medical procedure (i.e., how will it increase *this* patient's likelihood of having a healthy baby?), the reasons against, the possible alternatives. (See Appendix 5.) The following questions should be carefully considered when deciding about a diagnostic test or fertility treatment.

What is the source of the information you are gathering, and how might this source shape the message conveyed? Remember, media reports are likely to be superficial, at best, and may be misleading. Information from doctors often reflects less than straightforward medical considerations. In some instances, doctors divide into "camps" loyal to a particular treatment approach; recommendations may also vary along geographic lines. Doctors are subject to persuasion by drug manufacturers, who are in a no-lose situation—even if treatment fails, patients and doctors are likely to try again, perhaps with even greater amounts of medication.

How thoroughly has this condition or treatment been studied, and by whom? What types of research have been conducted? Most important, have well-designed randomized controlled trials demonstrated a treatment's benefits in patients similar to you?

Is there conflict or disagreement among physicians about this diagnosis or treatment? What are the controversies and how do they relate to your situation? What cautions do physicians express, especially regarding adequacy of existing studies and potential for harm? Do experienced, knowledgeable doctors recommend against a given procedure in cases like yours?

Does the weight of evidence lean one way or the other? As in many areas of medicine, fertility patients must often reach decisions based on partial and, perhaps, changing information. No single study provides full answers or certainty; rather, patients and doctors have to consider the accumulation of knowledge presently available. Based on current knowledge some medical decisions are, in effect, toss-ups; a patient's personal preferences and convenience can determine the actual choice. Some decisions do require more significant evidence than others. You might, for example, stop smoking or cut down on coffee on far less evidence that this action will improve your fertility than you would demand to justify undergoing surgery or in vitro fertilization. Preliminary suggestions of increased ovarian cancer risk may convince you *not* to take fertility drugs if your mother had this illness or if the benefits for you are questionable.

What individual risks must you balance against a procedure's benefits? A family history of ovarian or breast cancer is one such risk when considering fertility drugs. Women who have previously experienced blood clots (for example, when taking oral contraceptives or for no identifiable reason) may be at increased risk for developing clots during ovarian stimulation treatments.[14] Just as the success rate is 100 percent for the individual who has a healthy baby, so too is the incidence of a serious medical complication for the individual who has one.

Can you gain a sense of "where things are" in the development of a particular treatment for your fertility problem? Is an intervention a new, experimental procedure that is being aggressively applied? Or have doctors used this intervention over many years, developing less invasive modifications along the way?

If you decide on a fertility treatment, are there ways to minimize the risks? Your doctor should discuss with you the immediate and long-term risks of every medical procedure, and describe how he will watch for and handle side effects. Every patient should know the signs of treatment complications so that problems can be identified and responded to quickly. Patients can help doctors and medical staff avoid mistakes (for example, by double checking medication dosage and schedules, the number of embryos to be transferred or cryopreserved). Mistakes do happen. They are all the more likely when economic competition pressures physicians, nurses, pharmacists, and laboratory technicians to increase patient load and cut corners in an effort to reduce costs and enlarge profits. In addition, you can limit the number of attempts with a particular treatment (for example, not more than four to six months on clomiphene citrate; not more than four to six cycles of ovarian stimulation and egg retrieval) before reassessing or moving on to a next step. Subfertile couples—especially those with unexplained infertility of relatively short duration or with a diagnosis of mild abnormalities—may want to alternate treatment with no treatment cycles. Minimizing risks and maximizing benefits means individualizing your care—a process in which patient and doctor work together.

Recognizing Complications

Medical reports show that treatment complications can arise even after a doctor employs measures intended to avoid them—for example, severe ovarian hyperstimulation syndrome following preventive measures at the time of egg retrieval.[1] Complications can arise in women who have no known risk factors that might predict a bad reaction to a particular intervention.[2] One example from a published case report: following superovulation, a woman with none of the classic signs of ovarian hyperstimulation syndrome, as monitored through blood tests or ultrasound, suffers a stroke.[3] Since complications can become severe without typical warning signs, patients should report any troubling symptoms to their doctor.

If you do become pregnant after experiencing fertility problems, be sure to see a high-risk obstetrician and learn early signs of preterm labor. Women who conceive following fertility treatment have higher rates of obstetric complications, even with a single gestation; twin and larger pregnancies, of course, bring additional risk, often with different symptoms than in single gestations.[4] Be aware that most fertility patients have more than one characteristic associated with an increased risk of ectopic pregnancy.[5] Women who take ovarian stimulants—particularly followed by transfer of several embryos—also have an increased risk of heterotopic pregnancy (at least one embryo implanting within the uterus *and* at least one outside).[6] This risk may be as high as one out of every hundred pregnancies following hyperstimulated assisted reproduction, which is 100 times the naturally occurring rate.[7] Even after early ultrasound confirms a uterine pregnancy, alert your physician if you experience pelvic pain or pain shooting up toward your shoulder; to be on the safe side, if you do not receive an immediate response, you may need to seek attention at a hospital emergency room. The ectopic embryo must be removed, while attempting to preserve the uterine pregnancy.

---

1. Lewitt et al. 1996; Mukherjee et al. 1995; Orvieto et al. 1995.

2. Halme, Toma, and Albert 1995.

3. Inbar et al. 1994.

4. Dildy et al. 1996; Hardardottir et al. 1996; Tallo et al. 1995; Tan et al. 1992 (Obstetric outcome); Tanbo et al. 1995. The increased rate of complications during IVF pregnancies that are *not* multiples may be influenced by the woman's age and previous infertility history (Reubinoff et al. 1997).

5. Ankum et al. 1996; Scully 1996. The latter lists a number of causes of ectopic pregnancy, including ovulation induction, delayed ovulation, IVF, tubal damage from inflammation, previous surgery for ectopic pregnancy, prenatal DES exposure, and, perhaps, endometriosis.

6. Scully 1996; this clinical report describes a heterotopic pregnancy in a DES daughter. See also Tummin et al. 1994.

7. Tal et al. 1996.

Choosing and Working with Your Doctor

Choosing a physician, given recent health care trends, seems something of a luxury. The initial questions must now be "Do you have a choice?" and "Can you see a specialist?" Fertility medicine has always been subject to the provisions of an individual's health insurance, with some procedures covered, others not. For the increasing numbers of people enrolled in managed-care plans since the early 1990s, restrictions extend to choice of physician and to specialist referrals as well. In a divide more pronounced than ever, the fullest choice goes to patients who can afford it—who can shop around for a doctor who best meets their medical and personal needs, perhaps travel far from home, and, ultimately, pay their own bills. For other fertility patients, choice narrows to a list of doctors who meet an insurer's requirements.

To the extent that managed care eliminates unnecessary and overly specialized medical procedures, imposition of limits works toward the good. Nonetheless, I would argue that it is crucially important to find a highly qualified, knowledgeable, and skilled physician who respects the rights of individual patients, a
doctor with whom you feel comfortable and whose judgment you trust. This
emphasis does not imply that some doctors have all the answers or that patients
should leave decisions up to them. Rather it is because of fertility medicine's
uncertainties—the need to determine first *whether* an individual can benefit
from treatment and the specialty's convoluted measures of success—that finding a good doctor is so important. The fact is, fertility patients need to avoid inappropriate, exploitive, or unethical treatment that can take varying forms—
the overtreatment or undertreatment, the ineffective and futile—depending on
a patient's medical and financial condition and on her doctor's medical and
financial goals. Finding the right doctor—someone who will be involved with a
most intimate aspect of your life—should allow for individual preferences and
choice. If I were looking for such a physician once again, or choosing from an insurance plan's list, or deciding whether I needed to change doctors, I would be
most concerned with answers to the following questions.

*Does this doctor have the technical skill and experience necessary to address my fertil-
ity problem?* Most couples trying to conceive can begin with a general ob-gyn,
who should be willing to refer them to a specialist if and when initial, minimally
invasive treatments fail. Writing in the *Journal of the American Medical Association,*
one specialist suggests the following reasons to request such a referral: the couple has tried to conceive for more than three years or has tried one treatment
for six to twelve months, or the woman is over thirty-five.[15] For the more unusual, complex, or persistent problems, a fertility specialist with more extensive training, and with more sophisticated diagnostic and treatment abilities,
may be needed. If you have a well-identified problem (for example, certain hormonal or ovulation abnormalities, severe sperm deficits), you may want to look
for a specialist (an andrologist if initial testing suggests a male fertility problem)
with particular expertise in treating this condition. This advice may be difficult
to follow under many managed-care health plans. Patients may be offered treatments performed by doctors with little experience, even though a general rule
of thumb in medicine is that better outcomes are likely with a physician who
regularly performs a particular procedure.[16] At least, try to keep yourself off
the low end of a practitioner's learning curve. At the same time, with treatment
of men's fertility problems rapidly changing, couples may need to be particularly wary of physicians continuing to perform outdated procedures. Although

many gynecologists describe themselves as "specializing in infertility," the profession recognizes only those who have completed a certified two-year program in reproductive endocrinology after their ob-gyn residency; definition of a subspecialty in andrology (with training beyond general urology) is in great flux, as are the diagnostic and treatment techniques andrologists use.[17] While patients generally cannot evaluate directly a doctor's technical competence, they can find out how many times this doctor has performed a specific procedure, with what rates of success and complications. If possible, seek a consultation—and perhaps treatment—from a specialist at a medical school ob-gyn or urology-andrology department. Remember, the doctor who first evaluates your fertility does not necessarily have to be the doctor who provides treatment.

Is this doctor keeping up to date on current research in fertility medicine? This characteristic is also difficult to evaluate directly; however, a doctor may refer to recent studies that help to explain the risks and benefits of a treatment for your condition and age group. If you bring in an article from the newspaper or a medical journal, the doctor may—or may not—seem to be familiar with the relevant medical literature. Women and men with a complicated or severe fertility problem may want to find a physician who is actively involved in research related to this condition (for example, at a medical school with a strong ob-gyn/urology and reproductive endocrinology department) and who brings a broad scientific and biological understanding to the practice of medicine; this researcher must, however, be interested in providing direct care to patients as well. Whether he is involved directly in medical research or not, the doctor should be able to apply research findings in a way that makes sense for your individual case.[18]

What medical philosophy characterizes this doctor's recommendations, particularly regarding how aggressively to intervene? Given the considerable unknowns in fertility medicine, the respectable rates of treatment-independent pregnancies among subfertile couples, and the risks that come with medical interventions, I would look for a doctor who is generally cautious, who allows time for spontaneous pregnancies when chances are favorable, and starts treatment with the least invasive option. He—or she—would be oriented toward scientifically controlled studies demonstrating the benefits of a diagnostic or treatment procedure as a basis for employing that procedure. She would limit diagnostic testing to procedures shown to reliably identify abnormalities that actually lower fertility, procedures that contribute to reaching treatment decisions. I do not want a doctor who "throws everything" at a fertility problem—high doses of fertility drugs, immunotherapies, transfer of many embryos—in the hope that something will work. Nor do I want a doctor who is too eager to forge ahead with an unproven treatment when my health is at stake. Rather, she would recommend treatments shown to significantly improve chances for having a healthy baby in cases like mine, without bringing unacceptable risks; if no such treatment exists, she and I would agree to "try something new" only if there was a plausible biological rationale, given my fertility problem. Equally important, this doctor needs to be willing and able to adapt general medical philosophy to a patient's particular situation. For instance, the physician can maintain a conservative approach, yet recommend fairly aggressive treatment for women over forty, or in cases of long-standing infertility. A doctor can emphasize preventive measures, advise patients to stop smoking, ask about environmental or occupational exposures that may lower fertility, diagnose and treat reproductive tract infection, yet also apply fertility treatments proven effective for an individual's identified problem.

What are the incentives and rewards that could be influencing this doctor's medical recommendations? Fertility patients need to be aware especially of financial incentives that may lead a doctor to be overly aggressive with treatments (e.g., the patient is paying out of pocket for each procedure) or to withhold appropriate treatment (e.g., the patient receives treatment within a managed-care plan that gives bonuses to doctors with the least expenditures and fewest specialist referrals or penalizes doctors with the most). Ask a doctor if he is allowed to tell you about an outside specialist who has greater expertise with your condition and if he can refer you to that specialist. Whatever your health insurance plan, find out what procedures and medications are covered, what are not covered (or require you to pay a portion), what bonuses the doctor receives for not providing a medical service or referral (or penalties for providing same). If your fertility care is not within a managed-care plan (i.e., you are paying a fee for each medical service), be sure to discuss thoroughly the reasons for and against undergoing any recommended medical procedure. If the doctor recommends extensive diagnostic procedures (e.g., hysteroscopy, endometrial biopsies, immunologic tests, laparoscopy) that cost extra, find out how the results would affect your treatment plan. And, if you are considering a discounted treatment package, try to determine whether the terms (eligibility requirements, limitations, exceptions, and other fine print) in fact favor you or the fertility clinic.

A medical school faculty member may not be as influenced by personal financial incentives as some private physicians, although managed-care pressures are surely squeezing academic medicine as well. This doctor may, however, push patients toward a treatment he is developing or toward participating in clinical research that will further his career and prestige within the academic community. (Participation in a research project may certainly be reasonable, but only after thorough discussion of risks and benefits.)

Do you feel comfortable with the style and tone of the doctor and other staff? The sophistication of modern medical technology has not eliminated the importance of a doctor's "bedside manner." Some doctors are easy to talk with, others are not. Some doctors schedule enough time to clarify information, answer questions, discuss with patients their diagnosis and treatment; others do not. Unfortunately, since time during a doctor's day is money, time talking with patients can become one casualty of the managed-care era. However, I want to leave a medical appointment feeling the doctor answered my questions, took my comments seriously, and considered my concerns to be legitimate. I want a doctor with whom I can discuss alternatives and agree on a treatment plan that incorporates our assessment of benefits and risks for me. This doctor would not decree my treatment, saying, "This is how we do it," although she would tell me honestly if a treatment is likely to be futile. I want to feel that the doctor is more interested in medical problems and solutions than in business propositions. I do not want to feel the doctor and staff are inaccessible, that they are reluctant to give out information or to consult with colleagues, that I am participating in a cut-rate, high-volume assembly-line enterprise—or in a slick, pricey one.

All of these characteristics contribute to establishing and maintaining trust in a doctor, but this trust must flow two ways. Just as I need to feel confident about the doctor's medical judgment and skill, concern for patients' well-being, and desire to discuss openly medical reasoning and uncertainties, the doctor must know that I, too, will discuss and weigh the pros and cons of medical procedures, sharing my questions, concerns, and priorities in deciding about fertility treatment. (See Appendix 5.)

Some closing thoughts on choosing and working with doctors:

No doctor will have it all—personable, warm, supportive, with sound clinical judgment wedded to broad scientific understanding when making medical recommendations that involve incomplete knowledge and imperfect techniques. Your choice will require priorities and trade-offs. To make that choice, try to learn the strengths and weaknesses of individual doctors, fertility clinics, embryo laboratories. What are the reasons for *you* to choose one over another?

A higher reported treatment success rate, by itself, may not be very revealing when choosing between different fertility programs. Any group's statistics will vary year to year; since the latest annual SART Registry report of clinic-specific rates will always be more than a year old, you need to ask physicians about their outcomes with current staff and protocols. Even more important, success rates may reflect primarily the type of patients a doctor treats. Some doctors treat the easiest cases—women with well-defined conditions that have effective therapies (e.g., IVF for blocked fallopian tubes) or couples with minimal subfertility of short duration who might conceive without treatment as well. Others take patients with complex problems and lower chances of success, patients other physicians will not accept (a simple example is the upper age limit for women an assisted reproduction program will accept). This "patient selection" consideration can, of course, be tricky. Does refusal to treat result from a reasonable and honest assessment that treatment would be futile or harmful, or does it reflect a desire to maintain high success rates by treating only those with the best chance for success? Although a larger program generally means greater experience and skill, it can reflect indiscriminate use of medical procedures. Patients may not be receiving the individualized assessment and treatment they require; personnel may be working at a pace that is asking for mistakes.

There may be ways to fill in some gaps with the doctor you do choose. For example, if a research-oriented fertility clinic at a major medical center feels less personal than a private community practice, joining a small group of patients who meet to share their experiences may provide needed emotional support. To be more confident that you are getting the latest information while seeing a community physician, and that existing knowledge is interpreted most usefully for your individual case, you may want to schedule periodic consultations with a medical school specialist. And helping to establish new forums for discussing fertility medicine, as outlined in Chapter 8, can benefit patients of any doctor.

You need to let your doctor know how much information you want—for example, by asking questions, asking for reprints of medical articles, bringing medical articles or other relevant material to your appointment. For any medical procedure, discuss the reasons, pro and con, and the alternatives. Always ask about a less invasive option; some doctors backtrack readily from a more aggressive recommendation if a patient questions the need.[19] When considering a diagnostic procedure, be clear about how the results will affect treatment choices. If you will end up with the same treatment anyway, why is that diagnostic procedure necessary? Ask also about the ways you will be monitored for treatment complications.

With your doctor, think through the likely course of your fertility treatment. Be sure to focus on questions of time and age, as well as the type of fertility problem. Ask for an estimate of your chances of a pregnancy without treatment.[20] Can you wait before starting treatments or moving to more aggressive interventions? The goal is to avoid rushing into overly invasive procedures, while not delaying treatment too long. Be sure to focus on your own priorities and limits (emotional, physical, and financial) in setting and pursuing medical goals—not on priorities, enthusiasms, or achievements (financial, academic, or psychological) that may define a doctor's goals. Be sure you know all the procedures a doctor might perform if you are under anesthesia (for example, during a laparoscopy or hysteroscopy) and be explicit about when you are willing to rely on the doctor's judgment about a procedure in such circumstances. Discuss thoroughly with the doctor your goals, your consent to specific procedures toward these goals, your ways of confirming that your consent and your medical wishes more generally are being honored.

Create a tentative timeline that includes periodic review of procedures done, options still available, chances for success; consultations with another physician who is not affiliated with your own and who may advocate a different approach (patients enrolled in HMOs or other managed-care plans may need to insist on seeing a specialist); times when it may be appropriate to take a break from treatment cycles; a point at which you should stop fertility treatments. Agree on the number of attempts for a particular treatment ahead of time, so that you and your doctor are not pulled by momentum into prolonging ineffective treatments. Consider information from recent, well-designed studies about the maximum number of attempts after which a particular treatment is rarely successful. Your timeline should not lock you into a rigid plan, but should build in checkpoints for reassessing and moving on.

Although doctors have skills and expertise that people with fertility problems may need, their medical education generally does not devote much time to certain important topics. Many doctors receive only minimal training in statistics or research methods, training important not only for conducting clinical studies but for evaluating and applying findings reported in medical journals and continuing education courses. The medical education of ob-gyns and urologists pays scant attention to environmental and occupational health and the potential impact of daily physical settings on fertility. Nor does their medical education emphasize preventive steps throughout a patient's reproductive life, as suggested by epidemiological and biological studies. Doctors may not keep a woman's future fertility in mind when prescribing contraception or proposing a medical procedure (e.g., cryosurgery or cone biopsy of the cervix). In their role of informing patients about fertility diagnoses and treatments, doctors may not mention the harmful effects of smoking on fertility or the possibility that heavy caffeine intake lowers chances of conceiving and maintaining a pregnancy. Finally, although individual doctors are regularly making ethical judgments about their patients and reproductive interventions, they have no special expertise for solving ethical dilemmas. Medical students may take a course (or a unit in a course) on medical ethics; for the most part, however, they are kept busy learning what medical intervention can do and how it is done technically, rather than wrestling with the justification or wisdom of doing it.

As you consider a doctor's recommendation, remember both the ways physicians and laypeople may differ in perspective and the ways they may be similar. On the one hand, doctors and patients may share a desire to "do something" rather than allow time for a treatment-independent pregnancy. They may be similarly swayed more by advertisements and anecdotal success stories than by statistical probabilities. On the other hand, doctors may develop a different orientation toward the human body, allowing them to more easily accept experimenting with treatments and using invasive procedures. Remember also that doctors who become immersed in their careers, in the single-minded pursuit of a narrow medical (or financial) goal, may end up with a distorted view of your overall well-being.

What Else Can Individuals Do?

Women and men who experience fertility problems may feel they have their hands full gathering information and seeing doctors. However, a few additional steps can help round out fertility care; in many of these steps, fertility patients should not be alone but joined by anyone wanting to have a baby.

Prevention. In this book on infertility, as with most areas of medicine, the section on prevention is, unfortunately, relatively short. Although concern with costs has conferred greater medical respectability on a preventive emphasis in recent years, there have never been enough research or health care resources directed toward preventing fertility problems. Prevention is neither lucrative nor prestigious in a medical career (unless removing and freezing ovaries is considered "preventive"). Because there is still much unknown about causes of impaired fertility and because conceiving a pregnancy—even with effective treatment—is always a matter of probabilities, preventive measures (for example, not smoking) can benefit people already experiencing problems and undergoing treatment; it is never too late to give yourself the most favorable odds you can.

Stress. If anything is certain about fertility problems and their treatment, it is the stress they cause. Whether that very stress—or other life stresses—contributes to the problem is less clear. Doctors have long tended to cite stress or psychological factors as a catch-all explanation for their female patients' otherwise unexplained infertility—hence the decades-old advice to relax, with husband, on a long ocean cruise. Whether the body's response to stress interferes with pregnancy in some individuals and not others remains a physiological question in need of an answer. Nevertheless, finding ways to manage stress can have benefits independent of any direct impact on fertility, with truly no harm done.

Just what individuals find helpful varies, as do reactions to stress in the first place. You may find that meditation serves this purpose, or long walks, listening to music, talking with a therapist. Some fertility patients join support groups, meeting regularly with other women or men who share and understand this particular stress. While making a difficult situation more livable, the goal for any of these activities is not merely to cope and comply with whatever the doctor recommends. In fact, meeting with other patients can become a way not only to gain emotional support during a stressful time of your life but also to exchange information about diagnoses, treatments, and doctors.

Health care records. Attempts to become pregnant and have a healthy baby may span several years and many medical procedures. People forget, over time, which doctor did what diagnostic tests and with what results, how long they took what dosage of fertility drugs, which year the first surgery occurred, what exactly was the assisted reproduction protocol. Nor does anyone know all the causes and effects, interconnections, or long-term health consequences of today's medical intervention. For the good of your health now and in years to come, keep your own health records, including:

each doctor seen, with address and telephone number

diagnostic tests and results

all medications (name, dosage, dates taken, where purchased)

all surgical procedures and results (with name of doctor, where surgery performed)

any other treatments and results

information about your menstrual cycle over the years (for example, age of first period, regularity, length of cycle, pain or heavy bleeding, passing of large clots, noticeable changes) contraceptives used, for how long

environmental or occupational exposures (for example, to chemicals or radiation)

In addition, if you change doctors, ask for two copies of your medical file—one
for the new doctor, the other for you. Some doctors may say they will provide
files only to another doctor; however, a patient is entitled to see a copy of her
own medical records.

The bigger picture. Inevitably, when a couple is having difficulty conceiving a
pregnancy, their attention focuses on their own diagnosis and treatment. However, the wider politics and economics of health care do shape present medical
choices, care, and outcomes, and the choices made today will define essential
characteristics of the reproductive world in the decades to come. The direction
in which fertility medicine should move can perhaps best be imagined by answering this question: If the choice were up to them, how would women and
their partners prefer to experience childbearing? For many people, that choice
does not match today's increasing pull toward in vitro fertilization, cryopreserved embryos and ovaries, and laboratory-matured eggs. Fertility medicine
appears headed toward a generic solution to all manner of fertility problems.
The move is away from diagnostic procedures, because of their inadequacy and
cost, rather than toward improving diagnostic abilities and corresponding treatments. Although high-tech fertility medicine may provide the only pregnancy
option for a relatively few individuals with severe abnormalities, decisions
about the reproductive lives of many more women and men are also being
pushed toward highly technological, invasive, and uniform medical interventions. The daily focus of doctors on attaining pregnancies case by case cannot address the broader need for redoubling scientific research and redefining goals—
steps that lead to enhanced choices for everyone.

With government attuned to religious-political voices and a health care system driven toward financial profit, the buyers within this system need to do
more than beware. It is no coincidence that when governmental agencies and
the medical profession have finally taken actions to protect fertility patients
from deceptive success claims and incompetent and unethical physicians or to
move toward allowing scientific research to proceed, or to curb extreme excesses in HMO cost-cutting, it has been in the aftermath of public congressional
hearings or publicized medical wrongdoing.[21] Individuals cannot afford—in all
meanings of the word—to lose sight of the bigger picture. Through consumer
organizations, as constituents of elected government representatives, as patients

living in local communities where fertility specialists need to maintain a clientele, individuals can exert their own political and economic pressure. To the extent they have a choice, people can take their health care dollars to physicians with demonstrated skill and commitment to patient well-being—including, when appropriate, to academic research centers. Patients may agree to participate in research, but should join only in the scientifically controlled, ethically justified studies so badly needed in fertility medicine. They can report adverse side effects of fertility treatment, as well as possibly related health problems, not only to their doctor, but to consumer organizations like Resolve, DES Action, the National Women's Health Network, and the Endometriosis Association; anecdotal cases and patterns can be the first hint of a problem needing more systematic study.[22] Patients can advocate (and support elected officials who advocate) for protective regulations (including enforceable quality standards and independent monitoring of doctors and fertility clinics), increased research, registries that facilitate follow-up studies, and access to high-quality fertility care that is not reserved only for people with financial means.

The bigger picture of fertility medicine fits within an even larger composite. One dimension is that of health care for society as a whole. The diagnosis and treatment of fertility problems take their place among other needs, including prenatal care for all pregnant women, primary and preventive care for children and adults (including the elderly), as well as treatment of various acute and chronic ailments. This country has yet to come to grips with the problem of assuring good, affordable health care for its population. Questions about the best use and distribution of medical resources—from the most basic to the highly technological—involve all segments of the population and all areas of medicine. So too does concern that people's reproductive and overall health needs should not have to compete in a medical marketplace with the financial needs of large insurance companies, drug manufacturers, or medical entrepreneurs.

A Canadian Perspective

Dr. Patricia Baird, chair of the Canadian Royal Commission on New Reproductive Technologies, offers a perspective that differs from the dominant U.S. point of view:

> In Canada, our view of the individual's relationship to the collective is that we are all equal and therefore that we have an obligation to support each other in the face of illness or disease, and so we have a publicly supported health care system. We recommended that IVF or

other safe and effective procedures be brought within that system because having children is extremely important to people's lives; it is not a frill or a luxury. If there are safe and effective ways to treat infertility, they should be provided within the publicly supported system. If they are not proven, they should be in research trials. If they are not safe and effective, they should not be done at all, privately or publicly. . . .

The marketplace is a major force in today's societies. Given the pervasiveness and strength of the market, controlling and counterbalancing commercial activity to protect vulnerable interests is essential. Commercial organizations are designed to make money, not to balance conflicting interests. In an open market, it is assumed buyers can protect their own interests—the basic protections being information and choice. It is assumed that these protections will lead to market competition so that the interests of consumers will be served. In the area of medical practice, these consumer protections are not sufficient, as the degree of vulnerability is much greater. Infertility is closer to what is individual, . . . and information is asymmetric, with the physician having a different kind of understanding. Consumers' interests are vulnerable whereas the interests of the providers (for example in a privately offered service with a potential for personal gain) are not. In Canada, we think government therefore has a responsibility to guard citizens' interests by ensuring mechanisms are in place for regulation and accountability in the field.

Not only individuals, but the wider community too, have vulnerable interests that need protection. We all have a stake in the nature of the society in which we live—that it not be one in which people or their reproductive capacities are treated as commodities.[1]

In the United States, the coming years may force the recognition that certain groups and interests are vulnerable and need protection in health care. As genetic and other biomedical tools can identify an growing list of physical and mental health risks in individuals, even before symptoms appear, concerns about guaranteed health care—and about safe, effective treatments—will spread throughout the population. While fertility specialists—and other physicians—scramble toward their immediate goal of staking out insurable treatments, what is needed is more far-sighted and wide-ranging efforts toward establishing universal and efficiently provided health care that will be there for everyone, whatever illnesses or abnormalities the fates (genetic and otherwise) may deal.

---

1. Baird 1996, 129, 157.

Fertility medicine also fits within the bigger picture of an individual's life-time. I add the following comments, in closing, with a view toward this longer dimension, especially for women, who at some point in their life, in various ways, face questions of fertility.

An Epilogue

The aging of the baby-boom generation has become a public phenomenon in re-cent years, with menopause and Medicare sharing center stage. However, the medical community—especially obstetrician-gynecologists—and the pharma-ceutical industry have been alert for quite some time to the sheer number of women passing through their reproductive years toward menopause. As is the case in much of reproductive medicine, there are both benefits and dangers in this increased attention to older women's health. Whether a woman has experi-enced fertility problems or not, she will need to make decisions about hor-monal medications.

The baby-boom generation has, in fact, been an irresistible market from its own conception. During the post–World War II years, drug manufacturers pro-moted diethylstilbestrol as a wonder drug that would prevent miscarriage and "make normal pregnancies more normal" for all those women eager to start families. Baby-boom daughters became an inviting target as they reached their own reproductive years; infertility became the market, fertility medicine the expansive gynecologic specialty. Now, the very definition of "reproductive years" is changing in concert with the demographics; the professional organiza-tion of fertility specialists has officially extended their definition of those years to include menopause.

A cynic might even claim that physicians, in collaboration with the pharma-ceutical industry, have found the perfect reproductive problem in a woman's age. No woman can avoid this condition (the one alternative is decidedly worse), and the prospects for medical intervention cover all contingencies. Social pressures women may feel to have children—always substantial and widespread—are now open-ended. Pressure to "at least" bear the genetic offspring of one's male partner are enlarged as well. After the age of about forty, women having difficulty con-ceiving can try assisted reproductive technologies; as their fertility declines into menopause and beyond, they can switch to donated eggs. Whether successful with pregnancy or not, they will have reached the age of hormone replacement ther-apy. The greater proportion of women—those who do not attempt pregnancy during or after their forties—can move directly onto hormone replacement at menopause, for many after a decade or more of taking oral contraceptives.

Indeed, in 1992 the American Society for Reproductive Medicine announced its largest grant ever received from a drug company ($400,000 from Parke Davis and Co.) to educate physicians and consumers "on the specific hormonal needs of the peri-menopausal woman, who often experiences psychological and physiological changes during these years of transition." The educational program was actually being devised within the New York offices of a public relations firm hired to push a new pharmaceutical product, a low-dose oral contraceptive. Once again, a drug manufacturer was defining women's specific needs and providing the solution—a prescription drug, physicians educated to prescribe it, and women educated to want it. The drug manufacturer was also carving its share of the aging market—forty-something women during the "transition years" of approaching menopause, before their decision about some other company's post-menopausal estrogen replacement.[23] With this generous grant, the baby-boom generation has now been targeted from cradle to grave.

Most disturbing is, once again, this question: Who is doing the informing about what options? Just what "specific hormonal needs" were they talking about? Given the tremendous gaps in knowledge about women's health, how did anyone know what to educate physicians and consumers about? Studies then being initiated might someday answer questions about whether there are special perimenopausal needs and about risks perimenopausal women must weigh when considering hormonal contraception. The only need certain for women approaching menopause was the need to fend off misleading, exploitive educational efforts that do not truly inform their individual decisions.

No one was hiding the directive hand of a drug manufacturer who profits from the baby boomer's perimenopausal prescriptions. As with DES for this generation's birth and interventions to combat their infertility—often portrayed misleadingly as an "epidemic"—mid-life medical problems were being created out of concern for market shares rather than for health. Then women could be convinced—or rather "educated"—as to the cure. Starting with aging baby boomers, women would again be showered with information. They would find brochures in doctors' waiting rooms. Ads would appear in medical journals and the lay press. Patients and doctors would attend industry-sponsored conferences on perimenopause and menopause.

The choices will be all the more complex because hormone replacement does appear to benefit some women after menopause. The data are not yet in—not on menopause, even less on the "transition years"—and never will be without well-designed studies and vigilant regulation of the pharmaceutical industry. If anything, scientists are learning that estrogens are more complex and have more wide-ranging physiological effects than previously recognized. What women should already know is that drug company promotions encouraging routine use of hormones only obfuscate considerations of risks and benefits as individuals approach and pass through menopause. (One advertisement for an oral contraceptive—appearing not only in journals but as an insert in the conference packet for the ASRM's annual meeting—reads: "TRY IT ON ALL YOUR PATIENTS . . . EVEN ON YOUR DIFFICULT PATIENTS." This message is from Ortho Pharmaceuticals, Inc., the physician's "partner in women's health.")

New Product, Old Promotions

An early hint of broader claims for low-dose oral contraceptives—beyond the FDA-approved use for preventing pregnancy—appeared in 1996 when a prominent fertility specialist reported possible "bone-sparing properties of oral contraceptives" for women who are approaching menopause. Osteoporosis—a decrease in bone density that can contribute to fractures and skeletal deformity—is a well-established risk for women after menopause. Research indicates that approximately 10 percent of bone loss occurs during the five years surrounding menopause, the decline accelerating immediately following a woman's actual cessation of menstruation; estrogen replacement, especially if started soon after menopause, helps slow this process. Citing an FDA assessment that newly formulated low-dose oral contraceptives bring minimal health risks, this fertility specialist suggests that using them for "earlier intervention" may also provide "early prevention" of osteoporosis; doctors might, therefore, want to consider the minimizing of bone loss as "an added benefit to their primary effect, contraception."[1]

Much remains unknown about the physiology of hormones and bone strength—as well as about the ways bone fractures due to osteoporosis might be minimized, if not prevented. Prevention is certainly a desirable goal, but earlier medical intervention does not always achieve prevention and has at times resulted only in harm. This first whiff of claims about added benefits from oral contraceptives for women in their forties prompts three immediate concerns.

First, there has not been enough research to amass any weight of evidence regarding risks and benefits (other than contraception) for women who take oral contraceptives during their forties. Yet physicians will surely cite prevention of osteoporosis as a selling point when they prescribe this type of hormone; too many doctors will take a blanket approach, prescribing birth control pills to just about any perimenopausal woman—even those not specifically seeking contraception—irrespective of individual risks and benefits. Among questions needing thorough study:

Does use of low-dose oral contraceptives before menopause result in the added benefit actually desired, reduction of bone fractures during women's postmenopausal years?

Assuming a bone-sparing effect proves to be real, which perimenopausal women will most benefit from hormonal contraception? Since post-menopausal women do not all have the same risk of developing osteo-porosis, not all women in their forties will gain the same added benefit from birth control pills. These hormones will bring risks, however, to all who take them, to some women more than to others.

What minimum hormone dose achieves enough added benefit to outweigh the risks of birth control pills (e.g., blood clots, stroke, possible increased chance of developing breast cancer)? What specific type of hormones?

Beyond immediate and long-term health risks of taking oral contraceptives for a few years before menopause, what about women who also used birth control pills at younger ages (e.g., starting in their late teens or twenties) and at higher doses, accumulating, say, ten or more years of hormone use by the time they reach menopause (women who may then change to hor-mone replacement therapy)? Does this patient history alter, for example, a woman's risks for developing breast cancer? What about women who, for varying amounts of time, used fertility drugs? Women who never had a successful pregnancy (and never breast-fed) or who became pregnant after the age of thirty-five—both of which raise the risk of breast cancer?

Can women gain similar benefits by other means than hormonal medications (for instance, exercise, calcium, other type of medication for bone strength; diet or exercise for risk of heart disease after menopause), thereby avoiding the increase of risks that are more difficult to lower (e.g., breast cancer)?

Second, in noting a need for reliable birth control in healthy women over the age of thirty-five, the report's author argues that oral contraceptives are espe-cially effective, because the women are less fertile anyway, they have sexual in-tercourse less often than younger women, and they are more likely to take the pills as prescribed ("better compliance"). However, these same characteristics support use of nonhormonal contraception (especially barrier methods, which also help protect against sexually transmitted diseases). There is no guarantee, moreover, that doctors will prescribe oral contraceptives only to healthy women with low risk of complications. Screening measures cannot always identify indi-viduals who will experience hormone-related problems; nor will doctors always take the time and expense, in this cost-cutting era, to conduct a thorough patient history and examination, to order screening tests that do exist, and to weigh thor-

---

1. DeCherney 1996.

Whether they have been fertility patients or sailed through those reproductive decades without a hitch, women considering their own hormonal needs as they approach menopause will need to shift their focus to a new set of questions:

When the drug company pushes doctors to prescribe the low-dose birth control pill, are nonhormonal contraceptive alternatives fairly compared?

Before widespread use of a new hormonal medication (whether a fertility drug, contraceptive, or menopausal hormone replacement) is promoted, has enough time elapsed and enough research been done to detect various potential problems? (For example, an oral contraceptive lower in hormone dosage may use a different type of hormone; this different hormonal type may increase risk of blood clots, stroke, or other harmful side effects, regardless of the pill's dosage.)

When educating physicians and consumers, does the drug manufacturer emphasize that women over thirty-five who smoke should not take oral contra-ceptives? Are women and their doctors informed that even though estrogen re-placement *after* menopause appears to have cardiovascular and bone-sparing benefits, there are demonstrated risks (e.g., heart attack, stroke, blood clots) from oral contraceptives in premenopausal women with a family history of car-diovascular disease, with other individual "risk factors," and in women over forty—the new pill's target age?

Are claims about benefits of oral contraceptives limited to the only one ap-proved—preventing pregnancy? Will it be clear that whatever the benefits of estrogen replacement after menopause—and the muddle of risks and benefits, especially when taking hormones for many years, needs at least a decade of study for clarification—a woman's perimenopausal physiology and the hormonal contraceptive regimen are a very different matter? (Any contraceptive dosage will be higher than postmenopausal hormone replacement therapy.)

If my own baby-boom generation has learned anything about reproductive medicine, I hope it is to be more astute in detecting manipulations that steer people to options that are not in their best interest and may even be hazardous to their health. And I hope our lesson becomes a legacy for the generations who follow, so that when they consider reproductive interventions, whether younger or older, they will already be wiser.

Appendix 1
Useful References and Resources

Resources and references on the diagnosis and treatment of fertility problems are available through a variety of sources, including books, libraries, online databases, advocacy groups, professional organizations, and government agencies. This listing includes many of the most prominent sources. Appendix 2 focuses on finding and reading medical journal articles.

Basic Resources

Extensive lists of resources are available in many published handbooks on infertility, which include topics not covered in this book (e.g., the emotional impact of infertility, adoption, pregnancy loss, deciding not to have a child). The following two books, written by former fertility patients in consultation with fertility specialists, are particularly helpful:

> C. Harkness. 1992. *The infertility book: A comprehensive medical and emotional guide.* Berkeley: Celestial Arts.
> P. Robin. 1993. *How to be a successful fertility patient.* New York: Morrow.

For a straightforward, low-key reference book written by three fertility specialists (Canadian, British, and American), with good photographs and diagrams, see:

> S. L. Tan, H. S. Jacobs, and M. M. Seibel. 1995. *Infertility: Your questions answered.* New York: Birch Lane Press.

To find a nearby medical library open to the public, call the National Network of Libraries of Medicine at 800–338–7657. Planetree Health Resource Centers, a national nonprofit consumer health organization with locations in several states (California, Colorado, Connecticut, Illinois, Nebraska, Oregon, Washington), maintains libraries that are free and open to the public. Planetree can also provide computer search services (approximately $15–$25) and individualized research reports on specific medical conditions (written reports of 50–150 pages, approximately $175 plus shipping). For further information, contact:

> Planetree Health Resource Center
> California Pacific Medical Center
> 2040 Webster Street
> San Francisco, California 94115
> 415-923-3680 (recorded information)
> 415-923-3681

Core Articles

The articles listed below can serve as a starting point for reading medical literature on fertility problems. Each of these articles includes a reference list of previous related articles; a Medline computer search is the most efficient way to find more recent articles (see Appendix 2). Within each section articles are listed in alphabetical order.

Classics

R. E. Blackwell, B. R. Carr, R. J. Chang, et al. 1987. Are we exploiting the infertile couple? *Fertility and Sterility* 48:735–39.

J. A. Collins, W. Wrixon, L. B. Janes, et al. 1983. Treatment-independent pregnancy among infertile couples. *New England Journal of Medicine* 309:1201–6.

S. Fishel and P. Jackson. 1989. Follicular stimulation for high tech pregnancies: Are we playing it safe? *British Medical Journal* 199:309–11.

Overviews

J. A. Collins. 1995. A couple with infertility. *Journal of the American Medical Association* 274:1159–64.

ESHRE Capri Workshop. 1996. Infertility revisited: The state of the art today and tomorrow. *Human Reproduction* 11 (suppl. 4):5–33.

E. Geva, A. Amit, L. Lerner-Geva, et al. 1997. Autoimmunity and reproduction. *Fertility and Sterility* 67:599–611.

M. G. Hull. 1992. Infertility treatment: Relative effectiveness of conventional and assisted conception methods. *Human Reproduction* 7:785–96.

R. P. Jansen. 1995. Elusive fertility: Fecundability and assisted conception in perspective. *Fertility and Sterility* 64:252–55.

H. W. Jones and J. P. Toner. 1993. The infertile couple. *New England Journal of Medicine* 329:1710–15.

Female Infertility

D. L. Healy, A. O. Trounson, and A. N. Anderson. 1994. Female infertility: Causes and treatment. *Lancet* 343:1539–44.

Male Infertility

D. M. de Krester. 1997. Male infertility. *Lancet* 349:787–90.

ESHRE Andrology Special Interest Group. 1996. Consensus workshop on advanced diagnostic andrology techniques. *Human Reproduction* 11:1463–79.

S. S. Howards. 1995. Treatment of male infertility. *New England Journal of Medicine* 332:312–17.

N. E. Skakkebaek, A. Giwercman, and D. de Kretser. 1994. Pathogenesis and management of male infertility. *Lancet* 343:1473–79.

Assisted Reproductive Technologies

M. Y. Dawood. 1996. In vitro fertilization, gamete intrafallopian transfer, and superovulation with intrauterine insemination: Efficacy and potential health hazards on babies delivered. *American Journal of Obstetrics and Gynecology* 174:1208–17.

G. D. Palermo, J. Cohen, and Z. Rosenwaks. 1996. Intracytoplasmic sperm injection: A powerful tool to overcome fertilization failure. *Fertility and Sterility* 65:899–908.

L. S. Wilcox, H. B. Peterson, F. D. Haseltine, et al. 1993. Defining and interpreting pregnancy success rates for in vitro fertilization. *Fertility and Sterility* 60:18–25.

C. A. Benadiva, I. Kligman, O. Davis, et al. 1995. In vitro fertilization versus tubal surgery: Is pelvic reconstructive surgery obsolete? *Fertility and Sterility* 64:1051–61.

A. S. Penzias and A. H. DeCherney. 1996. Is there ever a role for tubal surgery? *American Journal of Obstetrics and Gynecology* 174:1218–23.

Risks

R. E. Bristow and B. Y. Karlan. 1996. Ovulation induction, infertility, and ovarian cancer risk. *Fertility and Sterility* 66:499–507.

B. Eshkenazi. 1993. Caffeine during pregnancy: Grounds for concern? *Journal of the American Medical Association* 270:2973–74.

M. A. Rossing, J. R. Daling, and N. Weiss. 1994. Ovarian tumors in a cohort of infertile women. *New England Journal of Medicine* 331:771–76.

Z. Shoham. 1994. Epidemiology, etiology, and fertility drugs in ovarian epithelial carcinoma: Where are we today? *Fertility and Sterility* 62:433–48.

A. Shushan, O. Paltiel, J. Iscovich, et al. 1996. Human menopausal gonadotropin and the risk of epithelial ovarian cancer. *Fertility and Sterility* 65:13–18.

A. J. Whittemore, R. Harris, J. Itnyre, et al. 1992. Characteristics relating to ovarian cancer risk: Collaborative analysis of 12 United States case-control studies. II. Invasive epithelium ovarian cancers in white women. *American Journal of Epidemiology* 136:1184–1203.

How to Find and Use Medical Journal Articles

G. H. Guyatt, D. L. Sackett, D. J. Cook, et al. 1993. Users' guides to the medical literature. II. How to use an article about therapy or prevention. A. Are the results of the study valid? *Journal of the American Medical Association* 270:2598–2601.

H. J. Lowe and G. O. Barnett. 1994. Understanding and using the medical subject headings (MeSH) vocabulary to perform literature searches. *Journal of the American Medical Association* 271:1103–8.

C. D. Naylor, G. H. Guyatt, et al. 1996. Users' guides to the medical literature. X. How to use an article reporting variations in the outcomes of health services. *Journal of the American Medical Association* 275:554–58.

A. D. Oxman, D. L. Sackett, G. H. Guyatt, et al. 1993. Users' guides to the medical literature. I. How to get started. *Journal of the American Medical Association* 270:2093–96.

J. F. Peipert and P. J. Sweeney. 1993. Diagnostic testing in obstetrics and gynecology: A clinican's guide. *Obstetrics and Gynecology* 82:619–23.

D. B. Seifer, M. D. Adelson, R. W. Abdul-Karim, et al. 1989. Appraising a clinical journal article in obstetrics and gynecology. *American Journal of Obstetrics and Gynecology* 160:198–201.

R. Sikorski. 1997. Medical literature made easy. *Journal of the American Medical Association* 277:959–60.

Reprints of articles in the *Journal of the American Medical Association* "users' guides" series (including several not listed here) are available from:

> Dr. G. H. Guyatt
> Room 2C12 McMaster University Health Sciences Center
> 1200 Main Street West
> Ontario, Canada L8N 3Z5

Consumer and Advocacy Groups

> DES Action, National Office
> 1615 Broadway, Suite 510
> Oakland, California 94612
> 510-465-4011 or information hotline: 800-DES-9288;
> E-mail: desact@well.com

Medical information, doctor referrals, and support for DES mothers, daughters, and sons; local groups throughout the United States and western Europe.

> Endometriosis Association
> 8585 N. 76th Place
> Milwaukee, Wisconsin 53223
> 800-992-3636 (in North America)

Medical information, doctor referrals, and support for women with endometriosis. The association is listed as coauthor for Mary Lou Ballweg, *The endometriosis handbook* (Chicago: Contemporary Books, 1995).

> Health Research Group
> 1600 20th St. N.W.
> Washington, D.C. 20009

Affiliated with Ralph Nader's Public Citizen, this health subgroup investigates and advocates on a broad spectrum of health issues, including drug approval and safety; disciplinary actions against doctors; access to one's own medical records; HMOs and other health insurance issues.

National Women's Health Network
514 10th St. N.W., Suite 400
Washington, D.C. 20004
202–628–7814

A public interest organization focused on a range of women's health issues; maintains a clearinghouse distributing informational materials on various topics, including infertility and reproductive technologies, pelvic inflammatory disease, occupational and environmental health.

Resolve, National Office
5 Water St.
Arlington, Massachusetts 02174
617–643–2424

Medical information, doctor referrals, and support for women and men experiencing infertility; adoption information; local groups throughout the United States.

Professional Organizations and Government Agencies

American Society for Reproductive Medicine (ASRM)
409 12th St. S.W., Suite 203
Washington, D.C. 20024-2125
202-863-2439

The professional organization of fertility specialists, publisher of journal *Fertility and Sterility;* informational material for patients available.

National Advisory Board on Ethics in Reproduction (NABER)
409 12th St., S.W.
Washington, D.C. 20024-2188
202-863-2503

Established by the American Society for Reproductive Medicine and American College of Obstetricians and Gynecologists (ACOG), this panel organizes conferences and publishes a newsletter focused on ethical issues of fertility medicine.

National Institutes of Health–National Institute of Child Health and
Human Development (Reproductive Medicine Network)
Center for Population Research–Reproductive Sciences Branch
Bldg-Room: 6100-8B01
Bethesda, Maryland 20892
301-495-6515

Government agency funding clinical research on fertility treatments (the first set of studies is focusing on intrauterine insemination and controlled ovarian hyperstimulation for unexplained and male infertility); provides information on research centers needing participants and on eligibility requirements.

Reproductive Toxicology Center
Columbia Hospital for Women Medical Center
2440 M Street, N.W., Suite 217
Washington, D.C. 20037-1404
202-293-5137

A subscription service for health professionals; gathers and disseminates information about effects of the chemical and physical environment on fertility, pregnancy, and fetal development. In addition to having access to the center's regularly updated database, subscribing physicians can request information about specific exposures of particular patients.

Society for Assisted Reproductive Technologies (SART)
1209 Montgomery Highway
Birmingham, Alabama 35216-2809
205-978-5000

An affiliated subgroup of American Society for Reproductive Medicine that focuses specifically on assisted reproductive technologies; it prepares annual reports of fertility clinic success rates by geographic region, which are available for purchase.

Women's Occupational Health Resource Center
Columbia University School of Public Health
Health Policy and Management
600 W. 168th Street, 6th floor
New York, New York 10032
212-305-3724

Provides information about working conditions that may contribute to fertility problems.

Appendix 2
Finding and Using the Medical Literature

Finding Medical Articles

A good place to start is a medical school library, the library of a large hospital, or a university's science library. In some cities, a Planetree Health Library provides health and medical information specifically for the public (see Appendix 1). The Medline database—the National Library of Medicine's electronic bibliography, indexing thousands of articles and abstracts from medical and scientific journals each month—offers the most efficient way to conduct a computer search, especially to find recent research and review articles. A system of key terms, known as MeSH (Medical Subject Headings, based on 10–12 indexing terms that represent contents of the article), can help narrow a Medline search to relevant articles. There may be a charge for Medline searches if you are not affiliated with an institution (e.g., a university) that provides computer access; your doctor or a friend or acquaintance who is a doctor may be able to sponsor your access. Ask a librarian to help the first few times. Ask also about any special databases that may exist for your particular problem (e.g., articles on environmental, occupational, and medical exposures that may affect fertility). Consumer organizations, such as Resolve, DES Action, or the Endometriosis Association, often have their own collection of medical articles or can help you obtain particular articles (see Appendix 1).

Medline access is also available via the Internet through many sites on the web. For information about Internet access to Medline and other databases, see R. Sikorski 1997 ("Medical literature made easy," *Journal of the American Medical Association,* 277:959–60). A useful resource about medical information on the Internet more generally is "Finding medical help online," *Consumer Reports,* February 1997.

Types of Articles Published in Medical Journals

Clinical studies report on diagnostic tests or treatments doctors use in caring for patients. The most common types of studies are case reports, observational studies, and randomized controlled trials.

> *Case reports* present a single—or sometimes more than one—anecdotal description of a patient's diagnosis, treatment, and outcome; these reports can provide first hints of a problem needing more systematic study or of a new way to handle a medical problem.
>
> *Observational studies* accumulate data from a series of patients who have undergone the same medical intervention. A *prospective* study includes patients enrolled from a certain time forward; a *retrospective* study reviews interventions performed on patients in the past, commonly by reading medical records of all patients treated during a specified time period.
>
> *Randomized controlled trials* follow a formal research structure that most closely approaches a scientific experimental method and most adequately tests a treatment's efficacy.

Epidemiological studies trace patterns of health and illness in human populations, using statistical associations among various factors to suggest cause-and-effect relationships that increase or reduce health risks. These studies are either prospective or retrospective.

A *prospective study* follows groups of people over time to compare specified outcomes (e.g., a yearly examination of women exposed prenatally to DES and of similar women, not exposed, to compare frequency of cancer, reproductive problems, and other health conditions).

A *retrospective, or case-control, study* traces back in time, comparing people with a particular outcome (e.g., ovarian cancer "cases") to similar people without that outcome ("controls") to identify possible causes (e.g., diet, cigarette smoking, use of oral contraceptives, use of fertility drugs, endogenous hormone levels, number of pregnancies).

Laboratory research involves experiments with animals (ranging from microscopic creatures to mice to primates) or parts (tissue, cells) of human and other animals. In fertility medicine, laboratory experiments related to assisted reproduction most often use eggs, sperm, and embryos to study various aspects of the fertilization process.

In addition to reports of individual studies, medical journals publish articles that bring together findings of several studies.

Meta-analyses use statistical techniques to combine data from studies on the same topic (e.g., studies that compare pregnancy rates of various assisted reproductive technologies for treating unexplained infertility) in order to increase the strength of research findings and conclusions. Basic features of included studies must be comparable, using statistical methods appropriate for the types of data involved, and the authors of the meta-analysis should describe criteria used to select included studies.

Review articles present a more qualitative overview of existing research on a particular topic (e.g., the diagnosis and treatment of endometriosis; uses of assisted reproduction for male infertility) to describe the state of the art based on current knowledge. Again, selection criteria should be explicit. Conclusions reached in this type of overview may be more influenced by the author's interpretations than would be the case in a meta-analysis; however, review articles are generally easier to evaluate for readers who do not have much statistical training.

Reading through a Medical Article

For most patients and doctors, medical journal articles describing clinical and epidemiological studies are of greatest interest. These articles generally follow a standard format:

Abstract. Before the article's text begins, a brief summary presents the study's main purpose and design, findings, and conclusions; readers can gain an initial idea of the study's relevance to their own situation.

Introduction. Describes the purpose of the study, the questions addressed or hypotheses tested, and the importance of this study as a contribution to existing knowledge about the topic.

Materials and methods. Describes how the study was conducted—the number of participants (sample size), criteria for defining who was included and excluded as participants, details of interventions performed (e.g., specific medications, dosage, timing; type of surgical procedures), study's design (e.g., retrospective review of past medical records; observational series of patients treated from starting date to ending date; randomized controlled trial), and statistical tests performed to analyze findings.

Results. Presents this study's outcomes as numbers, percentages, or measures of statistical significance (which reveal whether differences in outcome were large enough that they did not likely happen by chance).

Discussion. Formulates and explains conclusions drawn from the results about the original hypotheses and questions stated in the introduction. Considers implications of the findings, more generally, for patients' health and medical care.

Evaluating Information

Published articles vary in the quality of reporting and of the research itself. Moreover, just as doctors need to evaluate journal articles with an eye toward applying the findings to their patients, laypeople reading medical articles need to ask what light a study sheds on their particular situation. Two basic questions frame these evaluations: *How valid are the results and conclusions?* (That is, is this a well-designed, well-executed study?) And *are the findings about a diagnosis or treatment useful for me?*

The following considerations can help as you read medical articles and discuss them with physicians.

How were study participants selected? Are they similar to me on key characteristics, such as duration and severity of fertility problems, woman's age, the type of problems in the woman and/or man of a couple? Are groups that a study compares similar to each other on these characteristics?

On what basis were individuals excluded from the study, and how might that affect the findings? For example, if research on a treatment excludes women who previously underwent a different treatment, the participants may have milder fertility problems and/or problems of shorter duration.

Is there a control group appropriately selected for comparisons this study makes?

Is the sample size—i.e., the number of participants—large enough to provide useful findings. Many clinical studies do not have enough participants to detect differences between comparison groups if such differences do exist (creating a "false negative" result). The methods section should report the study's statistical "power"—how large a difference between groups a study of this size can detect.

Were participants assigned to the study's groupings randomly, in order to avoid influences that might bias the results? For example, a report on women undergoing IVF during one year at a fertility clinic finds IVF with ovarian hyperstimulation to be twice as effective as natural-cycle IVF (approximately 16 percent vs. 8 percent). If groups were assigned through doctor-patient consultation, women in the natural-cycle group may be "poor responders" to previous attempts at ovarian stimulation; these women may have a more severe fertility problem, of longer duration, and may be older. In contrast, women assigned to the hyperstimulation group may be trying IVF for the first time; since the more fertile couples are likely to conceive first, overall results for stimulated IVF will be highest during the initial year. A different bias arises if younger women, trying IVF for the first time, choose to take no medications while those who have undergone previous unsuccessful IVF cycles use fertility drugs.

Were participants and researchers "blinded" (i.e., they did not know who was receiving what)? For example, a doctor performing a second laparoscopy to evaluate changes in a patient's endometriosis following treatment with hormones should not know what treatment the patient received or whether she was an untreated "control."

How thorough is the follow-up of participants? How many of the initial participants are not included in the results ("lost to follow-up" or dropped during the study), and what is the reason? How might their absence affect the findings? For example, when trying to document pregnancy rates up to four years after undergoing a surgical treatment, physicians cannot always locate past patients to update their records. Since patients who eventually have a successful pregnancy are more likely to contact the surgeon than are women who never do become pregnant, a study based on review of patient records over past years will be biased toward the successful outcomes. Did groups receive the same length and manner of follow-up? Was the time period long enough? For example, a study of birth defects in newborns of mothers given DES during pregnancy would not find the cancer or reproductive problems that became apparent only after DES-daughters reached adolescence. Women given fertility drugs must be followed over enough years to cover the latency period during which cancers could develop.

Was a no-treatment group or background pregnancy rate (an estimated likelihood of spontaneous pregnancy) included in comparisons when treatment involved subfertile rather than completely infertile patients?

Do reported results support the conclusions? (At times, the logic connecting the two is surprisingly unclear.) Are generalizations about applying findings to other patients justified? For example, proposing a treatment (e.g., immunotherapy) for all unexplained infertility based on a study of women who did not succeed with IVF seems a long stretch. Are there compelling reasons not to apply the findings to particular patients? For example, a fertility treatment proven to be effective but with considerable side effects would not be recommended if patients have a good prognosis for conceiving without treatment. Patients with particular characteristics might make a treatment too risk-laden (e.g., ovarian stimulation in a woman whose mother and aunt died of premenopausal ovarian cancer).

•

Evaluating statistical methods and results can be difficult for most laypeople (and many doctors). However, technical weaknesses of a study often center on two basic questions: Did the researchers choose correct statistical tests for this type of study? Did their research design eliminate, as much as possible, factors that would invalidate or bias the results? In addition, readers need to ask whether the results have *clinical significance*—that is, do the findings have an impact on actual diagnosis or treatment of patients? A clinical study may report results that are statistically significant (not likely due to chance) but that do not change the care of patients in a real-world clinical setting. For example, a statistically significant reduction of visible pelvic adhesions following surgery or lengthening of women's luteal phase following hormone treatment may not improve chances for having a successful pregnancy. A particular diagnostic test may provide a valid measure of hormone levels in the bloodstream but not change the treatment plan doctors would propose; what these blood hormone levels reflect about an individual's fertility may not be well understood.

Appendix 3

Elements of Informed Consent

To comply with federal regulations for the protection of human subjects in biomedical research, investigators conducting a study must provide the following when obtaining a participant's informed consent:[1]

1. A statement that the study involves research, an explanation of the purposes of the research and the expected duration of the human subject's participation, a description of the procedures to be followed, and identification of any procedures that are experiments.

2. A description of any reasonably foreseeable risks or discomforts to the participant.

3. A description of any benefits to participants or to others from the research.

4. A disclosure of appropriate alternative procedures or courses of treatment, if any, that might be advantageous to the participant.

5. A statement describing the extent, if any, to which confidentiality of records identifying the participant will be maintained.

6. For research involving more than minimal risk, an explanation of whether any compensation will be provided and whether any medical treatments are available if injury occurs; if so, what the treatments are or where further information can be obtained.

7. An explanation of whom to contact for answers to pertinent questions about the research and participants' rights and whom to contact in the event of a research-related injury.

8. A statement that participation is voluntary, refusal to participate involving no penalty or loss of benefits to which the patient is otherwise entitled, and that a patient may discontinue participation at any time without penalty or loss of benefits to which he or she is otherwise entitled.

Proposed research, with certain exemptions, is to be reviewed by a duly constituted institutional review board (IRB), which must be established locally and have a minimum of five members, including at least one scientist, one nonscientist, and one person not otherwise affiliated with that institution. The board reviews and has authority to approve, require modification in, or disapprove the proposed research. It also conducts continuing review of research at intervals appropriate to the degree of risk, but not less than once per year. Further, it has authority to observe or have a third party observe the consent process and research.

In order to approve research, the IRB must determine that all of the following requirements are met:

1. Risks to human participants are minimized.

2. Risks are reasonable in relation to anticipated benefits, if any, to human participants, and to the value of knowledge that may reasonably be expected to result.

3. Selection of human subjects is equitable.

4. Informed consent will be sought from each prospective human participant or the participant's legally authorized representative.

5. Informed consent will be appropriately documented in accordance with regulations.

6. When appropriate, the research plan makes adequate provision for monitoring the data collected to ensure the safety of human participants.

7. When appropriate, adequate provisions exist to protect the privacy of human participants and to maintain the confidentiality of data.

In addition, when some or all of the participants are likely to be vulnerable to coercion or undue influence, additional safeguards must be included in the study to protect the rights and welfare of these participants. In activities involving in vitro fertilization, for example, the IRB must determine that the investigator has provided for adequate monitoring of the actual informed consent process to verify that patients are not pressured into participating by family or medical personnel.

Appendix 4
Minimizing Fertility Problems

1. When trying *not* to conceive, choose contraception with an eye toward future fertility. It is especially important to avoid pelvic inflammatory disease (PID), a major cause of infertility in women, of ectopic pregnancy, of a need for assisted reproduction, and of lowered success with these treatments.[1] Barrier methods (condom, spermicide, diaphragm) can help prevent the category of PID known as sexually transmitted diseases (STDs), which are especially prevalent in women and men aged twenty to twenty-five and are the main cause of tubal infection and later infertility.[2] According to the American Society for Reproductive Medicine, STDs are the cause of infertility for approximately one-fourth of American couples unable to conceive. Sexually active women should be tested periodically for STDs (including chlamydia, an infection frequently missed by gynecologists), which can be symptomless even as they cause irreversible damage to the reproductive tract; if detected early, treatment with the proper medication can help preserve fertility.[3] According to the Centers for Disease Control, women are twice as likely as men to contract gonorrhea or chlamydia from a single incident of unprotected intercourse with an infected partner. Although most STDs are more easily transmitted to women than to men, most women do not seek medical care early enough (within two days of feeling abdominal pain) to avert damage from infection.[4]

Pelvic infections can also result from—or be aggravated by—use of intrauterine devices, which tend to cause problems particularly for women who have never been pregnant.

Although oral contraceptives are not linked to PID, they may aggravate fertility problems in some women. Overall, 20 percent of women do not ovulate for two to three months after stopping the use of birth control pills; and 20 percent of those seeking a pregnancy do not conceive within a year, due perhaps to irregular ovulation.[5] To be cautious, a woman who does not ovulate regularly, is "borderline" normal, or has irregular periods (when physicians often prescribe these hormones!) might choose to avoid hormonal contraception.

2. Certain common substances have been linked to difficulties in conceiving. In particular, while trying to conceive (and throughout pregnancy), do not smoke. In addition, avoid heavy use of caffeine (coffee, caffeinated soft drinks), alcohol, and recreational drugs.[6] Although the evidence is not definitive, several studies do link these substances (whether used by women or men) to lower pregnancy and birth rates, to a longer time before conceiving, and to increased rates of miscarriage. Douching may also lower a woman's fertility, perhaps by contributing to pelvic inflammatory disease.[7] In such instances of incomplete knowledge, taking preventive action will do no harm.

Also be sure the doctor knows what medications (prescription and over-the-counter) you and your partner take. In addition to possible effects on a woman's fertility, certain medications (including some ulcer, ulcerative colitis, and antifungal drugs) can impair sperm production. If you have any question, consult a pharmacist at a nearby medical center.

3. At any age, try to avoid medical interventions that might compromise present or future fertility—the "iatrogenic" causes. Women should be cautious, for example, about cervical conization (excising a cone-shaped wedge of the cervix to remove abnormal cells) and pelvic surgeries (for example, as a treatment for endometriosis) that cause scarring or adhesions, and about hormonal manipulations or inseminations of questionable benefit. Clearly, doctors must also play a role in this type of prevention, and they should emphasize other preventive steps women and men can take all along the way toward an eventual pregnancy.

4. Evaluate exposures where you live, work, and play that may lower fertility in women and men—including chemicals, metallic substances, physical exposures (e.g., heat, radiation), gases (e.g., anesthetics, carbon dioxide). Research now implicates a number of environmental and occupational "reproductive toxins" that interfere with sperm development in males and with egg development, ovulation, implantation, or success in carrying to term in females and that can contribute to genetic damage that leads to impaired fertilization, implantation, or miscarriage. In addition to their own exposure, women's fertility may be lowered by substances their partner brings home from work (e.g., toxic

residues on clothing.) The following tabulation lists known or suspected chemicals that may lower fertility:[8]

Chemicals harmful to males	Chemicals harmful to females
dibromochloropropane (DBCP, pesticide)	ethylene oxide (sterilizer)
lead and other heavy metals	lead and other heavy metals
chlordecone (Kepone, pesticide)	anesthetic gases
ethylene glycol ethers (electronics manufacturing; ink photo)	ethylene glycol
carbon disulfide (fumigant)	carbon disulfide
ethylene dibromide (fumigant)	cytotoxic drugs
vinyl chloride	plastics (polyurethane, styrene, polystyrene)
electromagnetic fields	

The possibility of increased risk of infertility in women (including miscarriage) from ionizing radiation of video display terminals remains controversial; women wanting to be cautious can try to limit their amount of time using a terminal and use equipment designed to minimize exposure.[9]

Unfortunately, too little scientific research has focused on such risks, nor does the medical education of doctors devote much attention to environmental and occupational health. State or federal regulations generally ignore reproductive hazards in defining safety standards for air quality, water, food, commercial products, or places of work. Acknowledging that current information remains inexcusably incomplete, however, does not mean ignoring exposures in daily life that may, to varying degrees, lower fertility. As part of a basic fertility evaluation, a doctor should discuss with patients environmental and occupational conditions that could make conception and pregnancy more difficult. Patients who suspect such an exposure can also consult an experienced occupational health physician. While keeping in mind that employee-employer relationships can be sensitive, a letter or phone call from a physician to a supervisor or employer can in some instances contribute to a mutually agreeable improvement of working conditions.

5. Additional factors that may lower fertility in women are very high-intensity physical activity and extreme weight loss (among those at risk are gymnasts, ballet dancers, severe dieters). The endocrine systems of adolescent girls and young adults may be particularly sensitive to these effects.

Patients—and their doctors—thus need to consider a variety of factors in evaluating their fertility risks. The following checklist provides a summary of information that should be provided to your doctor. [10]

Current work: employer, length of employment

Description of job tasks

Potential exposures: biologic (e.g., cytomegalovirus); chemical (e.g., vapors, fumes, solvents, dusts); psychological (e.g., stress); physical (e.g., noise, prolonged standing, heavy lifting)

Protective measures available to minimize exposures: personal protective equipment (gloves, respirator); engineering controls (ventilation, lifting devices, video terminal shields)

Any symptoms that relate to work exposures

Previous work: anything that may be relevant for exposures with possible long-term effects (lead, lipid-soluble substances)

Nonoccupational exposures: personal habits (e.g., smoking, caffeine use, drug use, douching); exposures in your community (e.g., air or water pollution); exposure to hazardous substances through a family member's exposure (e.g., lead, asbestos dust); hobbies (e.g., activities involving use of paint thinners or ceramic glazes, extreme physical activities); medications.

Just as individuals cannot prevent all that biology and genetics will bring, they can do only so much to avoid or remove harmful exposures throughout their lives; the preventive steps outlined here must also be backed by strong social and health policies from all levels of government, a prospect that seems to come and go with the political tides. [11]

Appendix 5
Doctors and Diagnoses

How to Get Information about Doctors

Consumer organizations—including Resolve, DES Action, the Endometriosis Association (see Appendix 1)—maintain doctor referral lists; ask how they evaluate physicians on their list. If you have a friend who is a doctor or nurse, you may be able to get an inside view of doctors in your community—particularly colleagues' assessments of a doctor's strengths and weaknesses. Ask non-specialist physicians about specialists (perhaps your general doctor can talk with a specialist at a nearby medical school about specialists in the community); arrange your own consultation with a medical school specialist about choosing a fertility clinic in your area; ask current and past fertility patients about their doctor, though be alert to the "halo" effect—seeing only the good—from patients who were successful or are in the midst of treatment, and the opposite from patients who were not successful.

Thinking about Diagnosis and Treatment

Just as an individual's fertility falls somewhere in a range between "normal" and complete infertility, many aspects of diagnosis and treatment of infertility can be seen as lying along a certain continuum. Initially devised for interviews with physicians, the following scheme can also help patients think about their own fertility problems and treatment options before discussing them with physicians.

Two important caveats: You and your partner may have more than one type of fertility problem and possible treatment. And for many diagnoses and treatments there are few firm answers and there may be conflicting information; you will need to evaluate the weight of existing information, both in quantity and quality.

Because doctors differ in their philosophies of diagnosis and of treatment, when you are choosing and working with a physician consider how both you and the doctor would answer the following questions: How certain and specific must a diagnosis be as a cause of lowered fertility before deciding about a treatment? How exhaustive should the diagnostic process be? How well proven must a treatment's efficacy be before using it? And how severe and how likely must a treatment's potential side effects be before eliminating that option?

Diagnoses

The following conditions can lower fertility and may be offered as "diagnoses" for failure to conceive or as the "problem" that must be treated:

Ovulation abnormalities: anovulation (abnormal endocrine function traced to hypothalamic region of brain; benign pituitary tumor); luteal phase defect; polycystic ovary syndrome

Tubal abnormalities: obstruction; damage; other

Endometriosis

Woman's age

Repeated spontaneous abortions

Male factor: sperm number; sperm motility; other

Immunologic problems

Both the ability to diagnose infertility and knowledge about its causes are limited. When a doctor gives a diagnosis as the reason for your fertility problem, the relationship may not be all that certain—and a diagnosis may not point to an effective treatment.

Indeed, more fertility problems may be "unexplained" than doctors care to admit. For example, a postcoital test shows the number of moving sperm, but cannot determine their ability to fertilize an egg. A hysterosalpingogram (an X-ray of the woman's reproductive tract after a dye has been injected into the uterus) shows whether fallopian tubes are open but reveals nothing about other tubal characteristics and functions, some as yet unknown, that may be important for conceiving. And a laparoscopy may show the presence of mild endometriosis, but it is not known whether that condition in fact lowers fertility.

You may wish to discuss with your doctor where your diagnosis falls on these continua:

Relationship to fertility well understood . . . . *Relationship very speculative*

Accurate diagnosis possible . . . . *Diagnosis uncertain*

Condition significant in lowering fertility . . . . . . *Condition probably not significant*

Effective treatment available . . . . *No effective treatment*

Treatments

Your doctor might recommend a number of treatments or combinations of treatments:

Surgeries: laparoscopy; laser or microsurgery; laparotomy

Medications: clomiphene citrate (Clomid); human chorionic gonadotropin (hMG; Pergonal); follicle-stimulating hormone (FSH); gonadotropin-releasing hormone agonist (GnRH-a; Lupron); other (e.g., GnRH ovulation pump)

Assisted reproductive technology: in vitro fertilization (IVF); gamete intrafallopian transfer (GIFT); zygote intrafallopian transfer (ZIFT); egg or sperm donation; micromanipulation (e.g., intracytoplasmic sperm injection or ICSI); surrogate gestation

Artificial insemination: intrauterine (IUI); vaginal

Immunotherapy: lymphocyte immunization; steroids; heparin/aspirin; intravenous immunoglobulin (IVIG)

Discuss with your doctor where your options lie along these continua:

Effectiveness demonstrated . . . . *Potential shown* . . . . *No evidence or negative evidence*

Physician agreement on usefulness . . . . *Controversy, disagreement*

Minimal risk . . . . *Significant risk*

Worth a try . . . . *Caution advised* . . . . *Don't do*

Be sure to ask for what patients and conditions a treatment has been shown to be effective. Get specific information about risks: What are they and how serious are they? How likely are they to occur? How much evidence is there? Remember that "no evidence of harm" does not necessarily mean the treatment is not harmful; often there is no evidence because no one has systematically recorded and studied immediate or long-term effects.

Warning Flags

While physicians vary in competence, knowledge, and manner, few are outright charlatans engaging in unethical practices. However, fertility patients should be alert to warning flags that may mean they should seek a different doctor:[1]

> extreme treatment recommendations, especially compared to what other doctors advise (for example, suggesting a surrogate pregnancy based on minimal diagnostic information about a woman's ability to carry a pregnancy herself)

> vague or diversionary responses when questioned about reasons or results (for example, about the number of viable eggs or embryos following superovulation and retrieval, about the outcome of a surgical procedure)

> repeated diagnosis of very early pregnancy loss without substantial evidence confirming there was a pregnancy

> resistance or unwillingness when asked to provide medical records, test results, sonograms to you or to other physicians

> refusal to provide an established procedure that is not experimental or is less aggressive (e.g., transfer fewer embryos) than what this doctor proposes

> restrictions on patient access to other medical and administrative staff in the office or clinic

> financial "deals" that seem too good to be true

If you have any question about a doctor, talk to other doctors and nurses in the community and to other patients. State medical licensing boards provide certain limited information to the public about previous disciplinary actions against a doctor. Greater public disclosure of such action has been a goal of the consumer-oriented Public Citizen Research Group. In 1996 Massachusetts passed legislation that includes a toll-free number for obtaining information about physician credentials and disciplinary history. Other states (including California, Florida, New York, and Wisconsin) are considering similar legislation.

Glossary

adhesions	Scar tissue at the site of a surgical or other wound, an infection, or an inflammation, which can form abnormal attachments between membranes and organs in a woman's pelvic area.
amenorrhea	Absence of menstruation.
andrologist	A urologist who specializes further in diagnosing and treating male fertility problems.
anovulation	Absence of ovulation.
ART	See *assisted reproductive technologies*
artificial insemination	A procedure that places sperm within a woman's reproductive tract (vagina, cervix, or uterus) without sexual intercourse in order to conceive a pregnancy; sperm may come from the husband (in which case the procedure is called AIH) or from a known or anonymous donor (AID).
assisted hatching	A laboratory process of thinning an embryo's outer layer before transfer to the uterus, in an attempt to improve the likelihood of implantation.
assisted reproductive technologies (ART)	Also known as advanced reproductive technologies; the category of fertility treatments that are based on extracting egg(s) from a woman's ovary to be combined with sperm for fertilization, usually in a laboratory dish, followed by return to the uterus or fallopian tubes.
azoospermia	Absence of sperm in ejaculated semen.
basal body temperature (BBT)	The body's first waking temperature (before any activity); recording of monthly patterns suggests whether ovulation occurs and, if so, on what day of the menstrual cycle.

bromocriptine (Parlodel)	A drug prescribed to lower levels of the hormone prolactin circulating in the blood; excess prolactin (sometimes suggested by milky discharge from a woman's nipples) can interfere with fertility.
catheter	Hollow tube that can be inserted into vessels or body cavities for moving and transferring fluids, gametes, and embryos.
cervical mucus	Secretions from glands in a woman's cervix that can help or hinder sperm movement into the uterus and that help filter out infectious agents; characteristics of this mucus change throughout a woman's menstrual cycle, most notably at the approach of ovulation.
cervix	The lower, usually elongated entrance to the uterus at the end of the vaginal canal.
chlamydia	A sexually transmitted infectious disease, often without symptoms, that can cause pelvic inflammatory disease, followed by infertility, in women.
cilia	Hair-like waving projections lining the inside of the fallopian tube, which normally help move an egg toward the uterus.
Clomid	See *clomiphene citrate.*
clomiphene citrate (Clomid, Serophene)	The most widely used fertility drug for stimulating ovulation; it is also used "empirically" (in a trial-and-error manner not based on scientifically demonstrated efficacy) in cases of "unexplained" infertility and luteal phase defect.
conception	Fertilization of a woman's egg by a single sperm, the initial step in pregnancy.
corpus luteum	The ovarian follicle just after it releases an egg for ovulation; during the next several days this body produces the hormone progesterone, which is essential in preparing the uterine lining for implantation of a fertilized egg.
cryopreservation	Freezing (usually in liquid nitrogen) and storing sperm, embryos, eggs, or ovarian tissue (with partially matured eggs).
danazol (Danocrine)	Drug derived from male hormones, used to treat endometriosis by altering a woman's natural hormone cycle.
Danocrine	See *danazol.*
DES	See *diethylstilbestrol.*
diethylstilbestrol (DES)	A synthetic estrogenic drug that was prescribed to pregnant women from 1940 to the early 1970s in an (ineffective) attempt to prevent miscarriage; harmful effects have been detected in offspring exposed to DES in utero (known as prenatal DES exposure).

donor egg or sperm	Gametes provided for assisted reproduction (ART) or (with sperm) for artificial insemination; in the United States, the donor usually receives a fee.
ectopic pregnancy	Implantation of an embryo outside the uterus, most often within a fallopian tube; can be life-threatening and must be removed (in very rare cases, an ectopic implantation that is not in a tube has developed into a viable pregnancy, which is delivered surgically).
embryo	The early stage of fetal development, generally considered to extend through the eighth week after fertilization.
endometrial biopsy	A procedure for evaluating fertility that extracts a small sample of inner uterine lining for analysis, to test whether the lining's monthly maturation is adequate for embryo implantation (the procedure is also used to detect abnormal cell growth in the uterus).
endometriosis	A condition in which tissue that normally lines the inner uterus migrates and implants elsewhere (e.g., behind the uterus, on ovaries or tubes); the abnormally located tissue swells in response to a woman's hormonal cycle, sometimes causing severe pain. The relationship of this condition to fertility remains unknown.
endometrium	The inner lining of the uterus, which monthly hormonal stimulation prepares for implantation of an embryo; if no pregnancy occurs, this lining is expelled through menstruation.
epididymis	Male duct system between testicle and penis, in which sperm mature and move out during ejaculation.
fallopian tubes	Two structures leading from ovaries to uterus, which normally transport ovulated eggs; sperm travel from the vaginal canal through the cervix and uterus into a tube to meet and fertilize an egg.
fecundity	A statistical measure of the chance that a woman will conceive during any single month and carry the pregnancy to a live delivery.
fertilization	Process during which a sperm penetrates an egg, setting off cellular activity and divisions that can lead to pregnancy and childbirth.
fimbria	Fringe-like structures at opening of fallopian tube near the ovary which capture an ovulated egg, bringing it into the tube and moving it toward the uterus.
follicle	Fluid-filled sac in the ovary that contains an egg; after ovulation, the corpus luteum that remains produces progesterone.

follicle-stimulating hormone (FSH)	Hormone released by pituitary gland, initiating egg maturation or sperm production; can be injected as a fertility medication.
FSH	See *follicle-stimulating hormone.*
gamete	The reproductive cell (or "germ cell") that is the female (egg) or male (sperm) contribution to conception; these cells carry the genetic information that governs development and defines characteristics of the individual offspring.
GIFT	Gamete IntraFallopian Transfer: Return of extracted eggs and sperm to a woman's fallopian tubes with the intent of gaining a more natural fertilization and implantation than with IVF; unlike in vitro procedures, GIFT does not allow confirmation of fertilization before transfer.
GnRH	See *gonadotropin-releasing hormone.*
GnRH-a, or agonist (Lupron)	A synthetic chemical that fills hormone receptors normally stimulated by GnRH; commonly used to suppress a woman's natural menstrual cycle before administering ovarian stimulants. Also used as a treatment for endometriosis.
GnRH pump	See *ovulation pump.*
gonadotropin-releasing hormone (GnRH)	Hormone produced and released into the bloodstream by the hypothalamus (a portion of the brain), stimulating the pituitary gland to release follicle-stimulating hormone (FSH) and luteinizing hormone (LH), for maturation of an egg or for sperm production.
hCG	See *human chorionic gonadotropin.*
heparin	A blood-thinning medication used in treatment of fertility problems that are believed to involve abnormalities of a woman's immune response to pregnancy.
heterotopic pregnancy	Implantation of at least one embryo normally, within the uterus, and one ectopically, outside the uterus.
hMG	See *human menopausal gonadotropin.*
hormones	Chemical substances produced by the body's endocrine glands, which travel through the bloodstream to target receptors, stimulating various physiological processes. Some hormones can be obtained from animals (including humans) and processed or can be synthesized through laboratory techniques, to be administered medically; these are known as "exogenous" hormones, in contrast to hormones produced "endogenously," that is, within the body.
human chorionic gonadotropin (hCG)	Hormone normally produced by the placenta during pregnancy, also commonly injected to trigger ovulation after use

of fertility drugs; residual levels after injection can result in an early false positive from a pregnancy blood test.

human menopausal gonadotropin (hMG, Pergonal)	A fertility drug (combining LH and FSH) that stimulates the ovaries to mature at least one and usually several eggs in a menstrual cycle.
hysterosalpingogram	X-ray of a woman's pelvic area, after dye is injected into the uterus, to evaluate whether fallopian tubes appear to be open (patent) and other organs appear normal.
hysteroscopy	Viewing within the uterus using a narrow scope through the vaginal canal.
ICSI (IntraCytoplasmic Sperm Injection)	A micromanipulation (technique using a microscope) procedure in which a single sperm (or head of a sperm) is injected into an egg for fertilization before transfer to the uterus or fallopian tube.
idiopathic	Without known cause or origin; used to describe certain fertility or other health problems.
immunization	As a fertility treatment, this procedure attempts to prevent immunologic "rejection" of a developing embryo or fetus by injecting the woman with cells drawn from her husband or another male.
implantation	Embedding of an embryo into the uterine lining early in a pregnancy.
institutional review board (IRB)	A committee of physicians, scientists, and ethicists at a hospital, medical, or research center who review proposals for studies using human subjects; before the study can begin, this committee must approve the research design and the process for obtaining informed consent.
intrauterine device (IUD)	A contraceptive device. A plastic or metal loop or shield inserted into the uterus, where it remains until removed. Some IUD models (e.g., the Dalkon Shield) have led to pelvic inflammatory disease and infertility.
intravenous immunoglobulin (IVIG)	A process for administering immune system proteins, through periodic intravenous infusions, in an attempt to prevent miscarriage in women thought to have abnormal immunologic responses to the fetus.
in vitro	Outside the body, in a laboratory dish: refers more specifically to fertilization of an egg for subsequent transfer to the uterus or fallopian tube.
in vivo	Within the body, referring more specifically to natural fertilization (in contrast to in vitro).
IUD	See intrauterine device.

IUI	IntraUterine Insemination: Placing specially prepared sperm past the cervix into the uterus.
IUI-COHS	IntraUterine Insemination with Controlled Ovarian Hyper-Stimulation: Intrauterine insemination following hormonal stimulation of the woman's ovaries to produce several ovulated eggs.
IVF-ET	In Vitro Fertilization with Embryo Transfer: The original and most commonly performed assisted reproductive technology, in which retrieved eggs are mixed with sperm in a laboratory dish. If fertilization occurs, embryos that appear to be developing well are returned to the uterus for implantation.
IVIG	See *intravenous immunoglobulin.*
laparoscopy	A surgical procedure in which the abdominal or pelvic organs are viewed through a small incision at the navel, using a laparoscope, a narrow telescope-like instrument; a small video camera can be attached to display an image on a video screen. In fertility treatment, diagnostic laparoscopy evaluates the condition of the uterus, fallopian tubes, and/or ovaries. During an operative laparoscopy, the doctor also attempts to correct observed abnormalities (e.g., remove adhesions or patches of endometriosis, or open blocked tubes); these procedures may require additional small incisions for surgical tools.
laparotomy	Surgery in which an abdominal incision allows more extensive access to reproductive organs than is possible during a laparoscopy; can be used for both diagnosis and treatment.
laser surgery	The use of an intense beam of light (laser) as the surgical tool to cut through or remove tissue.
LH	See *luteinizing hormone.*
Lupron	See *GnRH-a.*
luteal phase	The days following ovulation, during which the corpus luteum produces the hormone progesterone, ending with menstruation if no pregnancy occurs.
luteal phase defect (LPD)	A condition characterized by an inadequate amount or duration of progesterone, which may result in the part of the menstrual cycle following ovulation being shorter than normal (the norm is about fourteen days, followed by the onset of menstruation).
luteinizing hormone (LH)	The pituitary hormone that triggers release of a woman's mature egg through ovulation, followed by production of progesterone; in men, LH plays an important role in production of the hormone testosterone.

menopause	The cessation of menstruation, commonly occurring between the ages of forty-five and fifty-five; it may follow several years of irregular menstruation and declining fertility.
MESA	Microsurgical Epididymal Sperm Aspiration: An operation in which sperm are extracted from the epididymis of men with azoospermia.
micromanipulation	The technique of performing procedures directly upon eggs, sperm, and embryos viewed through a microscope (e.g., inserting a sperm into an egg).
microsurgery	A type of operation during which the surgeon looks through a microscope to perform delicate procedures (e.g., to repair damaged fallopian tubes).
miscarriage	See *spontaneous abortion*.
motility	Forward movement of sperm as observed during male fertility testing.
OHSS	See *ovarian hyperstimulation syndrome*.
oligospermia	Persistent low sperm counts on repeated semen analyses.
oocyte	An egg cell that matures in the ovary; also called an ovum (plural: ova).
ovarian hyperstimulation syndrome (OHSS)	A potentially dangerous side effect of fertility drugs (especially Pergonal, alone or in combination with others) during which too many eggs mature, enlarging the ovaries; the most severe cases—which can include ovarian rupture, abdominal bleeding, and liver, kidney, and/or lung failure—require in-hospital procedures and monitoring.
ovulation	Release of a mature egg from the ovary, approximately midway through a woman's menstrual cycle.
ovulation pump	Also known as GnRH pump; a small portable medication device (similar to an insulin pump for diabetes) that runs on batteries and is programmed to inject intermittent gonadotropin-releasing hormone dosages over several days; can be an effective and safe, if somewhat cumbersome, method for stimulating ovulation in women who do not ovulate on their own.
Parlodel	See *bromocriptine*.
patent/patency	Descriptive term for fallopian tubes that appear to be open and without obstructions when viewed during a hysterosalpingogram.
PCT	See *postcoital test*.
PDR	*See Physicians' Desk Reference*.

pelvic inflammatory disease (PID)	A general category of infections involving a woman's reproductive organs, most often the fallopian tubes; damage can lower fertility or cause complete infertility.
Physicians' Desk Reference (PDR)	Annual publication that compiles information from drug manufacturers about their medications, including approved uses, dosages, side effects, contraindications; generally available at pharmacies, large bookstores, and medical libraries.
PID	See *pelvic inflammatory disease.*
placebo	An inert substance with no medical effect (a "sugar pill") used in controlled experiments testing the efficacy of another substance.
postcoital test (PCT)	Also known as Huhner's test; evaluates a couple's fertility by examining a sample of vaginal secretions and cervical mucus several hours after intercourse, using a microscope to estimate the number of surviving sperm and their ability to move normally through the secretions.
pre-embryo	The earliest stage of development following fertilization, generally considered to span the first fourteen days; also called a zygote.
premature menopause	Also known as ovarian failure; a rare, abnormally early cessation of ovulation and menstrual cycles, occurring in a woman's late teens, twenties, or thirties.
salpingitis	Inflammation and/or obstruction of the fallopian tubes that may be acute (following recent infection) or chronic (persisting long after initial infection, sometimes without symptoms).
semen	Cloudy, thick secretions containing sperm that a male ejaculates during orgasm.
Serophene	See *clomiphene citrate.*
sexually transmitted disease (STD)	Any of several specific infections that spread between people through genital, oral, or anal sexual contact; in women, these infections can cause infertility, even without apparent symptoms.
sperm antibodies	Protein substances produced by a woman's or man's immune system in reaction to sperm; certain types may lower fertility in some couples.
sperm bank	A facility that stores frozen sperm for use in artificial insemination and assisted reproductive technologies.
sperm count	A rough evaluation of whether the quantity of sperm in a man's ejaculate is within normal range.

sperm penetration assay	Also known as hamster egg test; a male fertility test that attempts to evaluate sperm capacity to fertilize human eggs, based on demonstrated ability to penetrate eggs of a hamster.
sperm washing and "swim up"	A process of separating out the most active sperm from a semen sample in preparation for artificial insemination or assisted reproduction.
spontaneous abortion/ miscarriage	Loss of a pregnancy during the first (more frequently) or second trimester. In most cases, the woman's body expels or absorbs the remnants; if not, a medical procedure is needed.
sterility	Complete infertility that cannot be reversed by treatment.
stillbirth	A fetus that develops into the final trimester but dies before or during delivery.
superfetation	Implantation of several embryos following ovarian stimulation with fertility drugs, resulting in large multiple pregnancies.
superovulation	Maturation of several eggs in a single menstrual cycle by stimulating the ovaries with fertility drugs.
surrogacy	Carrying a pregnancy for another woman, following insemination with sperm or embryos.
SUZI	SUbZonal Insemination: A micromanipulation procedure in which several sperm are placed under the zona pellucida surrounding an ovulated egg, in the hope of assisting fertilization.
syphilis	One of the more common sexually transmitted or venereal diseases, with infection most easily spread from man to woman.
TESE	TEsticular Sperm Extraction: An operation in which immature sperm are extracted from the testicle of a man whose ejaculate contains no sperm.
testicle	Male reproductive organ that produces immature sperm and the hormone testosterone; also referred to in the plural as testes.
testicular biopsy	A surgical procedure that removes a tissue sample from a man's testicle; can be used to extract immature sperm for ICSI or to check for cancer.
TET	Tubal Embryo Transfer: Placement into the fallopian tubes of one or more fertilized eggs that have begun cell division; embryos must then travel to the uterus for implantation.
ultrasound	Technique through which high-frequency sound waves are reflected off internal organs, producing an image of these

structures; used commonly to monitor egg development in the ovaries, to confirm pregnancy, and to observe fetal growth.

unexplained infertility A general category describing couples who have not conceived but have no detectable or known cause of infertility. See also *idiopathic*.

urologist Physician specializing in processes and abnormalities involving the urinary tract (male and female) and the male reproductive tract.

varicocele A varicose vein in the testicle that may lower fertility in some men.

vasectomy A male sterilization procedure that severs the connecting ducts through which sperm normally reach the ejaculate; in some cases, surgical repair can reverse this procedure and restore a man's fertility.

venereal disease Another term for sexually transmitted diseases that can cause infertility; most commonly refers to syphilis and gonorrhea.

ZIFT Zygote IntraFallopian Transfer: Placement of one or more fertilized but undivided eggs into the fallopian tubes; embryos must then travel to the uterus for implantation. Differs from GIFT in allowing fertilization to be confirmed before transfer and from TET in using eggs at an earlier stage of development.

zona pellucida Outer corona-like structure surrounding a mature, ovulated egg that a sperm must traverse before fertilization can occur (unless sperm is injected into egg thorough ICSI).

Notes

Chapter 1

1. Grimaldi 1995.
2. Medical devices did not come under Food and Drug Administration (FDA) jurisdiction until 1976, when regulations were changed largely as a result of the Dalkon Shield injuries. Not until 1984, with increasing and irrefutable evidence of harm, did the manufacturer and the FDA announce that *all* women with Dalkon Shields should have a doctor remove the contraceptive device. See Mintz 1985.

Chapter 2

1. Taymor 1987, 206.
2. Wysowski 1993.
3. Collins 1995; Collins, Burrows, and Willan 1995; ESHRE Capri 1996.
4. Jaffe 1992a.
5. Jaffe 1992a.
6. Taymor 1987, 207.
7. Hsu et al. 1995.
8. Dickey et al. 1996; Hammond, Halme, and Talbert 1983; Shmidt et al. 1985; Wramsby, Fredga, and Liedholm 1987.
9. Cunha et al. 1987.
10. Herbst and Bern 1981.
11. DeCherney 1987.
12. Haney 1987, 453.
13. Bush et al. 1997; Collins et al. 1984; Glatstein et al. 1995; Griffith and Grimes 1990; Grimes 1993.
14. Blackwell et al. 1987; see also Soules 1985; and Younger 1989.
15. Blackwell et al. 1987, 735–36.

16. Benadiva et al. 1995. See also Bates and Bates 1996; Dubuisson et al. 1997; Penzias and DeCherney 1996; Tomaževič et al. 1996.

Chapter 3

1. Men unable to provide sperm through masturbation can undergo a minor surgical procedure to remove sperm from the testicles. Catholic couples wishing to meet a Vatican directive that fertility treatment can enhance but not replace natural conception must gather sperm for "assisted conception" in a perforated condom during conjugal intercourse; some sperm enter the woman in a "natural" manner while others are "assisted" by capture for in vitro fertilization.

Just who handles, counts, documents, and distributes embryos (e.g., to a woman or a freezer, or to be destroyed) became a very important issue with the revelation in 1995 that embryos had in effect been stolen at the Center for Reproductive Health at the University of California, Irvine.

2. American Society for Reproductive Medicine Ethics Committee 1994.

3. For some feminists, assisted reproduction is one more medical advance that can not only help women who experience fertility problems but can also provide more options regarding when and how women have children; for example, a woman who wants to establish her career first can rely on these technologies to enable pregnancy after the age of forty or to hire a surrogate who will carry the pregnancy. The opposing feminist analysis, however, sees these reproductive interventions as more technologically sophisticated methods for what a male-dominated medical specialty has always done—control women, turn their natural reproductive lives into medical "problems" and solutions, and reinforce childbearing as women's primary social role. In addition, these technologies exploit poorer, less powerful women who are providing such required body parts as fertile eggs or a surrogate uterus. See, for example: Klein 1989; Spallone and Steinberg 1987.

4. Kolata 1996.

5. Blackwell et al. 1987, 737.

6. American Fertility Society Ethics Committee 1990. See also Wagner and St. Clair 1989.

7. Schenker and Ezra 1994; Sher et al. 1993; Shushan, Eisenberg, and Schenker 1995; Wagner and St. Clair 1989; Wallach 1991.

8. Whittemore et al. 1992.

9. *Lancet* 1988.

10. Boulot et al. 1993; Evans et al. 1988; Hardardottir et al. 1996; Tabash 1993.

11. Grether, Nelson, and Cummins 1993. Statistics describing the increase in multiple births vary from country to country, as well as from one study to the next. However, a rough estimate of trends in the United States during the last twenty years indicates that twin births increased at twice the rate of singletons; triplets and higher at seven times the rate (Wright 1995). A study comparing 1990–92 with 1972–74 found triplet births up nearly 200 percent; approximately 38 percent of the increase was attributed to assisted reproductive technologies, 30 percent to ovarian stimulation drugs (without ART), and

30 percent to the pregnant women's increased age (Wilcox, Kiely, and Melvin 1996). A 1997 report from the National Center for Health Statistics at the Centers for Disease Control documents a threefold increase in deliveries of triplet or larger multiple births between 1980 and 1994, and a fourfold increase since 1971. During the past decade the increase has averaged 11 percent per year. These increases are most pronounced among married college-educated mothers over thirty—the women most likely to undergo fertility treatment. During 1994 there were 4,233 triplet births in the United States, 315 quadruplet births, and 46 with five or more babies. Infant mortality rates for these multiple births were twelve times the rate for single births (Martin, MacDorman, and Matthews 1997). In France, where careful birth records are kept, the late 1980s saw a tenfold increase in triplet births, thirtyfold in quadruplets (Rosenthal 1992). A Belgian study attributes one-fourth of the increase in multiple births to IVF, the rest to ovarian stimulation drugs with or without artificial insemination (Derom et al. 1993). See also Cefalo 1992; Jewell and Yip 1995; Powers and Kiely 1994.

12. Quoted in Roan 1996.

13. Garel and Blondel 1992; Garel, Salobir, and Blondel 1997; Wilcox, Kiely, and Melvin 1996. In a letter to *Lancet* a parent who has written about the lives of children born very prematurely conveys the stressful impact of so-called minor, as well as major, handicaps; see Harrison 1997.

14. Cefalo 1992, 398.

15. Statement of Dr. Mark Evans, interviewed on ABC television ("Turning Point") March 16, 1994.

16. Frederiksen, Keith, and Sabbagha 1992. See also Berkowitz et al. 1988; Evans et al. 1995; Lynch et al. 1990; Tabash 1993.

17. Berkowitz et al. 1996; Depp et al. 1996.

18. *Lancet* 1988. As of 1996, specialists were still citing a lack of adequate information about outcomes with and without fetal reduction, making patients' decisions all the more difficult (Haning et al. 1996). One comparison of twin pregnancies that had been reduced and pregnancies that originated as twins—all following fertility treatment—found more pre-term births and fetal growth restriction in the reduced pregnancies (Silver et al. 1997).

19. Boulot et al. 1993; Newman, Hamer, and Miller 1989; Smith-Levitin et al. 1996.

20. Evans et al. 1988, 296.

21. Bollen et al. 1993, 509. *Lancet* 1988, 774.

22. Weiner 1988, 821.

23. World Health Organization Technical Report Series 820, cited in Wilcox et al. 1993.

24. *Lancet* 1988, 774.

25. Roest et al. 1997 (Triplet pregnancy); see also Edwards, Lobo, and Bouchard 1997; ESHRE Capri 1996.

26. Seibel, Ranoux, and Kearnan 1989. Questions about repeated IVF attempts became even more pressing during the 1990s as concerns focused on costs and on insurance coverage. Many insurance plans refuse to pay for any assisted reproductive technologies,

and none will pay for an endless number of treatment cycles. Under capitated managed-care plans, in which doctors receive a set fee per patient regardless of medical services provided, it is in the doctors' interest to determine the likelihood of success for individual patients and a "reasonable" number of attempts.

27. Corfman et al. 1993.

28. Edwards, Lobo, and Bouchard 1997, 917, 919 (this print journal editorial was also the subject of online comments through the journal's web site); see also Seibel 1995.

29. Corfman et al. 1993.

30. Claman et al. 1993; Paulson et al. 1992; Seibel 1995.

31. Taymor, Ranoux, and Gross 1992.

32. Dodson et al. 1987.

33. Wagner and St. Clair 1989.

34. Jones 1996b; Jones, Jones, and Kolm 1997.

35. Clinic-specific success rates by geographic region are available to the public for purchase from the Society for Assisted Reproductive Technologies (see Appendix 1. Unfortunately, these volumes of statistics are unwieldy; a reader must plow through a massive quantity of numbers in search of useful comparisons). The SART Registry's methods of data collection and reporting continue to evolve and may eventually include data on the number of treatment attempts and number of transferred embryos resulting in success and failure. Annually compiled data from all reporting ART programs (75–80 percent of United States clinics) are published in *Fertility and Sterility*. Results obtained during 1994 were reported in 1996: approximately 85 percent of procedures were IVF, with success rates of 18 percent per initiated treatment cycle; 21 percent per egg retrieval; 23 percent per embryo transfer. Nineteen percent of confirmed pregnancies were lost, mostly as a result of first trimester miscarriage; the ectopic pregnancy rate was nearly 4 percent. Of the total pregnancies, 63.7 percent were singleton, 28.3 percent were twins, and 6.5 percent triplets or more; 1.4 were stillbirths. Sixteen programs reported a delivery rate of 30 percent or more per initiated cycle (Society for Assisted Reproductive Technologies, A.S.R.M. 1996).

36. Hershlag et al. 1991; Hershlag et al. 1992; Jones, Veeck, and Muasher 1993; Society for Assisted Reproductive Technologies, A.S.R.M. 1996.

37. Wilcox et al. 1993, 23. See also Tan et al. 1994 (Cumulative conception); Tan et al. 1994 (Pregnancy and birth); Tan et al. 1992 (Cumulative conception). One study of previously infertile women found that fetal loss *after* observing a heartbeat through ultrasound scan occurs more frequently in women over the age of thirty-six (Smith and Buyalos 1996).

38. Dawood 1996.

39. Martin 1993, 763. See also Seibel 1988.

40. Chapko et al. 1995.

41. For a journal debate on the usefulness of clinic-specific success rates, see Barri 1996; Deech 1996; Lobo 1996; Matthews 1996.

42. Hershlag et al. 1991; Hershlag et al. 1992; Jones, Veeck, and Muasher 1993.

43. Barabarino-Monnier et al. 1991; Check et al. 1994; Christiansen 1997; Gobert et al. 1990; Moncayo, Moncayo, and Dapunt 1990; Seibel, Ranoux, and Kearnan 1989;

Tan et al. 1992 (Cumulative conception); Templeton, Morris, and Parslow 1996; Wilcox et al. 1993.

44. Wagner 1996.

45. Jones, Veeck, and Muasher 1993. See also Jones 1996a.

Chapter 4

1. Richardson 1994, 5.

2. McDonough 1993, 1100.

3. Noting the enlarging number of laparoscopic procedures and of gynecologists performing them with no more than a two-day instructional course—as well as an absence of critical evaluation or quality assurance—a 1992 editorial asked whether operative laparoscopy is a "surgical advance" or "technological gimmick" (Pitkin 1992).

4. Grimes 1992, 1068.

5. *Am J Obstet Gynecol* 1992, 1062.

6. Gant 1992; Grimes 1992.

7. McDonough 1992; Smith, Donohue, and Waszak 1994.

8. McDonough 1992, 1086. A report on gynecological use of laparoscopy and hysteroscopy (viewing inside the uterus through a scope inserted vaginally) finds high rates of complications, especially with inexperienced doctors performing an increased number of techniques (Smith, Donohue, and Waszak 1994; see also Härkki-Sirén and Kurki 1997). Concerns over both laparoscopic and laser surgery are not limited to fertility medicine. In the early 1990s, laparoscopic gallbladder removal became popular among physicians; however, the widespread use of this procedure by inadequately trained doctors resulted in increased risks and reduced benefits for many patients compared to the standard surgery (Grundfest 1993). In 1995, heavy marketing of laser surgery to ophthalmologists and potential consumers began after the Food and Drug Administration approved a new type of laser machine for correcting nearsightedness. As with in vitro fertilization, independent clinics and for-profit chains proliferated; advertisements appeared in newspapers and on television. With nearly half of the U.S. population nearsighted, this high-tech procedure represented a highly lucrative way for specialists to make up losses from managed care. Although this surgery might be appropriate for a small proportion of nearsighted people, laser manufacturers and doctors were targeting millions more who would be willing and able to pay the approximately $4,000 cost of surgery instead of the price for eyeglasses or contact lenses (Hall 1995).

9. Bickell et al. 1994. This study compared rates of hysterectomy performed by gynecologists of varying age, gender, locale, and other characteristics.

10. Detsky 1995; Kolata 1996.

11. A mid-decade editorial written by the president of the Society of Reproductive Surgeons (a subgroup of the American Society for Reproductive Medicine) summarizes concerns about the rapid growth of new surgical techniques; these concerns include "the quality of the procedures, the indications for [using] these procedures, the selection of patients upon whom the procedures are performed, the complications that may occur . . . , and the techniques for training, certifying, and monitoring surgeons who use these techniques" (Keye 1994, 1115).

12. Donesky and Adashi 1995, 456. Even with the recent growth of managed care, many infertility services remain outside such insurance plans, with patients commonly paying our of their own pockets.

13. Bateman, Kolp, and Hoeger 1996, 35.

14. McDonough 1992, 1090. See also Grimes 1992.

15. The brief editorial appeared at the end of Dodson 1987, 445.

16. Wallach 1991, 478.

17. Nulsen et al. 1993.

18. Petersen et al. 1994.

19. Van Voorhis et al. 1997. It is important to note that cost-effectiveness comparisons are most useful when the treatments bring similar chances for success. A *cost-effective* fertility treatment (i.e., with lower costs per delivery) may not bring the greatest success rate per treatment cycle. Thus, intrauterine insemination is more cost-effective for some patients than IVF because each cycle costs so much less. However, patients undergo more treatment cycles and endure more failed attempts to reach success rates comparable to a single ART cycle. What is needed are better ways to identify patient subgroups for whom less invasive and less costly treatments bring pregnancy rates per cycle equivalent to ART, reserving the latter for individuals unlikely to become pregnant any other way.

20. Crosignani, Walters, and Soliani 1991.

21. Collins 1995.

22. Dawood 1996. This overview notes especially the need for studies with larger numbers of participants in order to obtain reliable, statistically significant results.

23. Corsan and Kemmann 1991, 469.

24. Martinez et al. 1993, 811. See also Corsan and Kemmann 1991; Dodson and Haney 1991.

25. Mascarenhas et al.1994.

26. Wright 1995, 46. In a different interview, Dr. Louis Keith, director of the Center for the Study of Multiple Births in Chicago, also states bluntly, "The human mother isn't meant to carry a litter" (Roan 1996).

27. Evans et al. 1995, 1753, 1755. Dr. Keith conveys the danger in doctors' narrow view of their own goals and accomplishments: "For the infertility specialist, his criteria for success is to get [the patient] pregnant. The perinatologist's criteria for success is to get the fetuses to viability [a chance to live at birth]. Success to the neonatologist is to get the kids out of the neonatal intensive care unit alive. The pediatrician's criteria for success is to see that the damage isn't too bad"(Roan 1996). The outcome of this chain of events, stemming initially from ovarian hyperstimulation, can be serious obstetric risks for the woman and lifelong health problems for her offspring. See also Craft et al. 1988; Derom et al. 1993; Wilcox, Kiely, and Melvin 1996; Wright 1995.

28. Corsan and Kemmann 1991, 470. Results of studies attempting to establish spontaneous pregnancy rates among "infertile" couples vary, depending on methodology and characteristics of the patient population. A classic study of "treatment-independent pregnancies" among couples labeled "infertile" found, in a two- to seven-year follow-up, an overall 61 percent pregnancy rate. By diagnosis, the pregnancy rates

were 44 percent for couples with ovulatory disorders; 61 percent for those with endometriosis, tubal defects, or semen deficiencies; and 96 percent for couples with cervical factor or unexplained infertility (Collins1983). See also Haney et al. 1987, a study
of couples on an IVF waiting list; Rousseau et al. 1983. More recent studies suggest an
approximately 15–17 percent livebirth rate after one year, 25–30 percent after two
years (Collins 1995; ESHRE Capri 1996; Gleicher 1996). The best prognosis for spontaneous pregnancies is for couples with unexplained infertility of less than three years
duration, the woman under thirty years of age or with a previous pregnancy.

29. Karlstrom, Bergh, and Lundkvist 1993, 558.

30. One exception is Dawood 1996, an overview of assisted reproduction studies
which concludes that, except for women with tubal blockage, "expectant management"—i.e., no treatment—*or* intrauterine insemination with superovulation should
be tried before IVF or GIFT.

31. Agarwal 1996.

32. Jaffe 1992b.

33. Hull 1992, 790. As with IUI, doctors sometimes prescribe clomiphene citrate
to subfertile men although this treatment has proven to be ineffective (ESHRE Capri
1996).

34. *Obstet and Gynecol Survey* 1989, 693. The article in question is Ho et al. 1989.

35. Jaffe 1994b, 418. See also Arici et al. 1994; Brook, Barratt, and Cooke 1994;
Peters et al. 1993; Ransom, Corsan, and Blotner 1994.

36. McNeely and Soules 1988, 2.

37. McNeely and Soules 1988, 6.

38. A subgroup of women with a luteal phase abnormality may have elevated levels
of a different hormone, prolactin; serum analysis of this hormone is hampered by timing problems similar to the progesterone test, because of prolactin's naturally fluctuat-
ing levels. A single test can give a misleading result of high, low, or normal, depending
on which part of the daily pattern happens to be caught.

39. McNeely and Soules 1988, 12.

40. Balasch et al. 1992, 973. See also Batista et al. 1993; Karamardian and Grimes
1992; Wentz, Kossy, and Parker 1990.

41. See Healy, Trounson, and Anderson 1994; Taymor 1987.

42. Quoted in Karamardian and Grimes 1992, 1396. See also Blacker et al. 1997.
No diagnostic test can currently confirm that a complete normal ovulation has occurred; pregnancy is the only definitive evidence (ESHRE Capri 1996).

43. Hull 1992.

44. Skakkebaek, Giwercman, and de Kretser 1994, 1478. See also Howards 1995.

45. Hull 1992, 789.

46. ESHRE Andrology 1996; ESHRE Capri 1996; Grimes 1993; Mao and Grimes
1988; O'Shea et al. 1993.

47. O'Donovan et al. 1993. This review of treatments for male infertility concluded that only 6 percent of infertile men have conditions for which a treatment has
been demonstrated to improve pregnancy rates. Although clinicians advocate various
interventions, such as intrauterine insemination or in vitro fertilization, the quality of

most studies is poor. More recent attempts that augment IVF with ICSI (see below) are raising pregnancy rates in some types of severe male infertility, although this procedure too is gaining popularity without systematic, scientifically controlled evaluation.

48. On varicocele, see Vermeulen and Vandeweghe 1984. On leukocytes, see Kiessling et al. 1995; Tomlinson, Barratt, and Cooke 1993.

49. Tucker et al. 1993, 325.

50. Silber, Van Stierteghem, and Zsolt 1996, 110.

51. Silber, Van Stierteghem, and Zsolt 1996.

52. Even leaving aside the technical details, lay readers may find themselves over-whelmed by the vast unknowns surrounding a treatment they may be offered. One urologist suggests the following (abbreviated) litany of possible reasons sperm may fail to fertilize an egg: "Lack of fertilization may be due to the impossibility of the sperm to bind to the zona pellucida due to a receptor defect in one or both of the gametes; it may be due to lack of sperm penetration into the zona pellucida after attachment due to ab-normalities in the glycosaminoglycans of the zona, or a mechanical or enzymatic defect of the sperm; it could be that the sperm has not been able to penetrate [the vitelline] membrane; it is also possible that due to intrinsic abnormalities of the chromatin or a defect in the [egg] the formation of the pronucleus has not been accomplished. It may be that . . . reconstitution of the male pronuclear membrane . . . has not been achieved due to either intrinsic sperm defects or extrinsic oocyte problems; or it is possible that . . . the male pronucleus has been formed normally while the female pronucleus has disappeared." After catching his (and the reader's) breath, he argues that efforts to "bypass these problems"—using techniques that help sperm penetrate an egg—require that "we better understand the abnormal physiology of the sperm unable to fertilize" (Acosta et al. 1988, 13–14). See also Engel, Murphy, and Schmid 1996; ESHRE An-drology 1996; Patrizio and Kopf 1997; Pryor et al. 1997.

53. Hull 1992, 790.

54. American Society for Reproductive Medicine Ethics Committee 1994.

55. Hervé and Moutel 1995.

56. Foresta et al. 1996 (Warning note). This same group would later elaborate on the Y chromosome defect in men with nonobstructive azoospermia (Foresta et al. 1996 [Use of]). See also Foresta et al. 1996 (Male infertility); Kremer et al. 1997.

57. Lundin, Sjögren, and Hamberger 1996.

58. Palermo et al. 1996.

59. Oehninger et al. 1995.

60. Palermo, Cohen, and Rosenwaks 1996.

61. Trip et al. 1997, 964.

62. ESHRE Andrology 1996; Jequier and Cummins 1997; Tournaye 1997; van der Ven and Haidl 1997.

63. Tucker et al. 1993.

64. Tucker et al. 1993, 330

65. Jaffe 1994a, 120.

66. Jequier and Cummins 1997; Tournaye 1997; van der Ven and Haidl 1997.

67. Patrizio and Kopf 1997.

68. Oehninger et al. 1995; Silber et al. 1996.

69. Byer 1994; Lundin, Sjögren, and Hamberger 1996.

70. Aboulghar et al. 1996; Oeihninger, Franken, and Kruger 1997.

71. Plouffe et al. 1992.

72. Branch et al. 1997; Christiansen 1997; Geva et al. 1997; Gleicher and Coulam 1997; Gleicher et al. 1997.

73. For example, critics of the use of intrauterine insemination with washed sperm in cases where blood tests reveal sperm antibodies are not surprised by poor success rates. The treatment's basic rationale is faulty, these specialists argue. For the vast majority of couples, washing sperm does not affect the specific type of antibody that may be lowering fertility; nor does bypassing the vagina and cervix with intrauterine insemination avoid the uterus, where a more formidable immune response may be awaiting the cleansed sperm (Adeghe 1993). See also Geva et al. 1997 and Gleicher et al. 1997 for discussion of anti-phospholipid antibodies.

74. Aoki et al. 1995. This mid-decade study suggests, for example, that lymphocyte immunization may help a small subgroup of couples with unexplained repeated miscarriages. One out of eleven couples may benefit, while the other ten will not; there is no way to predict which women the treatment will help. Other studies show benefit for an even smaller proportion of couples in which women receive this therapy.

75. Gill 1992; Simpson et al. 1996. Recent explanations focused on anti-phospholipid antibodies are now being questioned; see Bronson 1995; Denis et al. 1997; Gleicher 1997. Sher et al. 1994 explains infertility as resulting from these antibodies.

76. Scott 1984.

77. Bronson 1995; Christiansen et al. 1992; Denis et al. 1997; Fraser, Grimes, and Schulz 1993; Grimes, Fraser, and Schulz 1994; Moloney et al. 1989.

78. Bronson 1995; Coulam and Coulam 1992; Fraser, Grimes, and Schulz 1993; Geva et al. 1997; Moloney et al. 1989; Plouffe et al. 1992.

79. Coulam and Coulam 1992; ESHRE Capri 1996; Moloney et al. 1989; Scott 1984; Stray-Pedersen and Stray-Pedersen 1984.

80. For examples of alternate explanations for IVF failure, see Akman et al. 1996; Blazar et al. 1997; Paulson et al. 1997 (Cumulative conception).

81. Kwak et al. 1992. This study compares preconception with postconception treatment but does not compare these two approaches to placebo.

82. Aoki et al. 1995. In addition, women who take a long time to conceive—or who do not ever become pregnant—will be receiving this treatment for an extended period.

83. McDonough 1992, 1090; see also Van Voorhis et al. 1997. The same third-party pressure came to bear on training and monitoring gynecological surgeons. Insurance companies, concerned about liability and the costs of surgical complications, began pressing for improved instructional programs and credentialing (Keye 1994). Although some gynecologists had warned colleagues about performing large numbers of these procedures without sufficient attention to resulting complications or outcomes, or about trying to learn techniques in a weekend course, little was done to establish more formal training programs, credentialing requirements, or monitoring of such surgery. Whether cost concerns will provide needed impetus remains to be seen.

84. Check et al. 1994, 257; see also Templeton, Morris, and Parslow 1996.

85. Controversy over the safety of silicone breast implants presents a different form of this tendency to intervene medically now, ask questions later. Most telling are assertions about the need for scientific proof. For instance, Dr. Marcia Angell, editor of the *New England Journal of Medicine,* argues that women with breast implants, their lawyers, and the general public "have to wait for the science" before claiming silicone breast implants are causing debilitating illness in some women. A proportion of women who happen to have implants will also develop various unrelated health problems (generally the same proportion as in the wider population); that is, a certain number of women will experience both illness and implants. Only through "good science" can coincidence be "ruled out" (interview on PBS television, "Frontline," February 1996; the argument is developed more fully in Angell's 1996 book *Science on Trial: The Clash of Medical Evidence and the Law in the Breast Implant Case* [New York: Norton]). Without delving further into the breast implants story, what is striking is the presumption that silicone implants (or other medical devices such as early IUD models) are safe—at least, safe enough to insert into women's' bodies—until proven otherwise. Why not shift the initial burden of proof, with more stringent requirements for demonstrating safety (and efficacy) before exposing women to the always present potential for harm? It seems unfair to ask people to wait calmly for good science after the fact, once possible dangers have surfaced, if good science to better ensure safety beforehand is lacking.

86. Eimers et al. 1994a, 49. Although fertility clinic success rates, as discussed in Chapter 3, are now commonly divided into subgroups based on women's age, they do not incorporate information on patient's *duration* of infertility. Thus, they do not indicate to what extent a high success rate reflects an approach that jumps in quickly with aggressive treatment of couples who may not truly have much of a problem.

Chapter 5

1. L. Mastroianni, interviewed on NBC Nightly News, March 18, 1994.
2. McKaughan 1987.
3. Tan et al. 1992 (Cumulative conception).
4. Sauer, Paulson, and Lobo 1990.
5. Sauer, Paulson, and Lobo 1992. "Advanced reproductive age" is the tactful replacement for the obstetric term used more commonly in previous years (and still used by many physicians)—"elderly primagravida" (for a first pregnancy), a rather less appealing image, perhaps less encouraging of the prospect of pregnancy.
6. Sauer, Paulson, and Lobo 1993, 322.
7. Kolata 1994.
8. Interviewed on Public Broadcasting Service's *Nova,* "What's New about Menopause?" fall 1994.
9. Bopp et al. 1995; Wright 1995.
10. Scott and Hoffman 1995.
11. Maranto 1995.
12. Scott and Hoffman 1995.
13. Wallach 1995.

14. Bopp et al. 1995. A different study suggests that in women over forty, the response to ovarian stimulation (number and quality of eggs) is a better predictor of IVF success than is age or FSH level (Roest et al. 1996 [Ovarian response]).

15. Paulson and Sauer 1994, 572. See also Abdalla et al. 1997; Paulson et al. 1997 (Cumulative conception).

16. Wentz 1993.

17. Kolata 1995b, A1. The clinic excluded women with cancer of the ovary, cervix, or uterus (but not those with breast cancer).

18. Kolata 1995b, B8.

19. De Wilde and Hesseling 1995. The surgeons tied the ovaries away from irradiated areas; preliminary results showed that more of these women had normal menstrual cycles two years later than did controls. Developing such alternatives for more types of cancer and cancer treatments seems no less possible than reimplanting an ovary that can function adequately, though the potential market for cryopreserved ovaries may be considerably larger.

20. "ASRM Statement on Cryopreservation of Ovarian Tissue . . . in Women Undergoing Cancer Treatment," press releases, April 8 and 10, 1996.

21. Shaw and Trounson 1997, 403–4. See also Gosden, Rutherford, and Norfolk 1997.

22. Statistics on rates of perinatal death vary widely. One report states an increase from 25 per 1,000 in women between seventeen and nineteen, to 69 per 1,000 after the age of thirty-nine (Bopp et al. 1995). Another describes newborn infant deaths rising from 9.5 per 1,000 births in women ages thirty to thirty-four to 17 per 1,000 in women older than forty (ESHRE Capri 1996). See also Cunningham and Leveno 1995; Fretts et al. 1995; Smith and Buyalos 1996.

23. *Lancet* 1993. A French study found that maternal deaths were six times higher in women aged forty to forty-four than in women aged twenty-four to twenty-nine (ESHRE Capri 1996).

24. Quigly 1992. Complications of pregnancy and delivery are particularly high for the older egg recipients who conceive twins or greater multiples (Wolf et al. 1997).

25. Kolata 1995b.

26. Sauer, Paulson, and Lobo 1995a, 114.

27. Sauer, Paulson, and Lobo 1995b.

28. Borini et al. 1995.

29. This obstetrician had recently delivered the triplets of a 51-year-old woman who required three months in an intensive care unit after she gave birth; this woman had $1^1/_2$-year-old twins from previous fertility treatment. British physicians live in a different medical-political world. In 1993, a *Lancet* editorial asked whether helping women have a child after the age of fifty is a good use of medical technology. Their concern includes physical risks to the woman (including at what point a doctor's assessment of risks should lead to that doctor's refusal to arrange such a pregnancy), the long-term well-being of a child (which they consider to be "of overriding importance"), the impact on ovum donors, and the use of "scarce and expensive health resources." Particularly when treatment is covered by the National Health System, the editorial concludes, "jus-

tice demands that young infertile women should take precedence over those who are post-menopausal" (*Lancet* 1993).

30. Karlan, Marrs, and Lagasse 1994. This report is an important reminder of the concern about experiments with freezing ovarian tissue of women about to undergo cancer treatment.

31. Orwell et al. 1994.

32. Marcus and Edwards 1994, 817.

33. Halme, Toma, and Albert 1995.

34. Herman 1993. In some countries only women undergoing their own fertility treatment are eligible as egg donors, since they are taking on the risk of superovulation and egg retrieval anyway, with a chance of gaining benefits from these procedures.

35. Legro et al. 1995, 96.

36. Society for Assisted Reproductive Technologies, ASRM 1996.

37. Sauer 1996.

38. In the words of one response accompanying Sauer's article, from specialists in the United Kingdom, "It is one thing for the infertile to take these unavoidable risks, but quite another for a healthy fertile woman to do the same. No financial inducements can compensate for any adverse consequences" (Ahuja and Simons 1996, 1151).

39. Paulson et al. 1997 (Successful pregnancy).

40. This and other comments made in several news interviews, including the *News Hour* on PBS, April 25, 1997, as well as newspaper reports.

41. Paulson et al. 1997 (Successful pregnancy), 949.

42. McCarthy 1994.

43. American Society for Reproductive Medicine Ethics Committee 1994.

Chapter 6

1. Cunha et al. 1987.

2. Years later Bern expresses some chagrin that he and other basic scientists are still rarely invited to share their work in educational programs for medical students or practicing physicians. In an unusual collaboration, he and Herbst coedited a textbook on DES exposure (Herbst and Bern 1981).

3. Among the alternatives to experimenting on humans, research that uses animal models such as rodents or primates does bring its own controversies and trade-offs, arguments this discussion will not pursue. In addition to animal studies, however, a number of laboratory techniques (e.g., synthesizing and culturing tissue, bioengineering techniques) and computer modeling are increasingly feasible.

4. One study calculated the total cost of attaining a successful delivery with in vitro fertilization—including medications and monitoring, physician and laboratory charges, hospitalizations, complications, and loss of economic productivity. On average, the cost ranged from $66,667 for a success during the first IVF cycle to $114,286 by the sixth cycle; for older women or with a diagnosis of male infertility, a first-cycle success cost $160,000, rising to $800,000 for a successful delivery during the sixth cycle (Neumann, Gharib, and Weinstein 1994). The second study analyzed medical expenditures attached to multiple-gestation pregnancies, which have become increasingly frequent

with increasing use of fertility drugs and assisted reproductive technologies (Callahan et al. 1994). An analysis of costs during 1991–92 at one IVF program separated triplet or larger deliveries (about $340,000 per delivery) from singletons and twins (about $39,000). The authors recommended that physicians transfer fewer embryos, especially to younger women who are more likely to conceive large multiple pregnancies; that treatment plans include freezing of embryos for transfer during subsequent attempts; and that physicians discourage couples from repeated attempts if the likelihood of successful pregnancy is very low (Goldfarb et al. 1996). Another study calculated costs of excess hospital days for infants of multiple pregnancies following assisted reproduction (Wilcox, Kiely, and Melvin 1996). Comparisons of IVF to less invasive treatments increasingly focus on cost-effectiveness per cycle rather than medical efficacy (success rates) alone; see, e.g., Van Voorhis et al. 1997.

5. Collins 1994, 271.

6. See Tan et al.1994 (Cumulative conception). These authors note that a decade after adding GnRH-a to the superovulation process, sixteen years after the first IVF, no published reports compared rates of live birth following various ovarian stimulation regimens. See also Devreker et al. 1996; Feldberg et al. 1994; Fox et al. 1996; Harada et al. 1996; Lu at al. 1996; Manzi et al. 1994; Soliman et al. 1994; Stadtmauer et al. 1994.

7. The following studies deal with the issues in the order listed in the text: Seibel Kearnan, and Kiessling 1995; Seibel 1995; Harrison et al. 1994; Manzi et al. 1995; Dor et al. 1992; Check et al. 1994; Tan et al. 1994 (Pregnancy and birth rates); Svendsen et al. 1996; Aoki et al. 1995.

8. Fluker, Souves, and Bebbington 1993; Collins 1993. Interestingly, in this same issue of *Fertility and Sterility* in which these articles appeared, an overview of assisted reproductive technologies describes ZIFT as "well-accepted" (Mastroyannis 1993).

9. Fox et al. 1996; Harada et al. 1996; Miller, Goldberg, and Falcone 1996.

10. Sher et al. 1993; Tummin et al. 1994; Vauthier-Brouzes et al. 1994. And see Nazari et al. 1993, which stemmed from the observation that embryo transfers by different physicians within the same IVF program resulted in differing rates of clinical pregnancy and of ectopic/heterotopic pregnancy. This report identifies their differing techniques for releasing embryos into the uterus.

A similar trial-and-error process for determining how many embryos to transfer ensued when fertility efforts turned to older women; experimental efforts varied the number of embryos when using a woman's own eggs and using donor eggs (including for postmenopausal pregnancies). See Qasim et al. 1995; Sauer, Paulson, and Lobo 1995a; Sauer, Paulson, and Lobo 1995b; Svendsen et al. 1996; Yaron et al. 1997.

11. Agarwal 1996.

12. Tur-Kaspa et al. 1994. And see Wilcox, Weinberg, and Baird 1995. Other common medical views could change with greater biological knowledge. For example, physicians generally consider high levels of white blood cells in semen samples to be a cause of fertility problems; however, recent research suggests these leukocytes may actually be a normal component of semen, helping to eliminate abnormal sperm (Kiessling et al. 1995). Another example involves use of donor sperm for IVF in couples with unexplained infertility, a practice which, upon more systematic study, may not improve chances for conceiving beyond success rates using the partner's sperm (Azem et al. 1994).

13. Fluker et al. 1994, 195.

14. Taymor 1996, 242; see also Dickey et al. 1996. An entirely different therapy—a GnRH ovulation pump—is a safer and more effective method for overcoming the physiological abnormality in some women; see Tan et al. 1996.

15. D'Hooge et al. 1996; see also Guzick et al. 1997.

16. Healy, Trounson, and Anderson 1994.

17. Corsan and Kemmann 1991, 473. D'Hooge et al. 1996 suggests the laparoscopic procedure that detects mild endometriosis may result in inflammatory processes that promote further development of this condition.

18. Villa 1994. Since FDA approval of GnRH-a was as a treatment for prostate cancer, studies defining adverse side effects did not entail risks from *unapproved* uses in women (see Chapter 7).

19. Berga 1996.

20. Newton et al. 1996.

21. Jones 1995.

22. Guzick et al. 1994 (Endometriosis).

23. Shoham and Schacter 1996, 697.

24. Wentz 1989.

25. Dawood 1996, 1208.

26. Penzias and DeCherney 1996; Jequier and Cummins 1997; Tournaye 1997; Tripp et al. 1997; van der Ven and Haidl 1997.

27. Benrubi 1994.

28. Silverman and Altman 1996, 172.

29. Dieckmann et al. 1953.

30. Other young DES daughters (1 in 1,000) have developed a rare cancer, requiring hysterectomies and vaginectomies. The DES experience and the severe birth defects caused in Europe by the tranquilizer thalidomide—a medical disaster barely averted in this country when an FDA evaluator resisted pressure to approve the drug—revealed the profound impact of medications on a developing fetus. One result was exclusion of pregnant women from most drug research. The focus of medical research on men, however, left important questions of women's health largely ignored. With pressure growing to include women in medical studies, complex issues of risks and benefits for pregnant women require careful consideration by women and researchers alike.

31. Richardson 1994, 5. Among nonsurgical experiments during the 1980s was use of pituitary growth hormone in ovarian stimulation protocols; this human extract was later linked to the rare and devastating Creutzfeldt-Jakob disease (Edwards, Lobo, and Bouchard 1996). Physicians are beginning to experiment with a biosynthetic recombinant version of growth hormone that would not bring the same risk but shows no strong hints that it will improve pregnancy rates.

32. Weber and Marcus 1995.

33. According to a report on use of donor sperm, physicians performing artificial insemination in years past did, at times, use their own semen without telling the women, if no other source was available at the appointed time. See Orenstein 1995.

34. Ellis 1995.

35. Whittemore et al. 1992. Ovarian cancer is a rare but insidious disease. Approximately 1.5 percent of American women who live until the age of eighty-five will develop ovarian cancer; Whittemore's findings suggest an increase to approximately 4.5 percent if a woman takes fertility drugs. The lifetime risk for breast cancer for all women, by comparison, is 10 percent (Whittemore 1993). Ovarian cancer is extremely hard to detect until the disease has progressed too far for effective treatment; to date, specialists have not recommended general screening for ovarian cancer unless a woman's family history puts her in a very high risk category.

36. International Federation of Fertility Societies 1993 (adapted from Cohen et al. 1993).

37. Willemsen, Kruitwagen, and Bastiaans 1993. See also Goldberg and Runowicz 1992; Spirtas, Kaufman, and Alexander 1993.

38. Rossing, Daling, and Weiss 1994.

39. Wysowski 1993. According to Food and Drug Administration estimates, at least 12.5 million prescriptions of fertility drugs were filled between their introduction in the 1960s and the early 1990s (FDA media statement, January 13, 1993).

40. Brzezinski et al. 1994.

41. Arbour et al. 1994.

42. Shushan et al. 1996

43. Mosgaard et al. 1997.

44. Balasch and Barr 1993. At the close of the 1980s, two British gynecologists, writing about superovulation, posed the question, "Are we playing it safe?" (Fishel and Jackson 1989). They clearly think not, especially given the plausibility of an increased ovarian cancer risk. They note that early IVF treatments occurred during a woman's natural menstrual cycle; introduction of ovarian stimulation led quickly to expansion of fertility drug use, so that "almost invariably" women receive at least hMG, often in combination with clomiphene, FSH, and/or GnRH-a. These physicians argue against the usual "blanket approach" covering all patients who undergo assisted reproduction. Rather, fertility drug regimens should be individualized, to minimize a woman's risk, according to her particular medical characteristics and history. Another British specialist who urges flexibility in use of fertility drugs and number of embryos transferred has been attempting to predict the likelihood of complications from superovulation in order to reach more rational decisions about specific treatment protocols for individual patients; see Craft et al. 1988. See also Spirtas, Kaufman, and Alexander 1993.

45. Spirtas, Kaufman, and Alexander 1993.

46. Bristow and Karlan 1996; Chou, Lai, and Lai 1997.

47. Schildkraut, Bastos, and Berchuck 1997.

48. One technique specialists now cite as promising removes several immature eggs from a patient; the eggs can then mature in vitro before sperm are introduced for fertilization and transfer back to the woman. The ovary contains all of an individual's eggs at birth; they "rest" in a premature state until puberty, when the monthly maturation of an egg, leading to ovulation, begins. Approximately ten eggs reach the necessary stage of development each month. This technique was developed by Dr. Alan Trounson, in Australia (Trounson, Wood, and Kausche 1994). The first successful live birth occurred

in January of 1994. Removing individual eggs rather than ovarian tissue which contains eggs causes less injury to the woman. The initial effort was most successful in nonovulating women with polycystic ovarian syndrome. Experiments are continuing in an attempt to improve various aspects of the technique (e.g., Russell et al. 1997). If this process develops and becomes widely available in years to come, the superovulation and the precise timing and monitoring of current reproductive technologies will no longer be necessary, nor will the expense of fertility drugs. First reports of births after freezing and storing eggs, rather than ovary segments, appeared in October 1997.

49. Dawood 1996; Penzias and DeCherney 1996. Comparing the rate of obvious abnormalities at birth to the general population's rate of birth defects is inadequate even if done thoroughly. Had prenatal DES exposure not caused an exceedingly rare vaginal tumor in several girls during their teens—a startling condition gynecologists could not overlook—the medical profession and the public might never have recognized a DES-exposed population or the more frequent but less unusual reproductive problems caused by this medication given to pregnant women many years before.

50. Huggins and Wentz 1993.

51. Rossing et al. 1996.

52. Jaffe 1992b.

53. Endometriosis is one condition linked in some studies to environmental chemicals (see, e.g., Mayani et al. 1997).

54. Presented at "Environmental Estrogens: Pathway to Extinction?" (conference) May 13, 1995, Santa Rosa, Calif.

55. Skakkebaek, Giwercman, and de Kretser 1994, 1473.

56. Sher et al. 1993, 1011.

57. Gleicher et al. 1996.

58. Jequier and Cummins 1997; Tournaye 1997; van der Ven and Haidl 1997.

Chapter 7

1. Standards defining the legal safeguard of informed consent continue to evolve, particularly after revelations of consent that surely was not well enough informed (e.g., the Tuskegee syphilis studies; radiation experiments beginning in the mid-1940s; the recent assisted reproduction and research at the Irvine fertility clinic). Patients must understand how a procedure is performed, as well as its risks and benefits compared to available alternatives (see Appendix 3). Informed consent also provides a legal safeguard for doctors. Patients agree to a procedure "of their own free will" after the doctor meets the legal requirements of informed consent. Doctors can not only "let the patients decide" but also let patients take more of the legal responsibility.

2. Shanner 1995, 251.

3. Oxman et al. 1993. This review is the first of an ongoing series in *JAMA* (see Appendixes 1 and 2). Many published studies themselves use inappropriate, inadequate, or flawed statistics, according to a recent review (Welch and Gabbe 1996).

4. Jeyendran and Zaneveld 1993, 727.

5. Certainly, other personal characteristics of individual doctors, even less tangible, may shape the style and content of information they provide—for example, empathy

with what patients go through or concern with the ethics of fertility treatments. See Appendix 5 for additional considerations in choosing a doctor.

6. For discussion of this issue, see Collins 1995.

7. Bickell et al. 1994. A survey of board-certified reproductive endocrinologists found use of various fertility tests, beyond five "traditional" assessments (semen analysis, ovulation assessment, hysterosalpingogram, laparoscopy, and postcoital test), varied widely by physician age, sex, type of practice, and geographic location (Glatstein, Harlow, and Hornstein 1997).

8. Bickell et al. 1994; Detsky 1995; Lerner 1994. Lerner focuses on cancer treatments, including international variations in treatment.

9. Kolata 1996. This study was published as a book later that year: J. E. Wennberg, ed., *The Dartmouth Atlas of Health Care* (American Hospital Association). Specific surgeries studied were for breast cancer (in which the most extreme geographical variation was seen), prostate cancer, heart disease, and chronic back pain.

10. Pitkin 1992.

11. Woolhandler and Himmelstein 1995.

12. Pear 1995. One month later, the business section of *Time* magazine provided a vivid case in point. A 32-year-old woman diagnosed with metastatic breast cancer and her husband had to battle their managed care plan—Health Net—to obtain treatment they thought would, and should, be covered. In the process, they learned firsthand the limits not only on their choice of specialist but also on the treatment options offered by doctors adhering to managed-care "gag rules." An oncologist discussing the patient's treatment complained that he did not initially know she was a health plan member, prompting a colleague to ask, "If you know someone's a Health Net patient, do you talk to them differently than if they're somebody else?" See Larsen 1996.

13. Drake and Uhlman 1993; Moore 1995.

14. Wilkes, Doblin, and Shapiro 1992. According to a U.S. Senate staff report, pharmaceutical detail men spend $2.6 billion annually; drug manufacturers spend $10 billion per year overall for promotional activities. One study analyzed the accuracy of presentations by drug company representatives at university hospital presentations; not only did a considerable proportion of statements contradict readily available information, but doctors generally did not recognize that the information was inaccurate (Ziegler, Lew, and Singer 1995).

15. Chren and Landefeld 1994.

16. Wilkes, Doblin, and Shapiro 1992, 917.

17. Avorn et al. 1982.

18. Waud 1992.

19. Rawlins 1984.

20. Atkinson and Geiger 1991.

21. Brennan 1994. Interviewed in the *New York Times* (October 4, 1994) about ghostwritten medical journal articles for which the named "author" receives a fee, Brennan commented that "most physicians are unaware that there may be things in the published literature that are being paid for directly by pharmaceutical or public relations firms." Examples of topics in gynecology about which public relations firms have orchestrated "informational" campaigns for doctors and consumers: benefits of taking oral contraceptives;

osteoporosis and hormone replacement; low-dose oral contraceptives for peri-menopause.

22. Orwell et al. 1994.

23. Newton et al. 1996. The influence of drug manufacturers on research they fund is usually not as explicit as a 1995 incident reported by the *Wall Street Journal* (April 25, 1996). In this case, the maker of a thyroid replacement drug was unhappy with results of a study comparing its product with competing brands. Under pressure from this manufacturer, bound by a legal clause granting publication control to the funder, the re-searcher withdrew a report that was scheduled to be published in the *Journal of the American Medical Association*. The study was finally published a year later.

24. Moore 1995 tells the story of Tambacor. Eli Lilly and Company has a particularly poor track record of inadequate research and withholding of information from the FDA in seeking approval of DES, Oroflex, and Prozac (Cornwell 1996).

25. Examples of journal supplement topics sponsored by pharmaceutical companies include endometriosis, GnRH-a (Lupron), menopause and hormone replacement therapy, and ovulation induction. A report on the increasing number of drug company–sponsored symposiums published as medical journal supplements found that "such sponsorship, particularly by a single pharmaceutical company, is associated with a promotional orientation . . . and a distortion of the peer-review process" (Bero, Galbraith, and Rennie 1992). With the types of promotional activities for prescription drugs increasing (including press conferences by physician-researchers and television advertisements to consumers), the Food and Drug Administration may need to expand its regulatory efforts (Kessler and Pines 1990). Recently, the FDA focused on a new relationship drug manufacturers are developing to promote and steer patients toward their products—ownership of pharmacy-benefit management companies (PBMs) that provide medications to managed-care plans (Barnett 1995). Pharmacists, consumer advocates, and competing drug companies argue that FDA regulations should include these new arrangements in order to enforce existing rules about information and marketing. According to the president of a pharmacy trade group, PBM efforts to switch managed-care formularies to their product "undermine the patient-physician and patient-pharmacist relationship." Some PBMs deceive doctors and consumers by not disclosing their drug manufacturer ownership. One PBM, owned by Eli Lilly, gives pharmacists a small payment for patients successfully switched to an Eli Lilly drug (Barnett 1955, 1151).

26. Perlman 1994.

27. Orenstein 1995; Robin 1993.

28. The way patients interpret probability statistics is itself a topic of study; see, e.g., Woloshin 1994.

29. *All Things Considered,* July 20, 1995.

30. Fleming 1994, 116, 119. See also Shacochis 1996, a male journalist's account of the consuming power of the pregnancy quest, the taunt of unyielding hope.

31. Cha, Oum, and Kim 1997.

32. Aboulghar et al. 1996; de Kretser 1977; ESHRE Andrology 1996; Jequier and Cummins 1997; Pavlovich and Schlegel 1997; Tournaye 1997; van der Ven and Haidl 1997.

33. *Human Reproduction* 1995.

34. Grimes, Fraser, and Schulz 1994. See also Branch et al. 1997; Christiansen 1997; Denis et al. 1997; Geva et al. 1997; Gleicher and Coulam 1997; Kutteh et al. 1997.

35. Hill 1995.

36. James 1997; Yaron et al. 1995. The early weeks of a pregnancy, when women may still be taking hormonal medications, are a particularly sensitive period of fetal development. Many scientists are unimpressed by a frequent answer from physicians to questions about prenatal exposure—that the hormones they are giving pregnant women are harmless because there are such high levels of estrogen and progesterone during pregnancy anyway. This argument reflects little appreciation of the complex interplay of various endogenous hormones and the potential for disrupting processes of fetal development More generally, scientists are discovering that hormones—and particularly estrogens—have more complex, far-reaching functions and effects throughout the human life span than was previously known.

37. Smith and Buyalos 1996; see also Dildy et al. 1996.

Chapter 8

1. Greene 1995.

2. Katz 1995; see Blackwell et al. 1987. Interviewed in the *New York Times,* the same Federal Trade Commission staffperson noted the commercialism prevalent in fertility medicine: "You don't open your newspaper and see, 'We have a 21 percent success rate with transplantation of hearts.' This is the only branch of medicine doing success-rate advertising on this scale. It succeeds because of the desperation and emotional vulnerability of the patients" (Gabriel 1996).

3. Araneta et al. 1995.

4. In March 1995 the Food and Drug Administration proposed federal regulations setting specific guidelines for screening, processing, storing, and distributing reproductive tissue. Prospects for approving and enforcing these minimal standards, however, were not favorable in light of governmental attention to cutting the federal budget and reducing its regulatory efforts. The U.S. Public Health Service has also been drafting a new set of minimal standards. Some states, such as California, proceeded with laws aimed at protecting the tissue supply against sexually transmitted disease, though these regulations are fairly general, with no enforcement mechanisms.

5. Dr. L. Wilkening, interviewed on *All Things Considered,* National Public Radio, July 20, 1995.

6. Kelleher and Nicolosi 1995. This warning echoed statements from conventions past. Just as the cattle-breeding industry has pioneered reproductive technologies that later have been applied to humans, so too is this industry more advanced in protective regulations. For example, laws exist that prohibit and punish theft of cattle embryos— but not human ones. Among the complex legal questions arising from the Irvine clinic revelations was how to prosecute the accused physicians, given a lack of statutes or precedents defining what crime—in formal legal terms—they were accused of committing. Along with tightened university regulations, the California legislature began considering bills to establish laws governing aspects of fertility medicine. The American

Society for Reproductive Medicine and its affiliated subgroup, the Society for Assisted Reproductive Technology, issued a statement on November 21, 1995. After listing the societies' accomplishments in monitoring assisted reproduction, the statement continues: "Nevertheless, ASRM and SART believe that now is the time to consider establishing an independent licensing authority. Such an authority might oversee and validate the clinical and laboratory practice of the ART and function independently of and be funded separately from ASRM and SART. We are willing to assist in the development of this body."

7. Jones 1996a.

8. Nau 1994b. Earlier that year, France's senior health minister sought clarification of legal restrictions on IVF, with the aim of prohibiting postmenopausal pregnancies; see Nau 1994a.

9. Baird 1996. While the U.S. government was refusing any involvement with assisted reproduction, a Canadian royal commission was conducting a comprehensive review of research on in vitro fertilization, as a basis for reaching policy decisions at the provincial and national levels. This commission reported in 1993 that, except in cases of women with severely blocked fallopian tubes, "unproven and quite possibly ineffective procedures are being offered as medical treatment, and women are undertaking the risks of these procedures without knowing whether they are more likely to have a child than if they received no treatment" (Gabriel 1996). During the early 1990s, in contrast, the American Society for Reproductive Medicine defined IVF as appropriate therapy for *any* couples who failed with other treatments. This all-inclusive indication for treatment, however, could not withstand the pressure of financial constraints in a managed-care, cost-cutting medical world. By mid-decade, the society was promising new guidelines that would delineate which assisted reproductive technologies are appropriate for which fertility problems. The state of Oregon was even more restrictive than the Canadian province of Ontario when allocating medical resources for its low-income recipients of Medicaid. In Oregon's experimental program for prioritizing and rationing state-funded health care for the poor, treatment of infertility fell low on the priority list, below the cut-off for which services would be covered by Medicaid. In the Australian state of Victoria, an Infertility Treatment Act, implemented in 1996, includes measures to license and monitor fertility clinics and establish a central registry documenting pregnancies involving donor eggs, sperm, or embryos; see Cordner 1996.

10. Kondro 1996.

11. Montalbano 1995.

12. Annas, Caplan, and Elias 1996. The United Kingdom experienced its own controversy in 1997 when the HFEA allowed clinics to destroy "abandoned" frozen embryos—those left for more than five years with no communication from the couple and with no way for a clinic to locate the couple.

13. Dean 1994.

14. Dean 1994. In January 1994 the United Kingdom's HFEA issued a public consultation document—"Donated Ovarian Tissue in Embryo Research and Assisted Conception"—soliciting public comment, not as an opinion poll, in which the majority win, but as a way to obtain "considered views" that may influence policy decisions. This document asked: (1) Should ways be sought of increasing the supply of eggs for use in

research and infertility treatment? If so, what ways can be suggested? (2) Should ovarian tissue from live donors be used in research? (3) Should eggs or ovarian tissue from cadavers or fetuses be used in treatment? (4)If the view is that eggs or ovarian tissue from any of these sources should be allowed to be used in treatment or research, whose consent should be required, when should it be given, and in what form? Should there be any difference in the consents required for eggs or tissue used for research and eggs or tissue used for treatment? Additional comments were also invited on psychological effects, clinical and scientific issues, other moral and ethical issues, and any legal issues.

15. Skovmand 1995. Two years later Denmark's first legislation governing assisted reproduction established an age limit for women (forty-five) and restricted treatment to married heterosexual couples (Skovmand 1997).

16. Kondro 1995. Most of the nine procedures initially subject to the voluntary moratorium have never been used in Canada: sex selection for nonmedical reasons; commercial preconception or surrogacy arrangements; buying and selling eggs, sperm, and embryos; egg donation in exchange for in vitro fertilization services; germ-line genetic alteration; ectogenesis (mechanical, out-of-womb gestation); human embryo cloning; the creation of animal-human hybrids; and the retrieval of eggs from fetuses and cadavers for purposes of donation, fertilization, or research.

17. Kondro 1996.

18. IVF researchers were not alone in their efforts. Physicians and scientists wishing to experiment with tissue from aborted human fetuses—for example, transplanting fetal tissue as treatment for Parkinson's disease or diabetes—faced the same anti-abortion obstacle to government-funded research.

19. U.S. House of Representatives, Committee on Government Operations, 1989; U.S. House of Representatives, Subcommittee of the Committee on Government Operations, 1988. The Office of Technology Assessment (OTA) has been a useful government agency, providing Congress and the public with nonpartisan analyses on a range of technological developments. However, following the 1994 mid-term elections, Congress eliminated OTA funding.

20. Hilts 1989a; Hilts 1989b.

21. U.S. House of Representatives, Committee on Government Operations, 1989, 18.

22. That same summer, announcement of success with relatively easy medical, rather than surgical, abortions (i.e., taking certain medications, at home, early in pregnancy) suggested that the dispute over abortion itself—at least, as performed at clinics or doctors' offices—may be defused somewhat in coming years. The controversy over research using human embryos or fetal tissue, however, will remain.

23. Marshall 1997.

24. The Irvine clinic violations included insurance fraud—reporting a different, but insurable procedure when billing to an insurance company (for instance, instead of egg retrieval, which might not be covered by a patient's insurance, using the billing code for a surgical procedure to remove an ovarian cyst). Physicians were noticeably silent about this particular violation; the coding game for insurance claims is common across the medical spectrum, as insurers well know; see Bates and Bates 1996. Another allegation against Dr. Asch involved importing a fertility drug not approved by the FDA.

Other fertility specialists have developed inventive ways to circumvent the excessive price of fertility drugs—for example, facilitating patients' efforts to bring medications from countries where the cost is much lower.

25. Woolhandler and Himmelstein 1995

26. Gabriel 1996. For a rather derisive depiction of the focus on costs, see DeCherney 1995.

27. For example, the notable increase in multiple gestations is occurring disproportionately among more highly educated, middle-class, white women, as did exposure to DES, the baby-boom generation's wonder drug (Jewell and Yip 1995).

28. Bates and Bates 1996, 1205.

29. Bates and Bates 1996, 1203, 1202. See also Rabin, Qadeer, and Steir 1996, in which the "main outcome measure" of the study is "break-even capitation rate." According to an accompanying editorial, publication of this article addressing economic issues was the first time *Fertility and Sterility* diverged from publishing only "scientific" papers (Bates 1996). As if to defend this new focus, the editorial names several leading American journals that had already done the same.

30. Penzias and DeCherney 1996, 1218.

31. Bates and Bates 1996, 1202; Penzias and DeCherney 1996, 1223.

32. Penzias and DeCherney 1996, 1222.

33. Bates and Bates 1996, 1202, 1204.

34. Benadiva et al. 1995; Tan et al. 1996; Taymor 1996.

35. That lines are being drawn between general ob-gyns and fertility specialists is evident in Gleicher et al. 1996. This comparison of a Chicago managed-care infertility program and fee-for-service finds greater waste of resources (i.e., patients dropping out after initial diagnostic and treatment) with general ob-gyns than with the specialists' program. Added to the fray now are urologists and andrologists seeking to establish their foothold on the male infertility front (see, e.g., Jequier and Cummins 1997; van der Ven and Haidl 1997).

36. Stolberg 1997.

37. Logan and Scott 1996.

38. Abdalla et al. 1997.

Chapter 9

1. One coauthor of the 1987 "exploitation" editorial writes nearly a decade later of unacceptably high rates of multiple pregnancies (30–35 percent), with 60–80 percent of high-risk multiple deliveries the result of assisted reproductive technologies. He also described the "marketplace feel" of ART, where "patients generally pay cash in advance for a procedure that most likely [about 75 percent of the time] will fail" (Soules 1996, 695). See also Wagner 1996.

2. Begley 1995.

3. Consumers' Union 1996.

4. Collins et al. 1983, 1204.

5. Gabriel 1996.

6. Krieger 1996.

7. Clearly, ovarian hyperstimulation is more than an "annoyance." The disturbing eclipse of ethical questions by financial concerns appears in medical reports that address only the cost-effectiveness of shared-egg options for women who cannot otherwise afford IVF; see, e.g., Peskin et al. 1996.

8. Jansen 1995.

9. Jansen 1995, 253.

10. Jansen 1995, 253. Iatrogenic risks are obviously too great in the absence of countervailing benefit. For example, the belief that DES daughters and sons would never have been born at all if their mothers had not taken this medication is incorrect; taking diethylstilbestrol did not increase women's chances for a successful pregnancy and may even have increased chances of miscarriage.

11. Benadiva et al. 1995, 1059.

12. Agarwal 1996; Collins 1995; Nulsen et al. 1993; Seibel, Ranoux, and Kearnan 1989.

13. McCarthy 1993.

14. Kligman et al. 1995.

15. Collins 1995.

16. Naylor et al. 1996. An obvious question is how doctors learn a new technique and improve their skill. Some patients will be low on the learning curve (a position poor patients often occupy at public or medical school clinics). Fertility specialists need to develop better mechanisms for training and supervising less experienced physicians until they demonstrate the skill to perform well a particular procedure on their own. Certain procedures should be restricted to a few specialty centers (e.g., ICSI and other gamete micromanipulations; well-designed clinical studies of immunologic tests and treatments; preimplantation genetic testing; immature egg retrieval; egg and ovary cryopreservation).

17. ESHRE Andrology 1996; Jequier and Cummins 1997; Tournaye 1997; van der Ven and Haidl 1997.

18. To identify medical centers with active research programs on various fertility problems, check with the National Institutes of Health and the American Society for Reproductive Medicine (see Appendix 1).

19. Bickell et al. 1994.

20. Recent reports on making such estimates for individual couples include Collins 1995; Eimers et al. 1994a; ESHRE Capri 1996; Gleicher et al. 1996; Templeton, Morris, and Parslow 1996.

21. By the mid-1990s, several states were beginning to respond to complaints from consumers, doctors, and nurses by enacting or proposing restrictions on the most abusive HMO cost-cutting practices.

22. During the 1970s, for example, DES Action began receiving anecdotal reports of fertility and pregnancy problems from DES daughters, reports later confirmed in clinical and epidemiological studies.

23. The most prominent, the maker of Premarin (the most commonly used estrogen and the top-selling prescription drug in the United States), mounts promotional activities of its own—for example, a supplement to *Obstetrics and Gynecology* (February 1996) on "Menopause and Hormone Replacement," published with a grant from Wyeth-Ayerst Laboratories.

Appendix 3

1. Information in this appendix is based on U.S. Department of Health and Human Services, Title 45 Code of Federal Regulations, Part 46 (45 CFR Part 46), as summarized in G. Ellis 1995.

Appendix 4

1. During the early 1990s, the Centers for Disease Control estimated that 1 million women per year developed PID. For approximately 25 percent of these women, PID will result in infertility or ectopic pregnancy. After a second bout of PID, the proportion rises to 50 percent (Hillis et al. 1993).

2. Healy, Trounson, and Anderson 1994.

3. Centers for Disease Control 1997; Hillis et al. 1993; Hillis and Wasserheit 1996; Witkin et al. 1993; Witkin et al. 1994.

4. Hillis and Wasserheit 1996.

5. McKaughan 1987.

6. Numerous reports now link smoking to lowered fertility in women and men, including lowered success when undergoing fertility treatment. One study analyzed "time-till-pregnancy" (one of the more useful measures of a couple's relative fertility) in women who did become pregnant; women who smoked (even low levels of 1–9 cigarettes a day) took twice as long to conceive as nonsmokers (Alderete, Eshkenazi, and Scholtz 1995). Interviewed about these findings, coauthor Brenda Eshkenazi, an epidemiologist, elaborated: "If you are thirty-five years old when you try to conceive, this additional insult to the fertility system may be enough to make you infertile." See also Baird and Wilcox 1985; Parkhouse et al. 1992; Rosevear et al. 1992; Van Voorhis et al. 1992; Van Voorhis et al. 1996; Vine et al. 1994. Interestingly, some data suggest that offspring of women who smoke during pregnancy may have lowered fertility as adults (Joffe 1996).

Studies of caffeine intake are less clear-cut than smoking, though several reports suggest that women trying to conceive (or to maintain an early pregnancy) should limit, if not eliminate, coffee and other sources of caffeine. See Eshkenazi 1993; Infante-Rivard et al. 1993; Stanton and Gray 1995.

Whatever the particular substance under question, determining whether any safe level of exposure exists, showing no negative effects on fertility, is more difficult. A decision to err on the side of caution regarding these preventive measures can be based only on the weight of existing evidence and the biological plausibility of a connection to fertilization or early embryo development.

7. Baird et al. 1996.

8. Based on Giacoia 1992.

9. One recent study did report an increased risk for women from VDTs, as well as from volatile organic solvents, chemical dusts, and pesticides; differing exposures may result in different fertility problems (Smith et al. 1997; see also Paul 1997). Both of these articles provide a useful discussion of occupational exposures.

10. Based on Paul and Himmelstein 1988, 928.

11. Though iatrogenic exposures disproportionately affect middle-class women who seek out fertility specialists, lower-income women and men are more likely to experience hazardous conditions where they work and live. One exception may be 15,000 female dentists who—along with 80,000 dental assistants and 175,000 dental hygienists—work in settings not adequately equipped to remove nitrous oxide, an anesthetic gas that lowers women's fertility (Rowland et al. 1992). Whatever the occupation, controversy arises over how to protect workers' reproductive health. Federal regulations require that employers provide workplaces free from recognized hazards to employee health and safety. For many employers, the solution is to remove the employee rather than improve working conditions. Some companies exclude all women who might possibly become pregnant from jobs involving suspected reproductive dangers. Beyond violating sex discrimination laws, these policies ignore the fact that hazardous conditions often affect women's *and* men's fertility (as well as their more general health); in addition, of course, excluding workers from certain occupations or work sites can cause economic and personal hardship.

Appendix 5

1. See also Robin 1993.

Works Cited

The following abbreviations of journal names are used:

Am J Epidem	American Journal of Epidemiology
Am J Human Genetics	American Journal of Human Genetics
Am J Med	American Journal of Medicine
Am J Obstet Gynecol	American Journal of Obstetrics and Gynecology
Am J Public Health	American Journal of Public Health
Am J Reprod Immunol	American Journal of Reproductive Immunology
Fertil Steril	Fertility and Sterility
Gynecol Oncol	Gynecologic Oncology
Human Reprod	Human Reproduction
JAMA	Journal of the American Medical Association
J Reprod Med	Journal of Reproductive Medicine
New Engl J Med	New England Journal of Medicine
Obstet Gynecol	Obstetrics and Gynecology
Obstet Gynecol Survey	Obstetrical and Gynecological Survey

Abdalla, H. I., M. E. Wren, A. Thomas, et al. 1997. Age of the uterus does not affect pregnancy or implantation rates: A study of egg donation in women of different ages sharing oocytes from the same donor. *Human Reprod* 12:827–29.

Aboulghar, M. A., R. T. Mansour, G. I. Serour, et al. 1996. Prospective controlled randomized study of in vitro fertilization versus intracytoplasmic sperm injection in the treatment of tubal factor infertility with normal semen parameters. *Fertil Steril* 66:753–56.

Acosta, A. A., S. Oehninger, M. Morshede, et al. 1988. Assisted reproduction in the diagnosis and treatment of the male factor. *Obstet Gynecol Survey* 44:1–18.

Adamson, G. D., S. J. Hurd, D. J. Pasta, et al. 1993. Laparoscopic endometriosis treatment: Is it better? *Fertil Steril* 59:35–44.

Adeghe, J. H. 1993. Male subfertility due to sperm antibodies: A clinical overview. *Obstet Gynecol Survey* 48:1–8.

Agarwal, S. K. 1996. Clomiphene citrate with intrauterine insemination: Is it effective therapy in women above the age of 35 years? *Fertil Steril* 65:759–63.

Ahuja, K K., and E. G. Simons. 1996. Oocyte donation: Anonymous egg donation and dignity. *Human Reprod* 67:1151–54.

Akman, M. A., J. E. Garcia, M. D. Damewood, et al. 1996. Hydrosalpinx affects the implantation of previously cryopreserved embryos. *Human Reprod* 11:1013–14.

Alderete, E., B. Eshkenazi, and R. Scholtz. 1995. Effects of cigarette smoking and coffee drinking on time to conception. *Epidemiology* 6:403–8.

American Fertility Society Ethics Committee. 1990. Ethical considerations of assisted reproductive technologies. *Fertil Steril* 53 suppl. 2.

American Journal of Obstetrics and Gynecolgy. 1992. Laser surgery-operative laparoscopy: Technology assessment (editorial). 166:1062.

American Society for Reproductive Medicine Ethics Committee. 1994. Ethical considerations of assisted reproductive technologies. *Fertil Steril* 62 supplement.

Ankum, W. M., B. W. Mol, F. Van der Veen, et al. 1996. Risk factors for ectopic pregnancy: A meta-analysis. *Fertil Steril* 65:1093–99.

Annas, G. J., A. Caplan, and S. Elias. 1996. The politics of human-embryo research—Avoiding ethical gridlock. *New Engl J Med* 334:1329–32.

Aoki, K., S. Kaijura, N. Gleicher, et al. 1995. Pre-conceptual NK cell activity as a predictor of miscarriage. *Lancet* 345:1340–41.

Araneta, M. R., L. Mascola, A. Eller, et al. 1995. HIV transmission through donor artificial insemination. *JAMA* 273:854–58.

Arbour, L., S. Narod, G. Glendon, et al. 1994. In vitro fertilization and family history of breast cancer (letter). *Lancet* 344:610.

Arici, A., W. Byrd, K. Bradshaw, et al. 1994. Evaluation of clomiphene citrate and human chorionic gonadotropin treatment: A prospective, randomized, crossover study during intrauterine insemination cycles. *Fertil Steril* 61:314–18.

Arnold, S. F., D. M. Klotz, B. M. Collins, et al. 1996. Synergistic activation of estrogen receptor with combinations of environmental chemicals. *Science* 272:1489–91.

Atkinson, C., and J. Geiger. 1991. Just say no? When drug companies make offers doctors can't refuse. *Public Citizen,* March/April, 12–14.

Auger, J., J. M. Kuntsmann, F. Czyglik, et al. 1995. Decline in semen quality among fertile men in Paris during the past 20 years. *New Engl J Med* 332:281–85.

Avorn, J., M. Chen, R. Hartley, et al. 1982. Scientific versus commercial sources of influence on the prescribing behavior of physicians. *Am J Med* 73:4–8.

Azem, F., A. Botchan, Y. Yaron, et al. 1994. Outcome of donor versus husband insemination in couples with unexplained infertility treated by in vitro fertilization and embryo transfer. *Fertil Steril* 61:1088–91.

Bahadur, G., K. L. King, and M. Katz. 1996. Statistical modeling reveals demography and time are the main contributing factors in global sperm count changes between 1938 and 1996. *Human Reprod* 11:2635–39.

Baird, D. D., C. R. Weinberg, L. F. Voight, et al. 1996. Vaginal douching and reduced fertility. *Am J Public Health* 86:844–850.

Baird, D. D., and A. J. Wilcox. 1985. Cigarette smoking associated with delayed conception. *JAMA* 253:2979–83.

Baird, P. 1996. Assisted reproduction: A process ripe for regulation? (Conference proceedings). *Women's Health Issues* 6.

Balasch, J., and P. N. Barr. 1993. Follicular stimulation and ovarian cancer? *Human Reprod* 8:990–96.

Balasch, J., F. Fabregues, M. Creus, et al. 1992. The usefulness of endometrial biopsy for luteal phase evaluation in infertility. *Human Reprod* 7:973–77.

Barabarino-Monnier, P., B. Gobert, F. Guillet, et al. 1991. Antiovary antibodies, repeated attempts, and outcomes of in vitro fertilization. *Fertil Steril* 56:928–32.

Barnett, A. A. 1995. FDA scrutinizes drug firms' new connections. *Lancet* 346:1151.

Barri, P. N. 1996. Procreatics and honesty. *Human Reprod* 11:1368–69.

Bateman, B. G., L. A. Kolp, and K. Hoeger. 1996. Complications of laparoscopy—Operative and diagnostic. *Fertil Steril* 66:30–35.

Bates, G. W. 1996. Economic issues in *Fertility and Sterility*. *Fertil Steril* 66: 885–86.

Bates, G. W., and S. R. Bates. 1996. The economics of infertility: Developing an infertility managed-care plan. *Am J Obstet Gynecol* 174:1200–1207.

Batista, M. C., T. P. Cartledge, M. J. Merino, et al. 1993. Midluteal phase endometrial biopsy does not accurately predict luteal function. *Fertil Steril* 59:294–300.

Bayer, S. R., M. M. Seibel, D. S. Saffan, et al. 1988. Efficacy of danazol treatment for minimal endometriosis in infertile women. *J Reprod Med* 33:179–83.

Becker, S., and K. Berhane. 1997. A meta-analysis of 61 sperm count studies revisited. *Fertil Steril* 67:1103–5.

Begley, S. 1995. The baby myth. *Newsweek,* September 4, 38–47.

Benadiva, C. A., I. Kligman, O. Davis, et al. 1995. In vitro fertilization versus tubal surgery: Is pelvic reconstructive surgery obsolete? *Fertil Steril* 64:1051–61.

Benrubi, G. 1994. Guest editorial. *Obstet Gynecol Survey* 49:801.

Berga, S. L. 1996. A skeleton in the closet? Bone health and therapy for endometriosis revisited. *Fertil Steril* 65:702–3.

Berkowitz, R. L., L. Lynch, U. Chitkara, et al. 1988. Selective reduction of multifetal pregnancies in the first trimester. *New Engl J Med* 318:1043–46.

Berkowitz, R. L., L. Lynch, R. Lapinski, et al. 1993. First-trimester transabdominal multifetal pregnancy reduction: A report of 200 completed cases. *Am J Obstet Gynecol* 169:17–21.

Berkowitz, R. L., L. Lynch, J. Stone, et al. 1996. The current status of multifetal pregnancy reduction. *Am J Obstet Gynecol* 174:1265–72.

Bero, L. A., A. Galbraith, and D. Rennie. 1992. The publication of sponsored symposiums in medical journals. *New Engl J Med* 327:1135–40.

Bickell, N., J. Earp, J. Garrett, et al. 1994. Gynecologists' sex, clinical beliefs, and hysterectomy rate. *Am J Public Health* 84:1649–52.

Blacker, C. M., K. A. Ginsburg, R. E. Leach, et al. 1997. Unexplained infertility: Evaluation of the luteal phase; results of the National Center for Infertility Research at Michigan. *Fertil Steril* 67:437–42.

Blackwell, R. E., B. R. Carr, R. J. Chang, et al. 1987. Are we exploiting the infertile couple? *Fertil Steril* 48:735–39.

Blazar, A. S., J. W. Hogan, D. B. Seifer, et al. 1997. The impact of hydrosalpinx on successful pregnancy in tubal factor infertility treated by in vitro fertilization. *Fertil Steril* 67:517–20.

Bollen, N., M. Camus, H. Tournaye, et al. 1993. Embryo reduction in triplet pregnancies after assisted procreation: A comparative study. *Fertil Steril* 60:504–9.

Bopp, B. L., M. M. Alper, I. E. Thompson, et al. 1995. Success rates with gamete intrafallopian transfer and in vitro fertilization in women of advanced maternal age. *Fertil Steril* 63:1278–83.

Borini, A., G. Bafaro, F. Violini, et al. 1995. Pregnancies in postmenopausal women over 50 years old in an oocyte donation program. *Fertil Steril* 63:258–61.

Boulot, P., B. Hedon, G. Pelliccia, et al. 1993. Effects of selective reduction in triplet gestation: A comparative study of 80 cases managed with or without this procedure. *Fertil Steril* 60:497–503.

Branch, D. W., R. Silver, S. Pierangeli, et al. 1997. Antiphospholipid antibodies other than lupus anticoagulant and anticardiolipin antibodies in women with recurrent pregnancy loss, fertile controls, and antiphospholipid syndrome. *Obstet Gynecol* 89:549–55.

Brennan, T. A. 1994. Buying editorials. *New Engl J Med* 331:673–75.

Bristow, R. E., and B. Y. Karlan. 1996. Ovulation induction, infertility, and ovarian cancer risk. *Fertil Steril* 66:499–507.

Bronson, R. 1995. Immunology and reproductive medicine. *Human Reprod* 10:755–57.

Brook, P. F., C. L. Barratt, and I. D. Cooke. 1994. The more accurate timing of insemination with regard to ovulation does not create a significant improvement in pregnancy rates in a donor insemination program. *Fertil Steril* 61:308–13.

Brzechffa, P. R., and R. P. Buyalos. 1997. Female and male partner age and menotrophin requirements influence pregnancy rates with human menopausal gonadotropin therapy in combination with intrauterine insemination. *Human Reprod* 12:29–33.

Brzezinski, A., T. Peretz, S. Mor-Yosef, et al. 1994. Ovarian stimulation and breast cancer: Is there a link? *Gynecol Oncol* 52:292–95.

Bush, M. R., D. K. Walmer, G. M. Couchman, et al. 1997. Evaluation of the PCT in cycles involving exogenous gonadotropins. *Obstet Gynecol* 89:780–84.

Byer, J. 1994. In vitro fertilization at the time of diagnostic laparoscopy—Utility? (letter). *Fertil Steril* 63:1350.

Callahan, T. L., J. E. Hall, S. L. Ettner, et al. 1994. The economic impact of multiple-gestation pregnancies and the contribution of assisted reproduction techniques to their incidence. *New Engl J Med* 331:244–49.

Cefalo, R. C. 1992. Editor's comment. *Obstet and Gynecol Survey* 47:397–98.

Centers for Disease Control. 1997. *Chlamydia trachomatis* genital infections—United States, 1995. *JAMA* 277:952–53.

Cha, K. Y., K. B. Oum, and H. G. Kim. 1997. Approaches for obtaining sperm in patients with male factor infertility. *Fertil Steril* 67:985–95.

Chapko, K. M., M. R. Weaver, M. K. Chapko, et al. 1995. Stability of in vitro fertilization—embryo transfer success rates from the 1989, 1990, and 1991 clinic-specific outcome assessments. *Fertil Steril* 64:757.

Chaput de Saintonge, D. M., and A. Herxheimer. 1994. Harnessing placebo effects in health care. *Lancet* 344:995–98.

Check, J. H. 1984. Improvement of cervical factor by high-dose estrogen and human menopausal gonadotropin therapy with ultrasound monitoring. *Obstet Gynecol* 63:179.

Check, J. H., D. Lurie, C. Callan, et al. 1994. Comparison of the cumulative probability of pregnancy after in vitro fertilization–embryo transfer by infertility factor and age. *Fertil Steril* 61:257–61.

Chetkowski, R. J., R. J. Kruse, and T. E. Nass. 1989. Improved pregnancy outcome with the addition of leuprolide acetate to gonadotropins for in vitro fertilization. *Fertil Steril* 52:250.

Chou, H. H., Y. M. Lai, C. H. Lai, et al. 1997. Sertoli-Leydig cell tumour in an infertile patient after stimulated ovulation. *Human Reprod* 12:1021–23.

Chren, M. M., and C. S. Landefeld. 1994. Physicians' behavior and their interactions with drug companies. *JAMA* 271:684–89.

Christiansen, O. B. 1997. Immunologic causes of ovarian infertility and repeated implantation failure—Two aspects of the same problem? *Human Reprod* 12:638–39.

Christiansen, O. B., B. S. Christiansen, M. Husth, et al. 1992. Prospective study of anticardiolipin antibodies in immunized and untreated women with recurrent spontaneous abortions. *Fertil Steril* 58:328.

Claman, P., M. Domingo, P. Garner, et al. 1993. Natural cycle in vitro fertilization–embryo transfer at the University of Ottawa: An inefficient therapy for tubal infertility. *Fertil Steril* 60:298–302.

Cohen, J., R. Forman, S. Harlap, et al. 1993. IFFS expert group report on the Whittemore study related to the risk of ovarian cancer associated with the use of infertility agents. *Human Reprod* 8:996–98.

Colborn, T., and C. Clement, eds. 1992. *Chemically induced alterations in sexual and functional development: The wildlife / human connection.* Princeton, N. J.: Princeton Scientific Publishing Co.

Colborn, T., D. Dumanoski, and J. P. Myers. 1996. *Our stolen future: Are we threatening our fertility, intelligence, and survival? A scientific detective story.* New York: Dutton.

Collins, J. A. 1993. New treatments, preliminary results, and clinical practice. *Fertil Steril* 60:403–4.

———. 1994. Reproductive technology—The price of progress. *New Engl J Med* 331:270–71.

———. 1995. A couple with infertility. *JAMA* 274:1159–64.

Collins, J. A., E. A. Burrows, and A. R. Willan. 1995. The prognosis for live birth among untreated infertile couples. *Fertil Steril* 64:22–28.

Collins, J. A., Y. So, E. H. Wilson, et al. 1984. The postcoital test as a predictor of pregnancy among 355 infertile couples. *Fertil Steril* 41:703–8.

Collins, J. A., W. Wrixon, L. B. Janes, et al. 1983. Treatment-independent pregnancy among infertile couples. *New Engl J Med* 309:1201–6.

Consumers' Union. 1996. Fertility clinics: What are the odds? *Consumer Reports,* February, 51–54.

———. 1997. Finding medical help online. *Consumer Reports,* February, 27–31.

Cordner, S. 1996. Infertility treatment centre for Victoria, Australia. *Lancet* 347:684.

Corfman, R. S., M. P. Milad, T. L. Bellavance, et al. 1993. A novel ovarian stimulation protocol for use with the assisted reproductive technologies. *Fertil Steril* 60:864–70.

Cornwell, J. 1996. *The power to harm: Mind, medicine, and murder on trial.* New York: Viking.

Corsan, G. H., and E. Kemmann. 1991. The role of superovulation with menotropins in ovulatory infertility: A review. *Fertil Steril* 55:468–74.

Coulam, C. B., and C. H. Coulam. 1992. Update on immunotherapy for recurrent pregnancy loss. *Am J Reprod Immunol* 27:124–27.

Coulam, C. B., J. J. Stern, and M. Bustillo. 1994. Ultrasonographic findings of pregnancy losses after treatment for recurrent pregnancy loss: Intravenous immunoglobulin versus placebo. *Fertil Steril* 61:248–51.

Cowchock, F. S., and J. B. Smith. 1992. Predictors for live birth after unexplained spontaneous abortions: Correlations between immunologic test results, obstetric histories, and outcome of next pregnancy without treatment. *Am J Obstet Gynecol* 167:1208–12.

Craft, I., T. Al-Shawaf, P. Lewis, et al. 1988. Analysis of 1071 GIFT procedures—The case for a flexible approach to treatment. *Lancet* I:1094.

Crosignani, P. G., D. E. Walters, and A. Soliani. 1991. The ESHRE multicentre trial on the treatment of infertility: A preliminary report. *Human Reprod* 6:953–58.

Cunha, G. R., O. Taguchi, R. Namikawa, et al. 1987. Teratogenic effects of clomiphene, tamoxifen, and diethylstilbestrol on the developing human female genital tract. *Human Pathology* 18:1132–43.

Cunningham, F. G., and K. J. Leveno. 1995. Childbearing among older women—The message is cautiously optimistic. *New Engl J Med* 333:1002–3.

Darder, M. C., Y. M. Epstein, S. L. Treiser, et al. 1996. The effects of prior gravidity on the outcomes of ovum donor and own ooctytes. *Fertil Steril* 65:578–82.

Dawood, M. Y. 1996. In vitro fertilization, gamete intrafallopian transfer, and superovulation with intrauterine insemination: Efficacy and potential health hazards on babies delivered. *Am J Obstet Gynecol* 174:1208–17.

Dean, M. 1994. New controversies over assisted conception. *Lancet* 343:165.

DeCherney, A. H. 1987. Anything you can do I can do better . . . or differently! *Fertil Steril* 48:374–76.

———. 1995. Infertility: We're not taking new patients. *Fertil Steril* 64:470–73.

———. 1996. Bone-sparing properties of oral contraceptives. *Am J Obstet Gynecol* 174:15–20.

Deech, R. 1996. A patient's guide to donor insemination and in-vitro fertilization clinics. *Human Reprod* 11:1363–64.

de Kretser, D. M. 1997. Male infertility. *Lancet* 349:787–90.

Denis, A. L., M. Guido, R. D. Adler, et al. 1997. Antiphospholipid antibodies and pregnancy rates and outcome in in vitro fertilized patients. *Fertil Steril* 67:1084–90.

Depp, R., G. A. Macones, M. F. Rosen, et al. 1996. Multifetal pregnancy reduction: Evaluation of fetal growth in the remaining twins. *Am J Obstet Gynecol* 174:1233–40.

Derom, C., H. Maes, R. Derom, et al. 1993. Iatrogenic multiple pregnancies in East Flanders, Belgium. *Fertil Steril* 60:493–96.

Detsky, A. S. 1995. Regional variation in medical care. *New Engl J Med* 333:589–90.

Devreker, F., I. Govaerts, E. Bertrand, et al. 1996. The long-acting gonadotropin-releasing hormone analogues impaired the implantation rate. *Fertil Steril* 65:122–26.

De Wilde, R. L., and M. Hesseling. 1995. No more radiogenic castration in women with Hodgkin's disease (letter). *Am J Obstet Gynecol* 173:1639.

D'Hooghe, T. M., C. S. Bambra, B. M. Raeymaekers, et al. 1996. Development of spontaneous endometriosis in baboons. *Obstet Gynecol* 88: 462–66.

Diamond, M. P., B. C. Tarlatzis, and A. H. DeCherney. 1987. Recruitment of multiple follicular development for in vitro fertilization in the presence of a viable intrauterine pregnancy. *Obstet Gynecol* 70:498–99.

Dickey, R. P., S. N. Taylor, D. N. Curole, et al. 1996. Incidence of spontaneous abortion in clomiphene pregnancies. *Human Reprod* 11:2623–28.

Dieckmann, W. J., M. E. Davis, S. M.Rynkiewicz, et al. 1953. Does the administration of diethylstilbestrol during pregnancy have therapeutic value? *Am J Obstet Gynecol* 66:1062.

Dildy, G. A., G. M. Jackson, G. K. Fowers, et al. 1996. Very advanced maternal age: Pregnancy after age 45. *Am J Obstet Gynecol* 175:668–74.

Dodson, W. C., and A. H. Haney. 1991. Controlled ovarian hyperstimulation for treatment of infertility. *Fertil Steril* 55:457–67.

Dodson, W. C., D. B. Whiteside, C. L. Hughes, et al. 1987. Superovulation with intrauterine insemination in the treatment of infertility: A possible alternative to gamete intrafallopian transfer and in vitro fertilization. *Fertil Steril* 48:441–45.

Donesky, B. W., and E. Y. Adashi. 1995. Surgically induced ovulation in the polycystic ovary syndrome: Wedge resection revisited in the age of laparoscopy. *Fertil Steril* 63:439–63.

Dor, T., I. Ben-Shlomo, D. Levran, et al. 1992. The relative success of gonadotropin-releasing hormone-analogue, clomiphene citrate, and gonadotropin in 1,099 cycles of in vitro fertilization. *Fertil Steril* 58:986–90.

Drake, D., and D. Uhlman. 1993. *Making medicine, making money*. Kansas City, Mo.: Andrews & McMeel.

Dubuisson, J. B., C. Chapron, Y. Ansquer, et al. 1997. Proximal tubal occlusion: Is there an alternative to microsurgery? *Human Reprod* 12:692–98.

Edwards, R. G., R. Lobo, and P. Bouchard. 1997. Time to revolutionize ovarian stimulation (editorial). *Human Reprod* 12:917–19.

Eimers, J. M., E. R. te Velde, R. Gerritse, et al. 1994a. The prediction of the chance to conceive in subfertile couples. *Fertil Steril* 61:44–62.

———. 1994b. The validity of the postcoital test for estimating the probability of conceiving. *Am J Obstet Gynecol* 171:65–70.

Ellis, G. B. 1995. No news here. *Fertil Steril* 64:1062–63.

Engel, W., D. Murphy, and M. Schmid. 1996. Are there genetic risks with microassisted reproduction? *Human Reprod* 11:2359–70.

Eshkenazi, B. 1993. Caffeine during pregnancy: Grounds for concern? *JAMA* 270:2973–74.

ESHRE Andrology Special Interest Group. 1996. Consensus workshop on advanced diagnostic andrology techniques. *Human Reprod* 11:1463–79.

ESHRE Capri Workshop. 1996. Infertility revisited: The state of the art today and tomorrow. *Human Reprod* 11 (suppl. 4): 5–33.

Evans, M., J. Fletcher, I. Zador, et al. 1988. Selective first trimester termination in octuplet and quadruplet pregnancies: Clinical and ethical issues. *Obstet Gynecol* 71:289–96.

Evans, M. I., L. Littman, L. St. Louis, et al. 1995. Evolving patterns of iatrogenic multifetal pregnancy generations: Implications for aggressiveness of infertility treatments. *Am J Obstet Gynecol* 172:1750–55.

Evers, J. L. 1989. The pregnancy rate of the no-treatment group in randomized clinical trials of endometriosis therapy. *Fertil Steril* 52:906–7.

Feldberg, D., J. Farhi, J. Ashkenazi, et al. 1994. Minidose gonadotropin-releasing agonist is the treatment of choice in poor responders with high follicle-stimulating hormone levels. *Fertil Steril* 62:343–46.

Fisch, H., and E. T. Goluboff. 1996. Geographic variations in sperm counts; a potential cause of bias in studies of semen quality. *Fertil Steril* 65:1044–46.

Fisch, H., E. T. Goluboff, J. H. Olson, et al. 1996. Semen analyses in 1,283 men from the United States over a 25-year period: No decline in quality. *Fertil Steril* 65:1009–14.

Fishel, S., and P. Jackson. 1989. Follicular stimulation for high tech pregnancies: Are we playing it safe? *British Medical Journal* 199:309–11.

Fleming, A. T. 1994. *Motherhood deferred.* New York: Ballantine.

Fluker, M. R., C. G. Souves, and M. W. Bebbington. 1993. A prospective randomized comparison of zygote intrafallopian transfer and in vitro fertilization–embryo transfer for nontubal factor infertility. *Fertil Steril* 60:515–19.

Fluker, M. R., B. Urman, M. Mackinnon, et al. 1994. Exogenous gonadotropin therapy in World Health Organization groups I and II ovulatory disorders. *Obstet Gynecol* 83:189–96.

Foresta, C., A. Ferlin, C. Galeazzi, et al. 1996. Warning note on male infertility treatment. *Lancet* 347:618.

Foresta, C., A. Garolla, A. Ferlin, et al. 1996. Use of intracytoplasmic sperm injection in severe male factor infertility. *Lancet* 348:59.

Foresta, C., M. Rossato, A. Garolla, et al. 1996. Male infertility and ICSI: Are there limits? *Human Reprod* 11:2347–48.

Fox, J. H., K. V. Jackson, M. S. Rein, et al. 1996. A randomized clinical trial to evaluate the clinical effects of split- versus single-dose human menopausal gonadotropins in an assisted reproductive technology program. *Fertil Steril* 65:598–602.

Fraser, E. J., D. A. Grimes, and K. F. Schulz. 1993. Immunization as therapy for recurrent spontaneous abortion: A review and meta-analysis. *Obstet Gynecol* 82:854–59.

Frederiksen, M. C., L. Keith, and R. E. Sabbagha. 1992. Fetal reduction: Is this the appropriate answer to multiple gestation? *International Journal of Fertility* 37:8–14.

Fretts, R. C., J. Schmittdiel, F. H. McLean, et al. 1995. Increased maternal age and the risk of fetal death. *New Engl J Med* 333:953–57.

Gabriel, T. 1996. High-tech pregnancies test hope's limit. *New York Times,* January 7, 1.

Gant, N. F. 1992. Infertility and endometriosis: Comparison of pregnancy outcomes with laparotomy versus laparoscopic techniques. *Am J Obstet Gynecol* 166:1072–81.

Garel, M., and B. Blondel. 1992. Assessment at 1 year of the psychological consequences of having triplets. *Human Reprod* 7:729–32.

Garel, M., C. Salobir, and B. Blondel. 1997. Psychological consequences of having triplets: A 4-year follow-up study. *Fertil Steril* 67:1162–65.

Geva, E., A. Amit, L. Lerner-Giva, et al. 1997. Autoimmunity and reproduction. *Fertil Steril* 67:599–611.

Giacoia, G. P. 1992. Reproductive hazards in the workplace. *Obstet Gynecol Survey* 47:679–87.

Gill, T. S. 1992. Invited editorial: Influence of MHC and MHC-linked genes on reproduction. *Am J Human Genetics* 50:1–5.

Gindoff, P. R., J. L. Hall, and R. J. Stillman. 1994. Utility of in vitro fertilization at diagnostic laparoscopy. *Fertil Steril* 62:237.

Ginsburg, J., S. Okolo, G. Prelevic, et al. 1994. Residence in the London area and sperm density. *Lancet* 343:230.

Glatstein, I. Z., L. B. Craig, A. Palumbo, et al. 1995. The reproducibility of the postcoital test: A prospective study. *Obstet Gynecol* 85:396–400.

Glatstein, I. Z., B. L. Harlow, and M. D. Hornstein. 1997. Practice patterns among reproductive endocrinologists: The infertility evaluation. *Fertil Steril* 67(3): 443–51.

Gleicher, N. 1997. Antiphospholipid antibodies and reproductive failure: What they do and what they do not do; how to and how not to treat! *Human Reprod* 12:13–16.

Gleicher, N., and C. Coulam. 1997. Are we overlooking (auto)immune ovarian infertility? *Human Reprod* 12:637.

Gleicher, N., B. Vanderlaan, V. Karande, et al. 1996. Infertility treatment dropout and insurance coverage. *Obstet Gynecol* 88:289–93.

Gleicher, N., B. Vanderlaan, D. Pratt, et al. 1996. Background pregnancy rate in an infertile population. *Human Reprod* 11:1011–12.

Gobert, B., P. Barabarino-Monnier, M. C. Bene, et al. 1990. Ovary antibodies after IVF. *Lancet* 335:723.

Goldberg, G., and C. Runowicz. 1992. Ovarian carcinoma of low malignant potential, infertility, and induction of ovulation—Is there a link? *Am J Obstet Gynecol* 166:853.

Goldfarb, J. M., C. Austin, H. Lisbona, et al. 1996. Cost-effectiveness of in vitro fertilization. *Obstet Gynecol* 87:18–21.

Gordts, S., G. Garcia, M. Vercruyssen, et al. 1993. Subzonal insemination: A prospective randomized study in patients with abnormal sperm morphology. *Fertil Steril* 60:307–13.

Gosden, R. G., A. J. Rutherford, and D. R. Norfolk. 1997. Transmission of malignant cells in ovarian grafts. *Human Reprod* 12:403.

Greene, J. 1995. British fertility clinics don't have free rein. *Orange County Register,* August 7, 1–2.

Grether, J. K., K. B. Nelson, and S. K. Cummins. 1993. Twinning and cerebral palsy: Experience in four northern California counties, births 1983 through 1985. *Pediatrics* 92:854–58.

Griffith, C. S., and D. A. Grimes. 1990. The validity of the postcoital test. *Am J Obstet Gynecol* 162:615–20.

Grimaldi, J. V. 1995. Panel wants new safeguards. *Orange County Register,* October 21.

Grimes, D. A. 1992. Frontiers of operative laparoscopy: A review and critique of the evidence. *Am J Obstet Gynecol* 166:1067–68.

———. 1993. Technology follies: The uncritical acceptance of medical innovation. *JAMA* 269:3030–33.

Grimes, D. A., E. J. Fraser, and K. F. Schulz. 1994. Immunization as therapy for recurrent spontaneous abortion (reply to letter). *Obstet Gynecol* 83:637–38.

Grundfest, W. S. 1993. Credentialing in an era of change. *JAMA* 270:2725.

Guyatt, G. H., D. L. Sackett, and D. J. Cook. 1993. Users' guides to the medical literature. II. How to use an article about therapy or prevention. A. Are the results of the study valid? *JAMA* 270:2598–2601.

Guzick, D., I. Grefenstette, K. Baffone, et al. 1994. Infertility evaluation in fertile women: A model for assessing the efficacy of infertility testing. *Human Reprod* 5:2306–10.

Guzick, D. S., N. P. Stillman, G. D. Adamson, et al. 1997. Prediction of pregnancy in infertile women based on the American Society for Reproductive Medicine's revised classification of endometriosis. *Fertil Steril* 67: 822–29.

Guzick, D. S., Y. Yao, S. L. Berga, et al. 1994. Endometriosis impairs the efficacy of gamete intrafallopian transfer: Results of a case-control study. *Fertil Steril* 62:1186–91.

Hall, C. T. 1995. Eye surgery industry ready to zap customers. *San Francisco Chronicle,* December 13, E1.

Halme, J., S. K. Toma, and L. M. Albert. 1995. A case of severe ovarian hyperstimulation in a healthy oocyte donor. *Fertil Steril* 64:857–59.

Hammond, C. G., J. K. Halme, and L. M. Talbert. 1983. Factors affecting the pregnancy rate in clomiphene citrate induction of ovulation. *Obstet Gynecol* 62:196.

Haney, A. F. 1987. What is efficacious infertility therapy? *Fertil Steril* 48:543–48.

Haney, A. F., C. L. Hughes, D. B. Whiteside, et al. 1987. Treatment-independent, treatment-associated, and pregnancies after additional therapy in a program of in vitro fertilization and embryo transfer. *Fertil Steril* 47:634–38.

Haning, R. V., D. B. Seifer, C. A. Wheeler, et al. 1996. Effects of fetal number and multifetal reduction on length of in vitro fertilization pregnancies. *Obstet Gynecol* 87:964–68.

Harada, T., C. Katagiri, N. Takao, et al. 1996. Altering the timing of human chorionic gonadotropin injection according to serum progesterone (P) concentrations improves embryo quality in cycles with subtle P rise. *Fertil Steril* 65:594–97.

Hardardottir, H., K. Kelly, M. D. Bork, et al. 1996. Atypical presentation of preeclampsia in high-order multifetal gestations. *Obstet Gynecol* 87:370–74.

Härkki-Sirén, P., and T. Kurki. 1997. A nationwide analysis of laparoscopic complications. *Obstet Gynecol* 89:108–12.

Harkness, C. 1992. *The infertility book: A comprehensive and emotional guide.* Berkeley: Celestial Arts.

Harrison, H. 1997. Counseling parents of extremely premature babies (letter). *Lancet* 349:289.

Harrison, R. F., U. Kondaveeti, C. Barry-Kinsella, et al. 1994. Should gonadotropin-releasing hormone down-regulation therapy be routine in in vitro fertilization? *Fertil Steril* 62:568–73.

Healy, D. L., A. O. Trounson, and A. N. Anderson. 1994. Female infertility: Causes and treatment. *Lancet* 343:1539–44.

Herbst, A. L., and H. A. Bern, eds. 1981. *Developmental effects of diethylstilbestrol (DES) in pregnancy.* New York: Thieme-Stratton.

Herman, R. 1993. Fertility treatment's long-term effects. *Washington Post,* January 12.

Hershlag, A., E. H. Kaplan, R. A. Loy, et al. 1992. Selection bias in in vitro fertilization programs. *Am J Obstet Gynecol* 166:1–3.

Hershlag, A., E. H. Kaplan, R. A. Loy, et al. 1991. Heterogeneity in patient populations explains differences in in vitro fertilization programs. *Fertil Steril* 56:913–17.

Hervé, C., and G. Moutel. 1995. Sex chromosome abnormalities after intracytoplasmic sperm injection. *Lancet* 346:1096–97.

Hill, J. A. 1995. Treatment questioned. *Resolve national newsletter,* winter, 3–4.

Hillis, S. D., R. Joesoef, P. A. Marchbanks, et al. 1993. Delayed care of pelvic inflammatory disease as a risk factor for impaired fertility. *Am J Obstet Gynecol* 168:1503–9.

Hillis, S. D., and J. N. Wasserheit. 1996. Screening for chlamydia—A key to the prevention of pelvic inflammatory disease. *New Engl J Med* 334:1399.

Hilts, P. J. 1989a. Abortion debate clouds research on fetal tissue. *New York Times,* October 16, A19.

———. 1989b. Citing abortion, U.S. continues ban on fetal tissue transplants. *New York Times,* November 2, A1.

Ho, P., I. Poon, S. Chan, et al. 1989. Intrauterine insemination is not useful in oligoasthenospermia. *Fertil Steril* 51:682.

Howards, S. S. 1995. Treatment of male infertility. *New Engl J Med* 332:321–17.

Hsu, C. C., H. C. Kuo, S. T. Wang, et al. 1995. Interference with uterine blood flow by clomiphene citrate in women with unexplained infertility. *Obstet Gynecol* 86:917–21.

Huggins, G., and A. Wentz. 1993. Contempo. *JAMA* 270:235–36.

Hughes, E. G., D. M. Fedorkow, and J. A. Collins. 1993. A quantitative overview of controlled trials in endometriosis-associated infertility. *Fertil Steril* 59:963–70.

Hull, M. E., K. S. Moghissi, and D. F. Magyar. 1987. Comparison of different treatment modalities of endometriosis in infertile women. *Fertil Steril* 47:40.

Hull, M. G. 1992. Infertility treatment: Relative effectiveness of conventional and assisted conception methods. *Human Reprod* 7:785–96.

Human Reproduction. 1995. Immunology and reproductive medicine (editorial). 10:755–57.

Inbar, O. J., D. Levian, S. Masbiach, et al. 1994. Ischemic stroke due to induction of ovulation with clomiphene citrate and menotropins without evidence of ovarian hyperstimulation syndrome. *Fertil Steril* 62:1075–76.

Infante-Rivard, C., A. Fernandez, P. Gauthier, et al. 1993. Fetal loss associated with caffeine intake before and during pregnancy. *JAMA* 270:2940–43.

International Federation of Fertility Societies. 1993. Fertility drugs and ovarian cancer. *Fertil Steril* 60:406–8.

Jaffe, R. B. 1992a. Editor's comment. *Obstet Gynecol Survey* 47:131.

———. 1992b. Editor's comment. *Obstet Gynecol Survey* 47:346.

———. 1993. Editor's comment. *Obstet Gynecol Survey* 48:483–84.

———. 1994a. Editor's comment. *Obstet Gynecol Survey* 49:119–20.

———. 1994b. Editor's comment. *Obstet Gynecol Survey* 49:417–18.

———. 1995a. Editor's comment. *Obstet Gynecol Survey* 50:125.

———. 1995b. Editor's comment. *Obset Gynecol Survey* 50:661–63.

James, W. H. 1997. Secular trends in monitors of reproductive hazards. *Human Reprod* 12:417–21.

Jansen, R. P. 1995. Elusive fertility: Fecundability and assisted conception in perspective. *Fertil Steril* 64:252–55.

Jequier, A. M., and J. M. Cummins. 1997. Attitudes to clinical andrology: A time for change. *Human Reprod* 12:875–76.

Jewell, S. E., and R. Yip. 1995. Increasing trends in plural births in the United States. *Obstet Gynecol* 85:229–32.

Jeyendran, S. J., and L. J. Zaneveld. 1993. Controversies in the development and validation of new sperm assays. *Fertil Steril* 59:726–28.

Joffe, M. 1996. Decreased fertility in Britain compared with Finland. *Lancet* 347:1519–22.

Jones, H. W. 1995. Who should treat the infertile couple? *Obstet Gynecol Survey* 50:251.

———. 1996a. The time has come. *Fertil Steril* 65:1090–92.

———. 1996b. HFEA's patient guidelines penalize the value of embryo preservation. *Human Reprod* 11:1364–65.

Jones, H. W., D. Jones, and R. Kolm. 1997. Cryopreservation: A simplified method of evaluation. *Human Reprod* 12:548–53.

Jones, H. W., and J. P. Toner. 1993. The infertile couple. *N Engl J Med* 329:1710–15.

Jones, H. W., L. L. Veeck, and S. J. Muasher. 1993. On reporting pregnancies by assisted reproductive technology. *Fertil Steril* 60:759–61.

Karamardian, L. M., and D. A. Grimes. 1992. Luteal phase deficiency: Effect of treatment on pregnancy rates. *Am J Obstet Gynecol* 167:1391–98.

Karlan, B. Y., R. Marrs, and L. D. Lagasse. 1994. Advanced-stage ovarian carcinoma presenting during infertility evaluation. *Am J Obstet Gynecol* 171:1377–78.

Karlstrom, P., T. Bergh, and O. Lundkvist. 1993. A prospective randomized trial of artificial insemination versus intercourse in cycles stimulated with human menopausal gonadotropin or clomiphene citrate. *Fertil Steril* 59:554–59.

Katz, M. A. 1995. Federal Trade Commission staff concerns with assisted reproductive technology advertising. *Fertil Steril* 64:10–12.

Kelleher, S., and M. Nicolosi. 1995. Fertility group drafting self-policing legislation. *Orange County Register,* October 10.

Kessler, D. A., and W. J. Pines. 1990. The federal regulation of prescription drug advertising and promotion. *JAMA* 264:2409–15.

Keye, W. R. 1994. Hitting a moving target: Credentialing the endoscopic surgeon. *Fertil Steril* 62:1115–17.

Kiessling, A. A., N. Camparelli, H.-Z. Yin, et al. 1995. Semen leukocytes: Friends or foes? *Fertil Steril* 64:196–98.

Klein, R. D., ed. 1989. *Infertility: Women speak out about their experiences of reproductive medicine.* Winchester, Mass.: Unwin Hyman.

Kligman, I., N. Noyes, L. A. Benadiva, et al. 1995. Massive deep vein thrombosis in a patient with anti-thrombine III deficiency undergoing ovarian stimulation for IVF. *Fertil Steril* 63:673–76.

Kodama, H., T. Matsui, and J. Fukada. 1996. Benefit of in vitro fertilization treatment for endometriosis-associated infertility. *Fertil Steril* 66:974–79.

Kolata, G. 1994. Reproductive revolution is jolting old views. *New York Times,* January 11, A1.

———. 1995a. Diagnosis: Treatment pending. *New York Times,* February 12, B1.

———. 1995b. New surgery procedure removes parts of ovary for later implant. *New York Times,* December 12.

———. 1996. Sharp regional incongruity found in medical costs and treatment. *New York Times,* January 30, C3.

Kondro, W. 1995. Canada calls for moratorium on IVF technologies. *Lancet* 346:367.

———. 1996. Canada gets tough with reproductive technologies. *Lancet* 347:1758.

Kremer, J. A., J. H. Tuerlings, E. J. Meuleman, et al. 1997. Microdeletions of the Y chromosome and intracytoplasmic sperm injection: From gene to clinic. *Human Reprod* 12:687–91.

Krieger, L. 1996. Pharmacists fear fast pace will cause deadly mistakes. *San Francisco Examiner and Chronicle,* January 14, A-1.

Kutteh, W. H., D. L. Yetman, S. J. Chantilis, et al. 1997. Effect of antiphospholipid antibodies in women undergoing in-vitro fertilisation: Role of heparin and aspirin. *Human Reprod* 12:1171–75.

Kwak, J. Y., A. Gilman-Sachs, K. D. Beaman, et al. 1992. Reproductive outcome in women with recurrent spontaneous abortions of alloimmune and autoimmune causes: Preconception versus postconception treatment. *Am J Obstet Gynecol* 166:1787–98.

Lancet. 1988. Selective fetal reduction (editorial). II:773–75.

Lancet. 1993. Too old to have a baby? (editorial). 341:344–45.

Lancet. 1995. Male reproductive health and environmental estrogens (editorial). 345:933–35.

Larsen, E. 1996. The soul of an HMO. *Time,* January 22, 45–52.

Lawton, A. 1994. Optic neuropathy associated with clomiphene citrate therapy. *Fertil Steril* 61:390–91.

Lee, P., and M. Silverman. 1974. *Pills, profits, and politics.* Berkeley, Calif: University of California Press.

Leeton, J. L., P. Rogers, C. Caro, et al. 1987. A controlled study between the use of gamete intrafallopian transfer (GIFT) and in vitro fertilization and embryo transfer in the management of idiopathic and male infertility. *Fertil Steril* 48:605–7.

Legro, R. S., I. L. Wong, R. J. Paulson, et al. 1995. Recipient's age does not adversely affect pregnancy outcome after oocyte donation. *Am J Obstet Gynecol* 172:96–100.

Lerner, M. 1994. *Choices in healing: Integrating the best of conventional and complementary approaches to cancer.* Cambridge, Mass.: MIT Press.

Lewitt, N., S. Kol, N. Ronen, et al. 1996. Does intravenous administration of human albumin prevent severe ovarian hyperstimulation syndrome? *Fertil Steril* 66: 654–56.

Lipshultz, L. I. 1996. "The debate continues"—The continuing debate over the possible decline in semen quality. *Fertil Steril* 65:909–11.

Lobo, R. A. 1996. ART reporting: The American view. *Human Reprod* 11:1369–70.

Logan, R. L., and P. J. Scott. 1996. Uncertainty in clinical practice: Implications for quality and costs of health care. *Lancet* 347:595–98.

Lowe, H. J., and G. O. Barnett. 1994. Understanding and using the medical subject headings (MeSH) vocabulary to perform literature searches. *JAMA* 271:1103–8.

Lu, P. Y., A. L. Chen, E. J. Atkinson, et al. 1996. Minimal stimulation achieves pregnancy rates comparable to human menopausal gonadotropins in the treatment of infertility. *Fertil Steril* 65:583–87.

Lundin, K., A. Sjögren, and L. Hamberger. 1996. Reinsemination of one-day-old oocytes by use of intracytoplasmic sperm injection. *Fertil Steril* 66:118–21.

Lynch, L., R. L. Berkowitz, U. Chitkara, et al. 1990. First trimester transabdominal multifetal pregnancy reduction: A report of 85 cases. *Obstet Gynecol* 75:735–38.

Manzi, D. L., S. Dumez, L. B. Scott, et al. 1995. Selective use of leuprolide acetate in women undergoing superovulation with intrauterine insemination results in significant improvement in pregnancy outcome. *Fertil Steril* 63:866–73.

Manzi, D. L., K. L. Thornton, L. B. Scott, et al. 1994. The value of increasing the dose of human menopausal gonadotropin in women who initially demonstrated a poor response. *Fertil Steril* 62:251–56.

Mao, C., and D. Grimes. 1988. The sperm penetration assay: Can it discriminate between fertile and infertile men? *Am J Obstet Gynecol* 159:279–86.

Maranto, G. 1995. Delayed childbearing. *Atlantic Monthly,* June, 55–66.

Marcoux, F., R. Maheux, S. Bérubé, et al. 1997. Laparoscopic surgery in infertile women with minimal or mild endometriosis. *New Engl J Med* 337:217–22.

Marcus, S. F., and R. G. Edwards. 1994. High rates of pregnancy after long-term down-regulation of women with severe endometriosis. *Am J Obstet Gynecol* 171:812–17.

Marshall, E. 1997. Embryologists dismayed by sanctions against geneticist. *Science* 275:472.

Martin, J. A., M. F. MacDorman, and T. J. Matthews. 1997. Triplet births: Trends and outcomes, 1971–94. *Vital and Health Statistics Series* 21 no. 55(PHS)97–1933.

Martin, M. C. 1993. Collection and report of assisted reproductive technology: Problems and solutions. *Fertil Steril* 60:762–63.

Martinez, A. R., R. E. Bernardus, J. P. Vermeiden, et al. 1993. Basic questions on intrauterine insemination: An update. *Obstet Gynecol Survey* 48:811–27.

Mascarenhas, L., G. Khastgir, W. Davies, et al. 1994. Controlled ovarian hyperstimulation: An adjunct to assisted reproductive technology. *Fertil Steril* 61:1158–60.

Mastroyannis, C. 1993. Gamete intrafallopian transfer: Ethical considerations, historical development of the procedure, and comparison with other advanced reproductive technologies. *Fertil Steril* 60:389–402.

Matthews, C. D. 1996. ART regulation: The Australian viewpoint. *Human Reprod* 11:1365–66.

Mau, U. A., I. T. Bäckert, P. Kaiser, et al. 1997. Chromosomal findings in 150 couples referred for genetic counseling prior to intracytoplasmic sperm injection. *Human Reprod* 12:930–37.

Mayani, A., S. Barel, S. Soback, et al. 1997. Dioxin concentrations in women with endometriosis. *Human Reprod* 12: 373–75.

McCarthy, K. 1993. Birth, fertility research emphasizes the negative. *American Psychological Association Monitor,* July, 12–13.

———. 1994. Infertile women need help accepting inability to conceive. *American Psychological Association Monitor,* July.

McDonough, P. G. 1992. The need for technology assessment in the reproductive sciences. *Am J Obstet Gynecol* 166:1082–90.

———. 1993. Dealing with uncertainty: The challenge of the decade? *Fertil Steril* 60:1100.

McKaughan, M. 1987. *The biological clock.* London and New York: Penguin Books.

McNeely, M. J., and M. R. Soules. 1988. The diagnosis of luteal phase deficiency: A critical review. *Fertil Steril* 50:1–15.

Miller, K. F., J. M. Goldberg, and T. Falcone. 1996. Follicle size and implantation of embryos from in vitro fertilization. *Obstet Gynecol* 88:583–86.

Mintz, M. 1985. *At any cost: Corporate greed, women, and the Dalkon Shield.* New York: Pantheon.

Moloney, M. D., J. N. Bulmer, J. S. Scott, et al. 1989. Maternal immune responses and recurrent miscarriage. *Lancet* I:45.

Moncayo, R., H. Moncayo, and O. Dapunt. 1990. Immunological risks of IVF. *Lancet* 335:180.

Montalbano, W. D. 1995. Italy's doctors ban "designer babies." *San Francisco Examiner and Chronicle,* April 16, A-5.

Moore, T. 1995. *Deadly medicine.* New York: Simon and Schuster.

Mosgaard, B. J., Ø. Lidegaard, S. K. Kjaer, et al. 1997. Infertility, fertility drugs, and invasive ovarian cancer: A case-control study. *Fertil Steril* 67:1005–12.

Mukherjee, T., A. B. Copperman, B. Sandler, et al. 1995. Severe ovarian hyperstimulation despite prophylactic albumin at the time of oocyte retrieval for in vitro fertilization and embryo transfer. *Fertil Steril* 64:641–43.

Nau, J. Y. 1994a. Debate about IVF in France. *Lancet* 343:166.

———. 1994b. Defence of medically assisted pregnancies in France. *Lancet* 344:606.

Naylor, C. D. 1995. Gray zones of clinical practice: Some limits to evidence-based medicine. *Lancet* 346:840–42.

Naylor, C. D., G. H. Guyatt, et al. 1996. Users' guides to the medical literature. X. How to use an article reporting variations in the outcomes of health services. *JAMA* 275:554–58.

Naz, R. K., and A. C. Menge. 1994. Antisperm antibodies: Origin, regulation, and sperm reactivity in human infertility. *Fertil Steril* 61:1001–13.

Nazari, A., H. A. Askari, J. H. Check, et al. 1993. Embryo transfer technique as a cause of ectopic pregnancy in in vitro fertilization. *Fertil Steril* 60:919–21.

Nettles, J. B. 1995. Support groups: A neglected resource in obstetrics and gynecology. *Obstet Gynecol Survey* 50:495–96.

Neumann, P. J., S. D. Gharib, and M. C. Weinstein. 1994. The cost of a successful delivery with in vitro fertilization. *New Engl J Med* 331:239–43.

Newman, R. B., C. Hamer, and C. Miller. 1989. Outpatient triplet management: A contemporary review. *Am J Obstet Gynecol* 161:547–55.

Newton, C., D. Slota, A. A. Yuzpe, et al. 1996. Memory complaints associated with the use of gonadotropin-releasing hormone agonists: A preliminary study. *Fertil Steril* 65:1253–55.

Novy, M. J. 1994. Concurrent tuboplasty and assisted reproduction. *Fertil Steril* 62:242.

Nulsen, J. C., S. Walsh, S. Dumez, et al. 1993. A randomized and longitudinal study of human menopausal gonadotropin with intrauterine insemination in the treatment of infertility. *Obstet Gynecol* 82:780–86.

Obstetrical and Gynecological Survey. 1989. Editor's comment. 44:692–93.

O'Donovan, P. A., P. Vandekerckhove, R. J. Lilford, et al. 1993. Treatment for male infertility: Is it effective? Review and meta-analysis of published randomized controlled trials. *Human Reprod* 8:1209–22.

Oehninger, S., D. Franken, and T. Kruger. 1997. Approaching the next millennium: How should we manage andrology diagnosis in the intracytoplasmic sperm injection era? *Fertil Steril* 67:434–36.

Oehninger, S., L. Veeck, S. Lanzendorf, et al. 1995. Intracytoplasmic sperm injection: Achievement of high pregnancy rates in couples with severe male factor infertility is dependent primarily upon female and not male factors. *Fertil Steril* 64:977–81.

Olsen, G. W., K. M. Bodner, J. M. Ramlow, et al. 1995. Have sperm counts been reduced 50 per cent in 50 years? A statistical model revisited. *Fertil Steril* 63:887–93.

Orenstein, P. 1995. Looking for a donor dad. *New York Times Magazine,* June 18, 35.

Orvieto, R., D. Dekel, D. Dicker, et al. 1995. A severe case of ovarian hyperstimulation syndrome despite the prophylactic administration of iv albumin. *Fertil Steril* 64:860–62.

Orwell, E. S., A. A. Yuzpe, K. A. Burry, et al. 1994. Nafarelin therapy in endometriosis: Long-term effects on bone mineral density. *Am J Obstet Gynecol* 171:1221–25.

O'Shea, D. L., R. R. Odem, C. Cholewa, et al. 1993. Long-term follow-up of couples after hamster egg penetration testing. *Fertil Steril* 60:1040–45.

Oxman, A. D., D. L. Sackett, G. H. Guyatt, et al. 1993. Users' guides to the medical literature. I. How to get started. *JAMA* 270:2093–96.

Palermo, G. D., J. Cohen, and Z. Rosenwaks. 1996. Intracytoplasmic sperm injection: A powerful tool to overcome fertilization failure. *Fertil Steril* 65:899–908.

Palermo, G. D., L. T. Colombero, G. L. Schattman, et al. 1996. Evolution of pregnancies and initial follow-up of newborns delivered after intracytoplasmic sperm injection. *JAMA* 276:1893–97.

Parkhouse, N., R. Crowe, D. A. McGrouther, et al. 1992. Smoking and decreased fertilisation rates in vitro (letter). *Lancet* 340:1409–10.

Patrizio, P., and G. S. Kopf. 1997. Molecular biology in the modern workup of the infertile male: The time to recognize the need for andrologists. *Human Reprod* 12:879–83.

Paul, M. 1997. Occupational reproductive hazards. *Lancet* 349:1385–88.

Paul, M., and J. Himmelstein. 1988. Reproductive hazards in the workplace: What the practitioner needs to know about chemical exposures. *Obstet Gynecol* 71:921–38.

Paulsen, C. A., N. G. Berman, and C. Wang. 1996. Data from men in greater Seattle area reveals no downward trend in semen quality: Further evidence that deterioration of semen quality not geographically uniform. *Fertil Steril* 65:1015–20.

Paulson, R. J., I. E. Hatch, R. A. Lobo, et al. 1997. Cumulative conception and live birth rates after oocyte donation: Implications regarding endometrial receptivity. *Human Reprod* 12:835–39.

Paulson, R. J., and M. V. Sauer. 1994. Pregnancies in post-menopausal women. *Human Reprod* 9:571–72.

Paulson, R. J., M. V. Sauer, M. M. Francis, et al. 1992. In vitro fertilization in unstimulated cycles: The University of Southern California experience. *Fertil Steril* 57:290–93.

Paulson, R. J., M. H. Thornton, M. M. Francis, et al. 1997. Successful pregnancy in a 63-year-old woman. *Fertil Steril* 67:949–51.

Pavlovich, C. P., and P. N. Schlegel. 1997. Fertility options after vasectomy: A cost-effectiveness analysis. *Fertil Steril* 67:133–41.

Pear, R. 1995. Physicians resent HMO "gag clauses." *New York Times,* December 21, A22.

Peipert, J. F., and P. J. Sweeny. 1993. Diagnostic testing in obstetrics and gynecology: A clinician's guide. *Obstet Gynecol* 82:619–23.

Penzias, A. S., and A. H. DeCherney. 1996. Is there ever a role for tubal surgery? *Am J Obstet Gynecol* 174:1218–23.

Perlman, D. 1994. It worked—Baby's due in February. *San Francisco Chronicle,* July 21, 1.

Peskin, B. D., C. Austin, H. Lisbona, et al. 1996. Cost analysis of shared oocyte in vitro fertilization. *Obstet Gynecol* 88:428–30.

Peters, A. J., B. Hecht, A. C. Wentz, et al. 1993. Comparison of the methods of artificial insemination on the incidence of conception in single unmarried women. *Fertil Steril* 59:121–24.

Petersen, C. M., H. H. Hatasaka, K. P. Jones, et al. 1994. Ovulation induction with gonadotropins and intrauterine insemination compared with in vitro fertilization and no therapy: A prospective, nonrandomized, cohort study and meta-analysis. *Fertil Steril* 62:535–44.

Pinchbeck, D. 1996. Downward motility. *Esquire,* January, 79–84.

Pitkin, R. 1992. Operative laparoscopy: Surgical advance or technical gimmick. *Obstet Gynecol* 79:441–43.

Plouffe, L., E. W. White, S. P. Tho, et al. 1992. Etiologic factors of recurrent abortion and subsequent reproductive performance of couples: Have we made any progress in the past ten years? *Am J Obstet Gynecol* 167:313–21.

Powers, W. F., and J. L. Kiely. 1994. The risks confronting twins. *Am J Obstet Gynecol* 170:456–61.

Pryor, J. L., M. Kent-First, A. Muallem, et al. 1997. Microdeletions in the Y chromosome of infertile men. *New Engl J Medicine* 336:534–39.

Qasim, S. M., M. Karacan, G. H. Corsan, et al. 1995. High-order oocyte transfer in gamete intrafallopian transfer patients 40 or more years of age. *Fertil Steril* 64:107–10.

Quigly, M. M. 1992. The new frontier of reproductive age. *JAMA* 268:1321–22.

Rabin, D. S., U. Qadeer, and V. E. Steer. 1996. A cost and outcome model of fertility treatment in a managed care environment. *Fertil Steril* 66:896–903.

Ransom, M. X., G. Corsan, and B. Blotner. 1994. Does increasing frequency of intrauterine insemination improve pregnancy rates significantly during superovulation cycles? *Fertil Steril* 61:303–7.

Rawlins, M. D. 1984. Doctors and the drug makers. *Lancet* II:276–78.

Reubinoff, B. E., A. Samueloff, M. Ben-Haim, et al. 1997. Is the obstetric outcome of in vitro fertilized singleton gestations different from natural ones? *Fertil Steril* 67:1077–83.

Richardson, D. A. 1994. Ethics in gynecologic surgical innovation. *Am J Obstet Gynecol* 170:1–6.

Roan, S. 1996. How many babies is too many? *Los Angeles Times,* May 14, A1.

Robin, Peggy. 1993. *How to be a successful fertility patient.* New York: Morrow.

Roest, J., A. M. van Heusden, H. Mous, et al 1997. The ovarian response as a predictor for successful in vitro fertilization treatment after the age of 40 years. *Fertil Steril* 66:969–73.

Roest, J., A. M. van Heusden, A. Verhoeff, et al. 1997. A triplet pregnancy after in vitro fertilization is a procedure-related complication that should be prevented by replacement of two embryos only. *Fertil Steril* 76:290–95.

Rosenthal, E. 1992. Cost of high-tech fertility: Too many tiny babies. *New York Times,* May 22, C1.

Rosevear, S. K., D. W. Holt, T. D. Lee, et al. 1992. Smoking and decreased fertilisation rates in vitro. *Lancet* 340:1195–96.

Rossing, M. A., J. R. Daling, and N. Weiss. 1994. Ovarian tumors in a cohort of infertile women. *New Engl J Med* 331:771–76.

———.1996. In situ and invasive cervical carcinoma in a cohort of infertile women. *Fertil Steril* 65:19–22.

Rousseau, S., J. Lord, Y. Lepage, et al. 1983. The expectancy of pregnancy for "normal" infertile couples. *Fertil Steril* 40:768.

Rowland, A. S., D. D. Baird, C. R. Weinberg, et al. 1992. Reduced fertility among women employed as dental assistants exposed to high levels of nitrous oxide. *New Engl J Med* 327:993–97.

Russell, J. B., K. M. Knezevich, K. F. Fabian, et al. 1997. Unstimulated immature oocyte retrieval: Early versus midfollicular endometrial priming. *Fertil Steril* 67:616–20.

Sauer, M. V. 1996. Oocyte donation: Reflections on past work and future directions. *Human Reprod* 11:1149–50.

Sauer, M. V., R. J. Paulson, and R. A. Lobo. 1990. A preliminary report on oocyte donation extending reproductive potential to women over 40. *New Engl J Med* 323:1157–60.

————. 1992. Reversing the natural decline in human fertility: An extended trial of oocyte donation to women of advanced reproductive age. *JAMA* 268:1275–79.

————. 1993. Pregnancy after age 50: Application of oocyte donation to women after natural menopause. *Lancet* 341:321–23.

————. 1995a. Pregnancy in women 50 or more years of age: Outcomes of 22 consecutively established pregnancies from oocyte donation. *Fertil Steril* 64:111–15.

————. 1995b. Triplet pregnancy in a 51-year-old woman after oocyte donation. *Am J Obstet Gynecol* 172:1044–45.

Schenken, R. S., and D. S. Guzick. 1997. Revised endometriosis classification: 1996. *Fertil Steril* 67:815–16.

Schenker, J. G., and Y. Ezra. 1994. Complications of assisted reproductive techniques. *Fertil Steril* 61:411–22.

Schildkraut, J. M., E. Bastos, and A. Berchuk. 1997. Relationship between lifetime ovulatory cycles and overexpression of mutant p53 in epithelial ovarian cancer. *Journal of the National Cancer Institute* 89:932–38.

Scott, J. S. 1984. Immunologic factors and recurrent pregnancy loss. *Lancet* I:1122.

Scott, R., and G. Hoffmann. 1995. Prognostic assessment of ovarian reserve. *Fertil Steril* 63:1.

Scully, R. E., ed. 1996. Case records of the Massachusetts General Hospital. *New Engl J Med* 33:255–60.

Seibel, M. M. 1988. In vitro fertilization success rates: A fraction of the truth. *Fertil Steril* 72:265–66.

————. 1995. Toward reducing risks and costs of egg donation: A preliminary report. *Fertil Steril* 64:199–201.

————. 1996. IRBs and hospital ethics advisory boards (letter). *Fertil Steril* 66:671.

Seibel, M., M. Kearnan, and A. A. Kiessling. 1995. Parameters that predict success for natural cycle in vitro fertilization–embryo transfer. *Fertil Steril* 63:1251–54.

Seibel, M. M., C. Ranoux, and M. Kearnan. 1989. In vitro fertilization: How much is enough? (letter). *New Engl J Med* 321:1052.

Seifer, D. B., M. D. Adelson, R. W. Abdul-Karim, et al. 1989. Appraising a clinical journal article in obstetrics and gynecology. *Am J Obstet Gynecol* 160:198–201.

Shacochis, B. 1996. Missing children: One couple's anguished attempt to conceive. *Harper's* 293:55–63.

Shanner, L. 1995. Informed consent and inadequate medical information. *Lancet* 346:251.

Sharpe, R. M., and N. E. Skakkebaek. 1993. Are oestrogens involved in falling sperm counts and disorders of the male reproductive tract? *Lancet* 341:1392–95.

Shaw, J., and A. Trounson. 1997. Oncological implications in the replacement of ovarian tissue. *Human Reprod* 12:403–4.

Sher, G., M. Feinman, C. Zouves, et al. 1994. High fecundity rates following in vitro fertilization and embryo transfer in anti-phospholipid antibody seropositive women treated with heparin and aspirin. *Human Reprod* 9:2278–83.

Sher, G., R. Salem, M. Feinman, et al. 1993. Eliminating the risk of life-endangering complications following overstimulation with menotropin fertility agents: A report on women undergoing in vitro fertilization and embryo transfer. *Obstet Gynecol* 81:1009–11.

Shmidt, G. E., D. Sites, R. Mausirer, et al. 1985. Embryo toxicity of clomiphene citrate on mouse embryos fertilized in vivo and in vitro. *Am J Obst Gynecol* 153:679.

Shoham, Z. 1994. Epidemiology, etiology, and fertility drugs in ovarian epithelial carcinoma: Where are we today? *Fertil Steril* 62:433–48.

Shoham, Z., and M. Schacter. 1996. Estrogen biosynthesis—Regulation, action, remote effects, and value of monitoring in ovarian stimulation cycles. *Fertil Steril* 65:687–701.

Shorr, R., and W. L. Greene. 1995. A food-borne outbreak of expensive antibiotic use in a community teaching hospital. *JAMA* 273:1908.

Shushan, A., V. Eisenberg, and J. Schenker. 1995. Subfertility in the era of assisted reproduction: Changes and consequences. *Fertil Steril* 64:459–69.

Shushan, A., O. Paltiel, J. Iscovich, et al. 1996. Human menopausal gonadotropin and the risk of epithelial ovarian cancer. *Fertil Steril* 65:13–18.

Siedentopf, F., B. Horstkamp, G. Stief, et al. 1997. Clomiphene citrate as a possible cause of a psychotic reaction during infertility treatment. *Human Reprod* 12:706–7.

Sikorski, R. 1997. Medical literature made easy. *JAMA* 277:959–60.

Silber, S. J., A. Van Steirteghem, and N. Zsolt. 1996. Normal pregnancies resulting from testicular sperm extraction and intracytoplasmic sperm injection for azoospermia due to maturation arrest. *Fertil Steril* 66:110–17.

Silver, R. K., B. T. Helfand, T. L. Russel, et al. 1997. Multifetal reduction increases the risk of preterm delivery and fetal growth restriction in twins: A case-control study. *Fertil Steril* 67:30–33.

Silverman, W. A., and D. G. Altman. 1996. Patients' preferences and randomised trials. *Lancet* 347:171–74.

Simpson, J. L., S. A. Carson, J. L. Mills, et al. 1996. Prospective study showing that antisperm antibodies are not associated with pregnancy loss. *Fertil Steril* 66:36–42.

Skakkebaek, N. E., A. Giwercman, and D. de Kretser. 1994. Pathogenesis and management of male infertility. *Lancet* 343:1473–79.

Skovmand, K. 1995. Danish artificial-fertilisation research faces threat. *Lancet* 346:629.

———. 1997. First-ever fertilisation bill passed in Denmark. *Lancet* 349:1678.

Smith, D. C., L. R. Donohue, and S. J. Waszak. 1994. A hospital review of advanced gynecologic endoscopic procedures. *Am J Obstet Gynecol* 170:1635–42.

Smith, E. M., M. Hammond-Ehlers, M. K. Clark, et al. 1997. Occupational exposures and risk of female infertility. *Journal of Occupational and Environmental Medicine* 39:138–47.

Smith, K. E., and R. P. Buyalos. 1996. The profound impact of patient age on pregnancy outcome after early detection of fetal cardiac activity. *Fertil Steril* 65:35–40.

Smith-Levitin, M., A. Kowalik, J. Birnholz, et al. 1996. Selective reduction of multifetal pregnancies to twins improves outcome over nonreduced triplet gestations. *Am J Obstet Gynecol* 175:878–82.

Society for Assisted Reproductive Technologies and American Society for Reproductive Medicine. 1995. Assisted reproductive technology in the United States and

Canada: 1993 results generated from the American Society for Reproductive Medicine/Society for Assisted Reproductive Technologies Registry. *Fertil Steril* 64:13–21.

———. 1996. Assisted reproductive technology in the United States and Canada: 1994 results generated from the American Society for Reproductive Medicine/Society for Assisted Reproductive Technologies Registry. *Fertil Steril* 66:697–705.

Soliman, S., S. Daya, J. Collins, et al. 1994. The role of luteal phase support in infertility treatment: A meta-analysis of randomized trials. *Fertil Steril* 61:1068–76.

Soules, M. R. 1985. The in vitro fertilization pregnancy rate: Let's be honest with one another. *Fertil Steril* 43:511–13.

———. 1996. Now that we have painted ourselves into a corner. *Fertil Steril* 66:693–95.

Spallone, P., and D. L. Steinberg, eds. 1987. *Made to order: The myth of reproductive and genetic progress.* New York: Pergamon Press.

Spirtas, R., S. C. Kaufman, and N. J. Alexander. 1993. Fertility drugs and ovarian cancer: Red alert or red herring? *Fertil Steril* 59:291–93.

Stadtmauer, L., E. C. Ditkoff, D. Session, et al. 1994. High dosages of gonadotropins are associated with poor pregnancy outcomes after in vitro fertilization–embryo transfer. *Fertil Steril* 61:1058–64.

Stanton, C. K., and R. H. Gray. 1995. Effects of caffeine consumption on delayed conception. *Am J Epidem* 142:1322–29.

Stevens, W. 1994. Industrial chemicals may disrupt reproduction of wildlife. *New York Times,* August 23, B5.

Stolberg, S. G. 1997. "Unchecked" research on people raises concern on medical ethics. *New York Times,* May 14, A1.

Stolwijk, S. M., G. A. Zielhuis, M. V. Sauer, et al. 1997. The impact of the woman's age on the success of standard and donor in vitro fertilization. *Fertil Steril* 67:702–10.

Stray-Pedersen, B., and S. Stray-Pedersen. 1984. Etiologic factors and subsequent reproductive performance in couples with a prior history of habitual abortion. *Am J Obstet Gynecol* 148:140–46.

Svendsen, T. O., D. Jones, D. Butler, et al. 1996. The incidence of multiple gestations after in vitro fertilization is dependent on the number of embryos transferred and maternal age. *Fertil Steril* 65:561–65.

Tabash, K. M. 1993. A report of 131 cases of multifetal pregnancy reduction. *Obstet Gynecol* 82:57–60.

Tal, J., S. Haddad, N. Gordon, et al. 1996. Heterotopic pregnancy after ovulation induction and assisted reproductive technologies: A literature review from 1971 to 1993. *Fertil Steril* 66:1–12.

Tallo, C. P., B. Vohr, and W. Oh. 1995. Maternal and neonatal morbidity associated with in vitro fertilization. *Journal of Pediatrics* 127:794–800.

Tan, S. L., P. Doyle, S. Campbell, et al. 1992. Obstetric outcome of in vitro fertilization pregnancies compared with normally conceived pregnancies. *Am J Obstet Gynecol* 167:778–84.

Tan, S. L., P. Doyle, N. Maconochie, et al. 1994. Pregnancy and birth rates of live infants after in vitro fertilization in women with and without previous in vitro fertilization pregnancies: A study of eight thousand cycles at one center. *Am J Obstet Gynecol* 170:34–40.

Tan, S. L., J. Farhi, R. Homburg, et al. 1996. Induction of ovulation in clomiphene-resistant polycystic ovary syndrome with pulsatile GnRH. *Obstet Gynecol* 88:221–26.

Tan, S. L., H. S. Jacobs, and M. M. Seibel. 1995. *Infertility: Your questions answered.* New York: Carol Publishing Group.

Tan, S. L., N. Maconochie, P. Doyle, et al. 1994. Cumulative conception and live-birth rates after in vitro fertilization with and without use of long, short, and ultrashort regiments of the gonadotropin-releasing hormone agonist buserelin. *Am J Obstet Gynecol* 171:513–20.

Tan, S. L., P. Royston, S. Campbell, et al. 1992. Cumulative conception and livebirth rates after in-vitro fertilization. *Lancet* 339:1390–94.

Tanbo, T., P. O. Dale, O. Lunde, et al. 1995. Obstetric outcome in singleton pregnancies after assisted reproduction. *Obstet Gynecol* 86:188–92.

Tanenbaum, S. J. 1993. What physicians know. *New Engl J Med* 329:1268–70.

Taymor, M. L. 1987. Use and abuse of clomiphene citrate. *Fertil Steril* 47:206–7.

———. 1996. The regulation of follicle growth: Some clinical implications in reproductive endocrinology. *Fertil Steril* 65:235–47.

Taymor, M. L., C. J. Ranoux, and G. L. Gross. 1992. Natural oocyte retrieval with extra vaginal fertilization: A simplified approach to in vitro fertilization. *Obstet Gynecol* 80:888–91.

Templeton, A., J. K. Morris, and W. Parslow. 1996. Factors that affect outcome of in-vitro fertilisation treatment. *Lancet* 349:1402–6.

Thomas, K. B. 1994. The placebo in general practice. *Lancet* 344:1066–67.

Tomaevi, T., M. Ribi-Pucelj, A. Omahen, et al. 1996. Microsurgery and in vitro fertilization and embryo transfer for infertility resulting from pathological proximal tubal blockage. *Human Reprod* 11:2613–17.

Tomlinson, M. J., C. L. Barratt, and I. D. Cooke. 1993. Prospective study of leukocytes and leukocyte subpopulations in semen suggests they are not a cause of male infertility. *Fertil Steril* 60:1069–75.

Toona-Kellam, T. 1994. Letterman's top ten?! *Resolve of Northern California newsletter,* winter, 17.

Tournaye, H. 1997. Declining clinical andrology: Fact or fiction? *Human Reprod* 12:876–79.

Tripp, B. M., T. F. Kolon, C. Bishop, et al. 1997. ICSI and potential transmission of genetic disease (letter). *JAMA* 277:963–64.

Trounson, A., C. Wood, and A. Kausche. 1994. In vitro maturation and the fertilization and developmental competence of oocytes recovered from untreated polycystic ovarian patients. *Fertil Steril* 62:353–62.

Tucker, M. J., S. R. Wiker, G. Wright, et al. 1993. Treatment of male infertility and idiopathic failure to fertilize in vitro with under zona insemination and direct egg injection. *Am J Obstet Gynecol* 169:324–32.

Tummin, I. S., N. A. Whitmore, S. A. Daniel, et al. 1994. Transferring more embryos increases risk of heterotopic pregnancy. *Fertil Steril* 61:1065–67.

Turiel, J. 1992. Social impact of diethylstilbestrol exposure on women in the United States. In *Clinical practice of gynecology—DES update,* edited by K. Noller. New York: Elsevier.

Tur-Kaspa, I., Y. Maor, D. Levan, et al. 1994. How often should infertile men have intercourse to achieve conception? *Fertil Steril* 62:370–75.

U. S. House of Representatives, Subcommittee of the Committee on Government Operations. 1988. *Medical and social choices for infertile couples and the federal role in prevention and treatment.* Washington, D.C.: U.S. Government Printing Office.

U.S. House of Representatives, Committee on Governmental Operations. 1989. *Infertility in America:Why is the federal government ignoring a major health problem?* Washington, D.C.: U.S. Government Printing Office.

van der Ven, H., and G. Haidl. 1997. Clinical andrology is important for treatment of male infertility with ICSI. *Human Reprod* 12:879.

Van Voorhis, B. J., J. D. Dawson, D. W. Stovall, et al. 1996. The effects of smoking on ovarian function and fertility during assisted reproduction cycles. *Obstet Gynecol* 88:785–91.

Van Voorhis, B. J., D. W. Stovall, A. E. Sparks, et al. 1997. Cost-effectiveness of infertility treatments: A cohort study. *Fertil Steril* 67:830–36.

Van Voorhis, B. J., C. H. Syrop, D. G. Hammitt, et al. 1992. Effects of smoking on ovulation induction for assisted reproductive techniques. *Fertil Steril* 58:981.

Vauthier-Brouzes, D., G. Lefebvre, S. Lesourd, et al. 1994. How many embryos should be transferred in in vitro fertilization? A prospective randomized study. *Fertil Steril* 62:339–42.

Venn, A., L. Watson, J. Lumley, et al. 1995. Breast and ovarian cancer incidence after infertility and in vitro fertilisation. *Lancet* 346:995–1000.

Verlaenen, H., H. Cammu, M. P. Derdre, et al. 1995. Singleton pregnancy after in vitro fertilization. *Obstet Gynecol* 86:906–10.

Vermeulen, A., and M. Vandeweghe. 1984. Improved fertility after varicocele: Fact or fiction? *Fertil Steril* 42:249.

Villa, M. L. 1994. Endometriosis (letter). *New Engl J Med* 330:70.

Vine, M. F., B. H. Margolin, H. I. Morrison, et al. 1994. Cigarette smoking and sperm density: A meta-analysis. *Fertil Steril* 61:35–43.

Wagner, M. 1996. IVF: Out-of-date evidence or not. *Lancet* 348:1394.

Wagner, M. G., and P. A. St. Clair. 1989. Are in-vitro fertilization and embryo transfer of benefit to all? *Lancet* II:1027–30.

Wallach, E. 1991. Gonadotropin for the ovulatory patient—The pros and cons of empiric therapy for infertility. *Fertil Steril* 55:478–80.

———. 1995. Pitfalls in evaluating ovarian reserve. *Fertil Steril* 63:12–13.

Waud, D. R. 1992. Pharmaceutical promotions—A free lunch? *New Engl J Med* 327:351–53.

Weber, T., and J. Marcus. 1995. In quest for miracles, did fertility clinic go too far? *Los Angeles Times,* June 4, A1.

Weiner, J. 1988. Selective first trimester termination in octuplet and quadruplet pregnancies (letter). *Obstet Gynecol* 72:821.

Welch, G. E., and S. G. Gabbe. 1996. Review of statistics usage in the *American Journal of Obstetrics and Gynecology. Am J Obstet Gynecol* 175:1138–41.

Wennberg, J. E., ed. 1996. *The Dartmouth atlas of health care.* Chicago, Ill.: American Hospital Publishing.

Wentz, A. C. 1989. Editor's comment. *Obstet and Gynecol Survey* 44:70.

———. 1993. Diagnosing infertility: Who is qualified? (reply to letter). *JAMA* 269:46.

Wentz, A. C., L. R. Kossy, and R. A. Parker. 1990. Impact of luteal phase defect in an infertile population. *Am J Obstet Gynecol* 162:937–45.

Whittemore, A. S. 1993. Fertility drugs and risk of ovarian cancer. *Human Reprod* 8:999.

Whittemore, A. S., R. Harris, J. Itnyre, et al. 1992. Characteristics relating to ovarian cancer risk: Collaborative analysis of 12 United States case-control studies. II. Invasive epithelium ovarian cancers in white women. *Am J Epidem* 136:1184–1203.

Wilcox, A. J., C. R. Weinberg, and D. D. Baird. 1995. Timing of sexual intercourse in relation to ovulation. *New Engl J Med* 333:1517–21.

Wilcox, L. S., J. L. Kiely, and C. L. Melvin. 1996. Assisted reproductive technologies: Estimates of their contribution to multiple births and newborn hospital stays in the United States. *Fertil Steril* 65:361–65.

Wilcox, L. S., H. B. Peterson, F. D. Haseltine, et al. 1993. Defining and interpreting pregnancy success rates for in vitro fertilization. *Fertil Steril* 60:18–25.

Wilkes, M. S., B. H. Doblin, and M. F. Shapiro. 1992. Pharmaceutical advertisements in leading medical journals: Experts' assessments. *Annals of Internal Medicine* 116:912–19.

Willemsen, W., R. Kruitwagen, and B. Bastiaans. 1993. Ovarian stimulation and granulosa-cell tumor. *Lancet* 347:986–88.

Wilshire, G. B., A. M. Emmi, C. C. Gagliardi, et al. 1993. Gonadotropin-releasing hormone agonist administration in early human pregnancy is associated with normal outcomes. *Fertil Steril* 60:980–83.

Witkin, S., J. Jeremias, J. A. Grifo, et al. 1993. Detection of *chlamydia trachomatis* in semen by the polymerase chain reaction in male members of infertile couples. *Am J Obstet Gynecol* 168:1457–62.

Witkin, S. S., K. M. Sultan, G. S. Neal, et al. 1994. Unsuspected *chlamydia trachomatis* infection and in vitro fertilization outcome. *Am J Obstet Gynecol* 171:1208–14.

Wolf, K. M., M. J. McMahon, J. A. Kuller, et al. 1997. Advanced maternal age and perinatal outcome: Oocyte recipiency versus natural conception. *Obstet Gynecol* 89:519–23.

Woloshin, K. K. 1994. Patients' interpretation of qualitative probability statements. *JAMA* 273:4e.

Woolhandler, S., and D. Himmelstein. 1995. Extreme risk—The new corporate proposition for physicians. *New Engl J Med* 333:1706–7.

Wramsby, H., K. Fredga, and P. Liedholm. 1987. Chromosome analysis of human oocytes recovered from preovulation follicles in stimulated cycles. *New Engl J Med* 316:120–24.

Wright, L. 1995. Double mystery. *New Yorker,* August 7, 45–62.

——— . 1996. Silent sperm. *New Yorker,* January 15, 42–55.

Wysowski, D. 1993. Use of fertility drugs in the United States, 1973 through 1991. *Fertil Steril* 60:1096–97.

Yaron, Y., A. Amit, A. Kogosowski, et al. 1997. The optimal number of embryos to be transferred in shared oocyte donation: Walking the thin line between low pregnancy rates and multiple pregnancies. *Human Reprod* 12:699–702.

Yaron, Y., A. Amit, A. Mani, et al. 1995. Uterine preparation with estrogen for oocyte donation: Assessing the effect of treatment duration on pregnancy rates. *Fertil Steril* 63:1284–86.

Young, D. C., M. C. Snabes, and A. N. Poindexter III. 1993. GnRH agonist exposure during the first trimester of pregnancy. *Obstet Gynecol* 81:587–89.

Younger, J. B. 1989. Truth in advertising. *Fertil Steril* 52:726–27.

Ziegler, M. G., P. Lew, and B. C. Singer. 1995. The accuracy of drug information from pharmaceutical sales representatives. *JAMA* 273:1296–98.

Index

Abortion, 49, 128, 233, 355nn18,22. *See also* Fetal reduction; Political arena

Adoption, 129, 306

Advanced reproductive technologies. *See* Assisted reproductive technologies

Age-related infertility, 121–22, 122–24, 344n5; and decision making, 115, 126–27, 144–46, 148–49; and diagnostic uncertainty, 125; and egg donation, 120, 121, 125–26; and fertility drugs, 124; and pressure on women, 118–19, 294–95; and treament success rates, 63, 122–23, 125, 272–73. *See also* Postmenopausal pregnancies

AIDS, 100

American College of Obstetricians and Gynecologists, 48, 89

American Gynecological and Obstetrical Society, 72–73

American Society for Reproductive Medicine (ASRM): on assisted reproductive technologies, 37, 39; on cancer risks, 168; on cryopreservation, 131–32; on egg donation, 149; on endometriosis, 32; and Internet, 264–65; on micromanipulation, 94; and monitoring, 41, 43, 225, 226, 229, 353–54n6; on pelvic surgery, 339n11; and success rates, 59; on unexplained fertility, 82

Anas, George, 121

Andrologists, 90, 283

Angell, Marcia, 344n85

Anti-abortion movement, 41, 234

Antinori, Severino, 231, 232

ART. *See* Assisted reproductive technologies

Artificial insemination, 25–26, 98, 227

Asch, Ricardo, 9–10, 148–49, 218, 260–61. *See also* Irvine clinic scandal

ASRM. *See* American Society for Reproductive Medicine

Assisted reproductive technologies (ART): and age-related infertility, 122–24, 125–26; conflicts within medical profession, 39, 66–67; and cost concerns, 53, 67, 337–38n26; decision making, 60–65; experimentation, 42, 161; feminists on, 41, 336n3; government research moratorium, 41–44, 166, 233, 234, 235, 236; and health insurance, 33, 67, 113, 337–38n26; and immunologic infertility, 107; incentives for, 40; moderation trend, 51–56, 155, 337–38n26, 347n10; monitoring, 40–41, 42–43, 113, 226; and multiple pregnancies, 46–51; and ovarian hyperstimulation, 33, 36–37, 43–46; risks/complications, 44–51; and stimulated intrauterine insemination, 80, 83; and treatment momentum, 53; unproven treatments, 39–40, 41–42, 43–44, 55–56, 66, 159, 161, 248–50; variations of, 37–39. *See also* Assisted reproductive technology success rates; GnRH-a; In vitro fertilization

Assisted reproductive technology success rates, 35, 40, 52, 56–60, 356n1; and age-related infertility, 63, 122–23, 125, 345n14; clinic-specific, 61–62, 64–65, 226, 338n35; definitions of, 30, 62–63, 338n37; and egg donation, 141; and moderation trend, 55; and multiple pregnancies, 46–47; stimulated IUI, 78–79; and treatment expansion pattern, 35–36

Australia, 354n9

Baby-boom generation, 294–95, 299

Basal body temperature (BBT) chart, 85, 86, 87, 88, 89

Bern, Howard, 152–53, 179, 346n2

Biochemical pregnancies, 58

Birth control pill, 45, 296–97

Bongaarts, John, 119

Breast cancer. *See* Cancer risks

Brennan, Troyen, 197–98, 351n21

Caffeine, 318, 358n6

Canada, 230, 233, 292–93, 354n9, 355n16